Methods in
Observational Epidemiology

MONOGRAPHS IN EPIDEMIOLOGY AND BIOSTATISTICS
Edited by Jennifer L. Kelsey, Michael G. Marmot, Paul D. Stolley, Martin P. Vessey

Monographs in Epidemiology and Biostatistics
Volume 26

Methods in Observational Epidemiology

SECOND EDITION

Jennifer L. Kelsey
Alice S. Whittemore
Alfred S. Evans
W. Douglas Thompson

New York   Oxford
OXFORD UNIVERSITY PRESS
1996

Oxford University Press

Oxford   New York
Athens   Auckland   Bangkok   Bombay
Calcutta   Cape Town   Dar es Salaam   Delhi
Florence   Hong Kong   Istanbul   Karachi
Kuala Lumpur   Madras   Madrid   Melbourne
Mexico City   Nairobi   Paris   Singapore
Taipei   Tokyo   Toronto

and associated companies in
Berlin   Ibadan

Published by Oxford University Press, Inc.,
198 Madison Avenue, New York, New York 10016

Oxford is a registered trademark of Oxford University Press

Library of Congress Cataloging-in-Publication Data
Methods in observational epidemiology / Jennifer L. Kelsey . . . [et
al.]. — 2nd ed.
p. cm. — (Monographs in epidemiology and biostatistics : v. 26)
Main entry of previous ed. under Kelsey.
Includes bibliographical references and index.
ISBN 0-19-508377-6
1. Epidemiology—Research—Methodology.   2. Epidemiology—
Statistical methods.   I. Kelsey, Jennifer L.   II. Series.
RA652.4.K45   1996
614.4'072—dc20   95-47816

9 8 7 6 5 4 3 2 1

Printed in the United States of America
on acid-free paper

Preface to Second Edition

The second edition of *Methods in Observational Epidemiology*, like the first edition, is written for those involved in the design, conduct, analysis, and interpretation of epidemiologic studies concerned with disease etiology. It has a practical orientation, and is meant to serve as both a textbook and a resource for persons who have had introductory courses in epidemiology and biostatistics.

Since the first edition was published in 1986, a variety of changes have taken place in the field of epidemiology. Additional sources of data are available, mainly because of the increasing use of computerized records for health-related purposes. The uses and limitations of certain epidemiologic concepts and techniques are now better understood. Modifications of traditional study designs, including nested case-control studies and case-cohort studies, are more frequently employed. Biologic markers of exposure, disease susceptibility, and disease are used in many studies. Methods of statistical analysis have been further developed.

In this second edition, *Methods in Observational Epidemiology* has been revised to take these developments into account. All chapters have been updated. Chapter 3, which summarizes sources of data on disease occurrence, has been expanded to include several additional sources of data. Chapter 5, which describes modifications of traditional study designs, now contains descriptions of nested case-control studies and case-cohort studies that are largely new to this second edition. Chapter 15, on other types of measurement, has been expanded to include sections on measurement in epidemiologic studies of the elderly and on biologic markers, since these have become major areas of epidemiologic research in recent years.

Much of the material in Chapters 6–9 on the analysis of data from epidemiologic studies is also new to this edition. Perhaps the greatest challenge in writing this second edition was trying to make some of the modern, frequently used methods of statistical analysis understandable to readers with limited mathematical or statistical background. We hope that most readers, even if they do not fully comprehend the theory behind some of the techniques, will understand the rationale for their use and be able to interpret results when they appear on a computer printout or in the literature. In particular, readers not familiar with maximum likelihood estimation and nested models should try to understand what these methods accomplish, but should not be concerned with acquiring an in-depth understanding of these techniques from this book alone. Alternatively, the sections on maximum likelihood estimation can be skipped without significant impact on comprehension of the rest of the material in the book. It is hoped that all readers will nevertheless be able to interpret the data presented in the exercises at the end of the chapters on data analysis.

In conclusion, we hope that this book will be useful to individuals from a variety of backgrounds undertaking epidemiologic studies in diverse settings, and that it will facilitate reading and interpreting the epidemiologic literature by people from many disciplines.

J.L.K.
A.S.W.
A.S.E.
W.D.T.

Preface to First Edition

This book is written for those wanting to design, conduct, analyze, and interpret epidemiologic studies concerned with disease etiology. It is meant to serve as a textbook for students who have already had courses in elementary epidemiology and biostatistics and as a resource for those actively engaged in epidemiologic research. Examples are taken from diseases of both non-infectious and infectious etiology, as it is the belief of the authors that many of the same approaches can be used in studies concerned with both non-infectious and infectious agents. Although the book focuses on observational, or non-experimental, epidemiologic studies, many of the procedures and concepts covered here also apply to experimental epidemiologic studies.

The first two chapters review elementary epidemiologic and biostatistical concepts and methods that are usually covered in introductory courses. Readers without background in these areas will probably need to supplement these chapters with introductory textbooks in epidemiology and biostatistics in order to understand fully the material in subsequent chapters.

Chapter 3 summarizes sources of data on disease occurrence. Chapters 4–8 describe the major types of study designs used in epidemiology, including the specific situations in which each is useful, the important issues to be considered in carrying them out, and methods of statistical analysis. Commonly employed multivariable statistical techniques such as logistic regression, proportional hazards models, and multiple regression are presented so as to give a reader with minimal background in statistical theory an idea of how these techniques are used in practice and how the statistics derived from them are interpreted. Chapter 9 discusses techniques of epidemic investigation. Chapter 10 describes common methods of sampling in epidemiologic studies and presents methods and tables used in the estimation of sample sizes needed in various types of investigations. The final three chapters cover issues related to measurement in epidemiology, including in-depth discussions of questionnaire design and the consequences of measurement error, and brief descriptions of the special issues of measurement that arise in studies of adverse reproductive outcomes, occupational exposures, and psychiatric and psychosocial epidemiology.

This book does not cover such important but highly specialized topics as genetic epidemiology and randomized trials. We nevertheless hope that a reader thoroughly familiar with the contents of this book will be able to apply epidemiologic methods to a variety of situations and to do so with both competence and confidence.

J.L.K.
W.D.T.
A.S.E.

Acknowledgments

Many people have generously assisted in the preparation of this book. We are especially indebted to Sander Greenland and Lorene Nelson, who carefully reviewed most of the book and made numerous helpful suggestions. Others who reviewed individual sections include Norman Breslow, Deborah Galuska, Ann Geiger, Maureen Hatch, Lisa Herrinton, Joseph Keller, Bruce Link, Richard Lipton, Susan Parker, Julie Parsonnet, and Emily White. Patricia Ford, Sarah Larson, and Ann Schein provided extensive and exceptionally cheerful typing assistance, Susanne Gnagy, Chantal Matkin, and Ann Schwartz played important roles in proofreading the final manuscript, and Mila Prill assisted in a variety of ways. Students in epidemiology classes at Columbia University and Stanford University offered numerous helpful suggestions. The encouragement of Jeffrey House of Oxford University Press was instrumental in bringing this second edition to completion. During the years of writing the first and second editions of the book, we have been most grateful for the support of Joseph B. Keller, Holly, Laurel, and Sunny Kelsey, and Gail Thompson, and also the support of persons no longer with us, including Brigette Evans, and Christy, Eppie, and Gwen Kelsey.

Contents

Methods in
Observational Epidemiology

1

Introduction

The connection between cause and effect has no beginning and can have no end.

Leo Tolstoy, *War and Peace*

Epidemiology, the study of the occurrence and distribution of diseases and other health-related conditions in populations, is used for many purposes. One is to determine the magnitude and impact of diseases or other conditions in populations or in selected subgroups of populations. This information can be used in setting priorities for investigation and for control, in deciding where preventive efforts should be focused, in evaluating the efficacy of therapeutic procedures, and in determining treatment facilities that are needed. Collecting information on disease frequency in populations is also an essential function of surveillance programs, which evaluate the efficacy of prophylactic and therapeutic measures and seek to detect unexpected changes in disease occurrence. Epidemiologic studies may also be used to learn more about the natural history and clinical course of diseases and of their pathogenesis in both the community and the individual. Perhaps most commonly, however, epidemiologic studies are undertaken to identify causes of disease, and it is this application of epidemiology that will be the focus of this book. Only observational epidemiologic studies will be emphasized because randomized trials are covered in Volume 8 of this series (Meinert, 1986).

The aims of the first two chapters are to give the reader an idea of the scope of observational epidemiologic studies concerned with disease etiology and to introduce some of the major issues and concepts in study design and analysis.

TYPES OF STUDIES

Learning about causes of disease through epidemiologic studies is generally a gradual process that requires different types of study designs, depending on the nature of the diseases and possible etiologic agents being considered, as well as on the current state of knowledge of the etiology of the disease. Epidemiologic studies are sometimes classified into *descriptive studies*, which are usually undertaken when little is known of the epidemiology of a disease, and *analytic studies*, which are carried out when leads about etiology are already available. Although considerable overlap exists between these two categories of studies, the distinction between them is nevertheless often useful.

Descriptive studies provide information on patterns of disease occurrence in populations according to such characteristics as age, gender, race, marital status, social class, occupation, geographic area, and time of occurrence. Usually, but not always, routinely collected data (covered in Chapter 3) are used to provide this information. The descriptive statistics thus generated can be used together with clinical observations, laboratory studies, and other sources of information (including analytic studies undertaken for other purposes) to generate hypotheses. *Analytic studies* are designed specifically to test causal hypotheses that usually have been generated from one or more of these sources. Because analytic studies often entail the collection of new data, they tend to be more expensive than descriptive studies, but, if properly designed and executed, they generally allow more definitive conclusions to be reached about causation.

For example, descriptive observations of the rapid increase in lung cancer death rates among males during the first half of the twentieth century together with clinical and autopsy studies led to the hypothesis that cigarette smoking is a cause of lung cancer (Doll, 1953). However, other factors besides cigarette consumption, such as the number of telephones, the number of automobiles, and diet, were also changing over this time period; conceivably, one or more of these factors could have been responsible for the increasing lung cancer death rates. Therefore, analytic studies were needed specifically to test the hypothesis that cigarette smoking was mainly responsible for this increase. If there had been genuine concern that telephones were really the cause of the increasing lung cancer death rates, and if in an analytic study an appropriate cohort of smokers and nonsmokers and of people who did and did not have telephones had been assembled and followed through time, then within this cohort smoking, and not telephone ownership, would have been found to be associated with an increased risk of lung cancer.

The discovery of an association between the use of oral contraceptives and venous thromboembolism provides another example of the gradual evolution of knowledge about the role of a suspected etiologic agent, first by means of clinical and descriptive epidemiologic studies and then by analytic epidemiologic studies. Suspicion that such an association might exist started with clinical case reports in the early 1960s that venous thromboembolism was occurring more frequently than previously among apparently healthy young women and that the affected women were almost always users of oral contraceptives (Jordan, 1961). An examination of routinely collected statistics showed that, in fact, mortality and hospitalization rates from venous thromboembolism had increased as oral contraceptive use had become more widespread (Markush and Seigel, 1969; Vessey and Inman, 1973). Meanwhile, analytic studies designed specifically to test the hypothesis that oral contraceptives were a cause of venous thromboembolism confirmed these preliminary leads (Royal College of General Practitioners, 1967; Sartwell et al., 1969; Vessey and Doll, 1968).

The clinical observation by Gregg, an Australian ophthalmologist, that mothers of infants with congenital cataracts often had a history of rubella (German measles) during pregnancy (Gregg, 1941) led to epidemiologic studies confirming the association between maternal rubella and congenital cataracts and identifying the first trimester as the time infections conferred the highest risk. Using both epidemiologic and laboratory techniques, prospective analyses of pregnant women defined the magnitude of the risk, the spectrum of congenital abnormalities associated with rubella infection, and the precise interrelationship between the time of infection and nature of the congenital abnormality (Siegel and Greenberg, 1960). These findings led to the development of rubella vaccine and the demonstration that its proper use decreased the frequency of congenital abnormalities. The discovery that cytomegalovirus, herpes simplex, and *Toxoplasma gondii* could also cause congenital defects illustrated that there may be several causes for the same clinical syndromes; thus, prevention of one exposure may not fully eliminate the disease but rather will affect only the portion due to the particular agent (Nahmias, 1974). This example also shows that epidemiologic evidence of causality does not always lead to fully effective preventive measures. Prevention of the other infectious causes of congenital abnormalities has not been successful because it has been impossible to implement practical ways of interrupting the chain of transmission or to overcome technical obstacles to the development of a safe and effective vaccine.

The geographic distribution of a disease may also provide clues to etiology. For example, maps with mortality rates for cancers of various sites by county in the United States (Mason et al., 1975; Pickle et al., 1987) have shown that certain geographic areas have especially high or low mortality rates. Analytic studies have been designed to examine the possible roles of specific industries or other factors in bringing about certain of the elevated rates.

Early in the twentieth century, observations on the prevalence of mottled enamel and of tooth decay in municipalities around the United States led to the discovery by analytic epidemiologic studies that fluoride in drinking water was responsible for the mottled enamel and also for the protection against tooth decay (McClure, 1970). Belief in the causal nature of the associations was further strengthened by studies showing that the frequency of mottled enamel decreased and the frequency of dental caries increased when communities changed from drinking water sources high in fluoride to sources low in fluoride. Finally, experimental studies in which fluoride (at levels below those at which mottled enamel develops) was added to the water of some communities but not others clearly established both the causal nature of the relation between lack of fluoride and tooth decay and the efficacy of fluoridated drinking water in reducing the frequency of dental caries.

Another example of how knowledge of the geographic distribution of a disease may eventually lead to identification of a causal association is the occurrence of a lymphoma (now known as Burkitt's lymphoma) in children in Africa. By trekking 10,000 miles by jeep through Africa and by using mailed questionnaires, Burkitt found that the disease occurred in central Africa only at altitudes below 3000 feet and only in localities with an annual rainfall of 40 inches or more. This observation reminded him of the similar distribution of vector-borne diseases such as yellow fever and malaria (Burkitt, 1969) and led to a vigorous search for an infectious agent; this effort eventually led to the identification by Epstein, Achong, and Barr (Epstein et al., 1964) of a herpes-like virus in cells grown from a tumor biopsy. The virus, now termed Epstein-Barr virus (EBV), turned out not to be vector-borne; however, malaria, which is carried by the *Anopheles* mosquito, can also contribute to the pathogenesis of African Burkitt's lymphoma. It is hypothesized that EBV infects and stimulates B lymphocytes into proliferation. The occurrence of malaria would greatly enhance the B-cell proliferation, and this cell proliferation would increase the likelihood of a cytogenetic change and the emergence of a malignant cell. In addition, malaria depresses the immune response to B-cell proliferation. In this instance, descriptive epidemiology led to the identification of the "cofactor" (malaria) and not the "cause" (EBV). However, prospective seroepidemiologic studies have established the causal nature of the association between EBV infection and Burkitt's lymphoma (de The et al., 1978).

Data routinely collected at the Centers for Disease Control and Prevention (CDC) also have uncovered epidemiologic leads. An observation derived from CDC data was the occurrence of the acquired immunodeficiency syndrome (AIDS), one of whose common manifestations is *Pneumocystis carinii* pneumonia (Centers for Disease Control, 1981). This disease was not reportable to CDC, but CDC controlled a drug (pentamidine) used for its therapy. A marked increase in demand for this drug piqued CDC's epidemiologic interest and led to confirmation of the increase of this infection and of other conditions associated with it, such as Kaposi's sarcoma, opportunistic infections, and immune deficiency. An intensive effort by CDC and other laboratories was mounted to determine those at high risk for AIDS in the United States (presently male homosexuals, hemophiliacs, intravenous drug users, and their sexual and other close contacts), the methods of transmission, and the causative agent(s). Epidemiologists, virologists, immunologists, clinicians, and personnel at blood banks engaged in investigations to understand the pathogenesis of this syndrome and ways to prevent its epidemic spread and high mortality. The causative agent was found to be the human immunodeficiency virus type 1 (HIV-1) (Gallo et al., 1984; Sarngadharan et al., 1984; Vilmer et al., 1984). This virus infects and destroys a subset of helper T lymphocytes (CD4 lymphocytes). Despite this knowledge of etiology, an effective vaccine has not been developed. Antiviral therapeutic agents have provided only moderate improvement in the course of the disease and have led to the emergence of resistant strains.

Descriptive data can also lead to "wild-goose chases." For instance, mortality rates from several other diseases in addition to venous thromboembolism were increasing during the 1960s, and in some instances these increases were attributed falsely to use of oral contraceptives. Sometimes differences in disease rates from one country to another or from one time period to another are really attributable to differences in diagnostic procedures or criteria. These and other problems that may arise in using descriptive statistics to generate hypotheses will be covered more fully in Chapter 3. However, the number of instances in which descriptive statistics provide false leads can be substantially reduced if thorough consideration is given to the biologic plausibility of any hypothesized association before more expensive and time-consuming analytic studies are undertaken.

When sufficient preliminary data from routinely collected and other sources indicate that a more detailed epidemiologic study should be undertaken to test a particular hypothesis, analytic epidemiologic studies are initiated. The three major types of analytic studies are *cohort* (or *follow-up*) *studies* (prospective and retrospective), *case-control studies,* and *cross-sectional studies.* The most definitive type of observational study is usually the *prospective cohort study,* discussed in detail in Chapters 4, 6, and 7. In a prospective cohort study, individuals, all of whom are initially free of the disease(s) under study, are classified according to whether they are exposed or not exposed to the factors of interest. The cohort is then followed for a period of time (which may be many years), and the incidence rates (number of new cases of disease per population at risk per unit time) or mortality rates (number of deaths per population at risk per unit time) in those exposed or not exposed are compared. For instance, in the Framingham Heart Study (Dawber et al., 1951), cholesterol levels, blood pressure levels, smoking habits, and other characteristics of the participants were determined at a time when they were apparently free of coronary heart disease. Members of the cohort have now been followed for more than 40 years after the baseline measurements were made. The incidence rates of coronary heart disease were determined according to cholesterol levels, blood pressure levels, smoking habits, and other characteristics (Kannel et al., 1961). Data from the Framingham study and other cohort studies undertaken in the 1950s and 1960s (The Pooling Project Research Group, 1978) provided the first definitive evidence that elevated blood pressure and cholesterol levels *predicted* coronary heart disease and were therefore involved in the etiology of the disease. Until such cohort studies were undertaken, it was considered possible that elevated blood pressure and cholesterol levels were a consequence of the disease. These data also permitted estimates of the risk of coronary heart disease at various levels of these factors (often called "risk factors" because they give some indication of a person's risk of developing disease). Since the study considered several possible risk factors, the associations between each of these factors and coronary heart disease could be estimated while taking into account in the statistical analysis the associations of the other possible risk factors for coronary heart disease (Truett et al., 1967). Cohort studies also frequently enable the investigators to study the relationship of the factors of interest to several different diseases at the same time. The Framingham study, for instance, has permitted examination of risk factors for stroke, gallbladder disease, cancer, hip fracture, and other diseases as well as heart disease.

Cohort studies can also focus on groups with particular exposures, such as those in certain occupational settings, those exposed to environmental hazards, those exposed to certain drugs or infectious agents, those with certain medical conditions, and those with certain psychological profiles.

Cohorts may also be assembled retrospectively. For instance, cohorts with specific exposures in the past, such as radium dial painters (Martland, 1931) and persons exposed to radiation in the course of air-collapse therapy for tuberculosis (MacKenzie, 1965), persons with certain characteristics when they were in college (Paffenbarger and Williams, 1967), and persons with antibodies to selected infectious agents (Evans et al., 1974; Evans et al., 1968), have been used in *retrospective* (or *historical*) *cohort studies*. Persons with these exposures and appropriate comparison groups are identified retrospectively and followed from the time of exposure up to the present to determine disease incidence or mortality rates in the presence or absence of the suspected risk factor. When suitable information on exposure and on other relevant variables is available and when follow-up of the cohort is feasible, retrospective cohort studies permit the same types of estimates as prospective cohort studies without the necessity of following cohort members for many years after the study is initiated. In other words, the follow-up period between the exposure to the risk factor and the development of disease has already occurred (or is still under way). For example, the cohort of persons in Hiroshima, Japan, who were within 2000 meters of the hypocenter of the atomic blast on August 6, 1945, has been followed to determine their risks for a variety of diseases as compared to the risks in "nonexposed populations" (those 2000 or more meters away from the hypocenter). These investigations have involved analysis of the immediate effects and the long-term consequences of exposure both in the exposed and in their progeny. A more detailed description of retrospective cohort studies is given in Chapter 5. Also described in Chapter 5 are nested case-control studies and case-cohort studies. These study designs involve making certain measurements in samples of cohort members and are therefore less expensive than traditional cohort studies that are based on measurements in all cohort members.

Most often, however, data on exposures that took place several years ago and on other relevant variables are not available. Prospective cohort studies are usually prohibitively expensive for studies of uncommon diseases or for situations when little preliminary information on possible risk factors is available. Therefore, *case-control studies,* discussed in detail in Chapters 8 and 9, are the most common type of epidemiologic study. In a case-control study (also called a case-comparison study, a case-referent study, or occasionally simply a retrospective study), persons with a given disease (the cases) and persons without the given disease (the controls) are selected; the cases are generally persons seeking medical care for the disease, whereas the controls may be selected from the general population, from the neighborhoods of the cases, from among other patients seeking medical care, or from other sources. The proportions of cases and of controls with certain background characteristics or exposure to possible risk factors are then determined and compared. The first analytic studies to test the hypothesis that smoking causes lung cancer, for instance, compared the proportion of smokers among lung cancer patients admitted to hospitals with the proportion of smokers in a control group comprising patients of the same gender and similar age admitted to the same hospitals with other diseases (U.S. Public Health Service, 1964). The proportion of smokers among lung cancer cases was found to be much higher than the proportion of smokers among the control subjects. Further, the cases tended to have smoked for much longer periods of time than the controls, and to have smoked more cigarettes per day. The associations between smoking and lung cancer were not attributable to effects of other variables measured in the studies. The smoking and lung cancer relationships found in case-control studies were in fact sufficiently strong that it was felt warranted to conduct more expensive, but more definitive, prospective cohort studies. Many other examples of case-control studies of disease etiology may be cited, such as studies concerned with the proportion of oral contraceptive users among women with and without thromboembolism (Royal College of General Practitioners, 1967; Sartwell et al., 1969; Vessey and Doll, 1968) or with the proportion of persons who recently went camping or who drank untreated mountain water among cases with *Giardia lamblia* infections and among controls (Wright et al., 1977).

Acute epidemics may be designed as either retrospective cohort or case-control studies. For instance, in an investigation of a food-borne outbreak, persons at a picnic might be divided into those who did and those who did not eat the potato salad, and the attack rates of disease (number of new cases occurring over a defined period of time per population at risk) determined in these two groups. On the other hand, picnickers could be divided into those with and without gastroenteritis, and the proportion of those who ate potato salad compared in these two groups. Because investigations of acute epidemics also present some specific features, such as the usually short time period between exposure and disease occurrence, they will be discussed specifically in Chapter 11.

Another study design is the *cross-sectional study,* or *prevalence study,* described in detail in Chapter 10. In a cross-sectional study, exposure to a possible risk factor and the occurrence of disease are measured at one point in time or over a relatively short period of time in a study population. Prevalence rates (number of cases of existing disease per population at risk in the given period of time) among those with and those without the exposure of interest are then compared. For instance, a prevalence study was undertaken to determine whether persons living in areas with high levels of air pollution were more likely to have chronic bronchitis than persons living in areas with low levels of air pollution (Ferris and Anderson, 1962). A prevalence study might be used to ascertain whether obese individuals are more likely to have osteoarthritis than nonobese individuals (Acheson and Collart, 1975). In prevalence studies, it is often difficult to differentiate between cause and effect. If obesity and osteoarthritis were associated, it would not be immediately apparent whether obesity predisposes to osteoarthritis or whether people with osteoarthritis tend to get less exercise and therefore become obese. It is only recently that cohort studies have shown that obesity in fact predicts subsequent osteoarthritis rather than osteoarthritis leading to obesity (Carman et al., 1994). Nevertheless, a prevalence study is often the most practical initial method of investigation for diseases with slow onsets, such as chronic bronchitis and osteoarthritis. For such diseases, it is difficult to define an incident case, and affected individuals often do not seek medical care until the symptoms become relatively severe. Another important use of prevalence studies is in serologic surveys of antibody patterns for evidence of previous exposure to a variety of infectious agents (Evans et al., 1974; Paul and White, 1973).

In cross-sectional studies as well as in other types of epidemiologic investigations, it is often not feasible to make measurements on an entire population; thus, samples of individuals are studied instead. In order to ensure that a sample is representative of the population as a whole and in order to obtain the most information for the least cost, various formal methods of sampling, described in Chapter 12, are used. Chapter 12 also gives procedures for estimating sample sizes needed to detect significant effects, using different types of study designs.

CONFOUNDING, INDIRECT AND DIRECT CAUSES OF DISEASE, AND EFFECT MODIFICATION

Three other major concerns of epidemiologists when designing, analyzing, and interpreting studies are controlling for *confounding variables,* identifying *indirect and direct causes* of disease, and detecting *effect modification.*

Confounding can perhaps best be introduced by an example. At one time there was concern that coffee consumption during pregnancy had an adverse effect on pregnancy outcomes, including birthweight. However, women who drink a great deal of coffee also tend to be heavy smokers of cigarettes, and cigarette smoking during pregnancy is known to increase the likelihood of delivering an infant of low birthweight. Therefore, although it might appear that coffee consumption increases the risk of delivering a low-birthweight infant, in fact this association occurs only because women who drink coffee during pregnancy tend to smoke cigarettes; it is really the cigarette smoking that brings about a lower birthweight. Coffee drinking is *not* associated with low birthweight once the mother's cigarette smoking habits are taken into account (Linn et al., 1982). In other words, unless cigarette smoking, the confounder, is taken into account either in the study design or the statistical analysis, misleading conclusions may be reached about the relationship between coffee consumption and low birthweight.

A *confounder* is a variable (e.g., cigarette smoking) that (a) is causally related to the disease or condition under study (e.g., low birthweight) independently of the exposure of primary interest (e.g., coffee consumption) or, as often occurs in practice, serves as a proxy measure for unknown or unmeasured causes, and (b) is associated with the exposure under study in the study population, but is not a consequence of this exposure. It follows from (a) that within each level of the exposure under study, the confounder is related to risk for disease, or in probabilistic terms, the confounder is related to the disease conditional on exposure level. Accordingly, cigarette smoking is a confounder for the association between coffee consumption and low birthweight because it is causally related to low birthweight, is associated with coffee consumption, but is not caused by coffee consumption. At each level of coffee consumption, cigarette smoking is positively associated with risk of delivering a low-birthweight infant. For instance, in the example mentioned above (Linn et al., 1982), among those with no coffee consumption, the relative risks for delivery of a low-birthweight infant according to cigarette smoking habits (risk of a low-birthweight infant for a mother in a given cigarette smoking category divided by the risk of a low-birthweight infant for a mother who does not smoke) are estimated to be as follows:

		Cigarette Smoking Status		
	Never smoked	Stopped smoking before or during pregnancy	Smoked <3 cigarettes per day during pregnancy	Smoked ≥3 cigarettes per day during pregnancy
Relative risk	1.0	1.6	1.3	2.2

For those who drink three cups of coffee per day during pregnancy, the relative risk estimates are as follows:

		Cigarette Smoking Status		
	Never smoked	Stopped smoking before or during pregnancy	Smoked <3 cigarettes per day during pregnancy	Smoked ≥3 cigarettes per day during pregnancy
Relative risk	1.0	1.1	1.4	2.1

Similarly, increasing relative risks for delivery of a low-birthweight infant with increasing cigarette consumption during pregnancy are seen at the other levels of coffee consumption considered. On the other hand, at a given level of cigarette smoking, no effect of coffee consumption can be detected. If cigarette smoking is taken into account in the statistical analysis (by methods described in Chapters 6, 7, and 9), the relative risks associated with various levels of coffee consumption (risk of delivery of a low-birthweight infant for mothers with a given level of coffee consumption divided by risk of a low-birthweight infant for a mother who drinks no coffee during pregnancy) are estimated to be (Linn et al., 1982)

	Number of Cups per Day of Coffee				
	0	1	2	3	≥4
Relative risk	1.0	1.1	1.2	0.9	0.9

In other words, the apparent relationship between maternal coffee consumption and delivery of a low-birthweight infant occurred only because women who drank coffee also tended to smoke cigarettes. Coffee consumption is not associated with risk of delivering a low-birthweight infant, once cigarette smoking is taken into account.

In many instances in which it is believed that a causal association exists, the possibility must be kept in mind that an unidentified confounder is in fact responsible for the association. For instance, many studies demonstrated a positive association between the presence of herpes simplex virus type 2 (HSV-2) and cervical cancer (Rawls et al., 1973). However, one of the main reasons that this association was not accepted as causal by many people was that the presence of HSV-2 is frequently associated with the presence of other sexually transmitted infectious agents; therefore, another as yet unidentified sexually transmitted agent might exist that (a) *is* causally associated with cervical cancer and (b) is associated with HSV-2 exposure only because HSV-2 and the unidentified agent are associated with multiple sexual partners and with early age at first intercourse. Certain human papilloma viruses are now thought to be such agents.

In addition to identifying confounding variables, which, if ignored, may cause the investigator to believe that an association exists when it does not or to believe that an association does not exist when in fact it does, an investigator also is concerned in the study design and analysis with *separating out indirect causes from more direct causes.* For instance, it is known that infants with congenital dislocation of the hip are more likely to have been firstborn than are other infants. This is shown using data from a hypothetical case-control study in Table 1–1. It is also recognized that infants with congenital dislocation of the hip are more likely to have been born by breech delivery than infants without congenital dislocation of the hip (Table 1–2) and that firstborn infants are more likely to have been born by

Table 1–1. Number and Percentage of Firstborn among Infants with Congenital Dislocation of the Hip (CDH) and among Control Infants, Hypothetical Data

	Cases (CDH)	Controls	Total
Number firstborn	100	80	180
Number not firstborn	100	120	220
Total	200	200	400
Percentage firstborn	50	40	

Table 1–2. Number and Percentage of Births by Breech Delivery among Infants with Congenital Dislocation of the Hip (CDH) and among Control Infants, Hypothetical Data

	Cases (CDH)	Controls	Total
Number born by breech	60	20	80
Number not born by breech	140	180	320
Total	200	200	400
Percentage born by breech	30	10	

breech delivery than other infants. Accordingly, the investigator wants to know (a) if infants with congenital dislocation of the hip are more likely to have been born by breech regardless of whether they are firstborn, and (b) if infants with congenital dislocation of the hip are more likely to be first-born regardless of whether they are born by breech. Table 1–3 shows that infants with congenital dislocation of the hip are more likely to have been born by breech regardless of whether they are firstborn, whereas Table 1–4 indicates that infants with congenital dislocation of the hip are not more likely to have been firstborn, once the association between breech delivery and congenital dislocation of the hip is taken into account. Breech malposition is not a confounder for the association between being firstborn and congenital dislocation of the hip because it is not an independent risk factor for congenital dislocation of the hip. One concludes that being firstborn is indeed a risk factor for congenital dislocation of the hip, but only because it increases the risk for breech malposition, which is the more direct cause of congenital dislocation of the hip. The sequence can be illustrated as follows:

Other factors
↓   ↘
Firstborn ⟶ Breech malposition ⟶ Congenital
dislocation
of hip

Obviously, other factors, many of which are not yet identified, also influence the likelihood of breech malposition. Sorting out such associations is a major concern in data analysis and interpretation.

In some instances it is not possible to determine whether a given variable is in fact a confounder, is a link in the causal chain, or is by chance associated with the risk factor and disease in a particular study. Generally, an understanding of the biologic relationships among the exposure, possible confounder, and disease is necessary to be certain of the true role of a given variable.

Effect modification, sometimes referred to as statistical interaction, also

Table 1–3. Number and Percentage of Births by Breech Delivery among Infants with Congenital Dislocation of the Hip (CDH) and among Control Infants According to Whether They Were Firstborn, Hypothetical Data

	Firstborn			Not Firstborn		
	Cases (CDH)	Controls	Total	Cases (CDH)	Controls	Total
Number born by breech	48	16	64	12	4	16
Number not born by breech	52	64	116	88	116	204
Total	100	80	180	100	120	220
Percentage born by breech	48	20		12	3	

needs to be considered when epidemiologic studies are designed, analyzed, and interpreted. Effect modification occurs when the magnitude of the chosen measure of association between a causal agent and a disease differs according to the level of a third variable (or according to the levels of two or more variables). For instance, when all age groups are considered together, females have two to three times the risk for hip fractures as males (Buhr and Cooke, 1959). However, this overall ratio disguises the fact that at young ages males are at higher risk than females, whereas at older ages females are at considerably higher risk than males. The association between gender and hip fracture is thus modified by age, which in this instance is a surrogate measure of the high prevalence of osteoporosis in older women and of the propensity to severe trauma in young males. The association between body build and breast cancer is modified by menopausal status; obesity is a risk factor for breast cancer among postmenopausal women but not premenopausal women (LeMarchand et al., 1988). The detrimental effect of cigarette smoking on birthweight may be greater at older than at younger maternal ages (Fox et al., 1994). The association between early infection with Epstein-Barr virus (EBV) and African Burkitt's lymphoma exists mainly in the presence of widespread malaria early in life (Miller, 1982),

Table 1–4. Number and Percentage of Births by Firstborn among Infants with Congenital Dislocation of the Hip (CDH) and among Control Infants According to Whether the Delivery Was Breech, Hypothetical Data

	Breach Delivery			Not Breech Delivery		
	Cases (CDH)	Controls	Total	Cases (CDH)	Controls	Total
Number firstborn	48	16	64	52	64	116
Number not firstborn	12	4	16	88	116	204
Total	60	20	80	140	180	320
Percentage firstborn	80	80		37	36	

which is generally designated a cofactor by infectious disease epidemiologists, but which could be considered an effect modifier as well.

MEASUREMENT

Another major concern of epidemiologists is measurement: measurement of exposures, measurement of diseases, measurement of confounding variables, and measurement of effect modifiers. Although some variables such as ABO blood groups or the occurrence of a hip fracture can be measured with a relatively high degree of accuracy, epidemiologic studies are often limited by inaccurate measurement. A great deal of interest currently exists in the role of diet in the etiology of many chronic diseases, but determining the foods consumed at the time the disease process actually began is often exceedingly difficult, since most people cannot remember what their diet was 20 or 30 years previously. Even the measurement of current dietary intake is difficult because of daily variations in the diet and memory problems. Thus, failure to find an association between diet and disease may indicate either that no relationship exists or that measurement is so poor that an association that does exist cannot be detected.

Failure to measure confounding variables accurately may mean that the confounder is not adequately taken into account. For instance, cigarette smoking and coffee drinking are highly correlated. If one wants to measure the association between coffee drinking and disease, smoking habits must be carefully taken into account; otherwise, an association may be found between coffee drinking and disease that is in reality attributable to the confounding effect of smoking, which has not been measured with sufficient precision.

Another concern is that ascertainment of exposure be comparable in diseased and nondiseased individuals and that ascertainment of disease occurrence be comparable in exposed and unexposed persons. Lack of comparability, frequently referred to as differential misclassification, can result in positive associations between exposure and disease when none exists and in failure to find associations when associations do in fact exist. The possible effects of measurement error thus need to be considered along with various other issues in designing and interpreting studies, and will be discussed in Chapters 13 through 15.

CONCLUSION

Major concerns of epidemiologists trying to learn about disease causation through observational studies include choosing the most reliable sources of data, the correct study designs, representative study populations, and the appropriate methods of measurement; quantifying the magnitude of various risks associated with exposures; controlling for confounding variables; identifying direct and indirect causes of disease; and detecting effect modification. In practice, it may be impossible to meet all these objectives to the extent desired because people may not choose to participate, optimal measurement may not be feasible, and a variety of other problems may arise. Therefore, it is important to recognize the effects of various inadequacies in different situations because specific inadequacies can affect the study results in different ways.

It is hoped that this introductory chapter indicates that conclusions drawn from epidemiologic studies, as with other types of scientific inquiry, are not always final. Many require additional confirmatory epidemiologic or laboratory studies, the experimental reproduction of the exposure-disease association, or ascertainment of the effect of removal or modification of the suspected risk factor. What was considered a direct cause of a disease at one time may later be found to be an indirect cause when more information has been obtained on biologic mechanisms. What was believed to be a causal association may be found to be attributable to a confounding variable recognized at a later time. A causal agent in one setting or population may not operate in another setting or population. The best method of measurement at one point in time may be supplanted by a better method developed subsequently. In any one study, a reported association may have occurred by chance, especially when many possible associations are being considered, and even a true association may not apply to all population groups.

Thus, although it is important to use the most appropriate methods in any one study, it is also essential to keep an open mind as new knowledge accumulates from further epidemiologic, laboratory, and other types of studies and as attempts are made to replicate the results of even the most carefully executed individual studies. It is in this way that knowledge of disease etiology generally evolves.

REFERENCES

Acheson RM, Collart AB. 1975. The New Haven survey of joint disease. XVII. Relationship between some systemic characteristics and osteoarthrosis in a general population. *Ann Rheum Dis* 34:379–387.

Buhr AJ, Cooke AM. 1959. Fracture patterns. *Lancet* 1:531–536.

Burkitt DP. 1969. A children's cancer dependent on climatic factors. *Nature* 194: 232–234.

Carman WJ, Sowers MF, Hawthorne VM, Weissfeld LA. 1994. Obesity as a risk factor for osteoarthritis of the hand and wrist: a prospective study. *Am J Epidemiol* 139:119–129.

Centers for Disease Control. 1981. *Pneumocystis* pneumonia. *MMWR* 30:250.

Dawber TR, Meadors GF, Moore FE Jr. 1951. Epidemiologic approaches to heart disease: the Framingham Study. *Am J Public Health* 41:279–286.

de The G, Geser A, Day NE, Tukei PM, Williams EH, Beir DP, Smith PG, Dean AG, Bornkamm GW, Feorino P, Henle W. 1978. Epidemiological evidence for causal relationship between Epstein-Barr virus and Burkitt's lymphoma from Ugandan prospective study. *Nature* 274:756–761.

Doll R. 1953. Bronchial carcinoma: incidence and aetiology. *Br Med J* 7:521–527, 585–590.

Epstein MA, Achong BG, Barr YM. 1964. Virus particles in cultured lymphoblasts from Burkitt's lymphoma. *Lancet* 1:702–703.

Evans AS, Cox F, Nakervis G, Opton E, Shope R, Wells AY, West B. 1974. A health and serological survey of a community in the Barbados. *Int J Epidemiol* 3:167–175.

Evans AS, Niederman JC, McCollum RW. 1968. Seroepidemiologic studies of infectious mononucleosis with EB virus. *N Engl J Med* 279:1121–1127.

Ferris BG, Anderson DO. 1962. The prevalence of chronic respiratory disease in a New Hampshire town. *Am Rev Respir Dis* 86:165–177.

Fox SH, Koepsell TD, Daling JR. 1994. Birth weight and smoking during pregnancy—effect modification by maternal age. *Am J Epidemiol* 139:1008–1015.

Gallo RC, Salahuddin SZ, Popovic M, Shearer GM, Kaplan M, Haynes BF, Palker TJ, Redfield R, Oleske J, Safai B, White G, Foster P, Markham PD. 1984. Frequent detection and isolation of cytopathic retroviruses (HTLV-III) from patients with AIDS and at risk for AIDS. *Science* 224:500–502.

Gregg NM. 1941. Congenital cataract following German measles in the mother. *Trans Ophthalmol Soc Aust* 3:35–46.

Jordan WM. 1961. Pulmonary embolism. *Lancet* 2:1146–1147.

Kannel WB, Dawber TR, Kagan A, Revotskie N, Stokes J III. 1961. Factors of risk in the development of coronary heart disease—six-year followup experience. *Ann Intern Med* 55:33–50.

LeMarchand L, Kolonel LN, Earle ME, Mi MR. 1988. Body size at different periods of life and breast cancer risk. *Am J Epidemiol* 128:137–152.

Linn S, Schoenberg SC, Monson RR, Rosner B, Stubblefield PG, Ryan KJ. 1982. No association between coffee consumption and adverse outcomes of pregnancy. *N Engl J Med* 306:141–145.

MacKenzie I. 1965. Breast cancer following multiple fluoroscopies. *Br J Cancer* 19:1–8.

Markush RE, Seigel DG. 1969. Oral contraception and mortality trends from thromboembolism in the United States. *Am J Public Health* 59:418–434.

Martland HS. 1931. The occurrence of malignancy in radioactive persons. *Am J Cancer* 15:2435–2516.

Mason TJ, McKay FW, Hoover R, Blot WJ, Fraumeni JF Jr. 1975. Atlas of Cancer Mortality for U.S. Counties: 1950–1969. Washington, D.C., U.S. Department of Health, Education, and Welfare. DHEW Publication No. (NIH) 75–780.

McClure FJ. 1970. Water Fluoridation. The Search and the Victory. Washington, D.C., U.S. Government Printing Office.

Meinert C. 1986. Clinical Trials: Design, Conduct, and Analysis. New York, Oxford University Press.

Miller G. 1982. Burkitt lymphoma. In: A S Evans, Ed. Viral Infections of Humans. Epidemiology and Control. New York, Plenum, pp 599–619.

Nahmias AJ. 1974. The torch complex. *Hospital Practice* 9:65–72.

Paffenbarger RS Jr, Williams JL. 1967. Chronic disease in former college students. V. Early precursors of fatal stroke. *Am J Public Health* 51:1295–1299.

Paul JR, White C, eds. 1973. Serological Epidemiology. New York, Academic Press.

Pickle LW, Mason TJ, Howard N, Hoover R, Fraumeni JF Jr. 1987. Atlas of U.S. Cancer Mortality among Whites: 1950–1980. Washington, D.C., U.S. Department of Health and Human Services. DHHS Publication No. (NIH) 87–2900.

Pooling Project Research Group. 1978. Relation of blood pressure, serum cholesterol, smoking habit, relative weight and ECG abnormalities to incidence of major coronary events: final report of the Pooling Project. *J Chron Dis* 31:201–306.

Rawls WE, Adam E, Melnick JL. 1973. An analysis of seroepidemiological studies of herpes virus type 2 and carcinoma of the cervix. *Cancer Res* 33:1479–82.

Royal College of General Practitioners. 1967. Oral contraception and thromboembolic disease. *J Roy Coll Gen Pract* 13:267–279.

Sarngadharan MG, Popovic M, Bruch L, Schupbach J, Gallo RC. 1984. Antibodies reactive with human T-lymphotropic retroviruses (HTLV-III) in the serum of patients with AIDS. *Science* 224:506–508.

Sartwell PE, Masi AT, Arthes FG. 1969. Thromboembolism and oral contraceptives: an epidemiologic case-control study. *Am J Epidemiol* 90:365–380.

Siegel M, Greenberg M. 1960. Fetal death, malformation and prematurity after maternal rubella. Results of prospective study. *N Engl J Med* 262:389–393.

Truett J, Cornfield J, Kannel W. 1967. A multivariate analysis of the risk of coronary heart disease in Framingham. *J Chron Dis* 20:511–524.

U.S. Public Health Service. 1964. Surgeon General's Advisory Committee on Smoking and Health. Washington, D.C., U.S. Government Printing Office.

Vessey MP, Doll R. 1968. Investigation of relation between use of oral contraceptives and thromboembolic disease. *Br Med J* 2:199–205.

Vessey MP, Inman WHW. 1973. Speculations about mortality trends from venous thromboembolic disease in England and Wales and their relation to pattern of oral contraceptive usage. *J Obstet Gynecol (Br Commonw)* 80:562–566.

Vilmer E, Barre-Sinoussi F, Rougloux C, Gazengel C, Brun FV, Daugnet C, Fischer A, Manigne P, Chermann JC, Griscelli G, Montagier L. 1984. Isolation of new lymphotrophic retrovirus from two siblings with hemophilia B, one with AIDS. *Lancet* 1:753–757.

Wright RA, Spencer HC, Brodsky RE, Vernon TM. 1977. Giardiasis in Colorado: an epidemiologic study. *Am J Epidemiol* 105:330–336.

Exercises

1. Observation A: The age-adjusted incidence rate for breast cancer in Japanese women is considerably lower than the age-adjusted incidence rate for breast cancer in North American women. The proportion of Japanese women who smoke cigarettes is also much lower than the proportion of North American women who smoke cigarettes.

Observation B: Within North America, cigarette smoking does not increase the incidence rate of breast cancer, and within Japan, smoking does not increase the incidence rate of breast cancer. Which of the answers given below do you believe is correct?

   a. Observation A provides better evidence as to whether or not a causal association between smoking and breast cancer exists than Observation B.

   b. Observation B provides better evidence as to whether or not a causal association between smoking and breast cancer exists than Observation A.

   c. Observations A and B provide equally good evidence as to whether or not a causal association between smoking and breast cancer exists.

   Give the reason for your answer.

2. Which type of analytic study is each of the following?

   a. The smoking histories of patients entering a hospital with lung cancer are compared with the smoking histories of patients entering for other conditions requiring surgery.

   b. Inductees into the army are asked about their smoking history and current habits. Smokers and nonsmokers are subsequently compared in relation to the development of lung cancer and other chronic diseases.

   c. In a study of the relationship between reproductive abnormalities and in utero exposure to diethylstilbestrol (DES), the incidence rates of reproductive abnormalities in individuals whose mothers were exposed to DES when they were pregnant 20–30 years previously are compared to the incidence rates of reproductive abnormalities in individuals who were not exposed to DES 20–30 years previously.

   d. Estrogen levels are measured in the blood of a sample of women in the age group 50–59 years. At the same examination, their bone mineral density is also measured. The proportion of women with low bone mineral density is compared in relation to estrogen level.

3. Which of the following are examples of prevalence data?

   a. All cases of tuberculosis found in a mass chest x-ray survey.

   b. All reported new cases of influenza in a one-month period.

   c. All reported new cases of cancer in a single year.

   d. All cases of coronary heart disease found during an initial examination of persons included in a community survey.

4. The incidence rate of cardiovascular disease is about three times greater in men than in women, but the prevalence rate shows no difference according to gender. One plausible explanation is that:

   a. The mortality rate is greater in women.

   b. The case fatality rate is greater in women.

   c. The duration of the disease is greater in women.

   d. Women receive less adequate medical care for the disease.

   e. The diagnosis is more often missed in women.

5. In a cross-sectional (prevalence) study, it is found that people getting little physical activity have higher prevalence rates for severe ulcers than those who get moderate or a lot of physical activity. The difference in prevalence rates is statistically significant.

Which of the following conclusions would you reach? (Circle one or more answers.)
   a. Lack of physical activity causes severe ulcers.
   b. Lack of physical activity protects against severe ulcers.
   c. Severe ulcers cause people to become physically inactive.
   d. None of the above.

6. In a prospective cohort study, it is found that men who drink alcoholic beverages are more likely to develop lung cancer than men who are not drinkers. However, among smokers the risk for lung cancer among drinkers and nondrinkers is the same. Also, among nonsmokers the risk for lung cancer among drinkers and non-drinkers is the same. In this example, smoking is a(n):
   a. Confounding variable.
   b. Effect modifier.
   c. Neither of the above.

7. In a case-control study, it is found that the percentage obese is higher among postmenopausal breast cancer cases than among postmenopausal controls, whereas the percentage obese is equal in premenopausal cases and controls. In this example, menopausal status is a(n):
   a. Confounding variable.
   b. Effect modifier
   c. Neither of the above.

2

Biologic and Statistical Concepts

In addition to the issues of study design reviewed in Chapter 1, designing, conducting, and interpreting epidemiologic studies requires an understanding of the biologic processes involved in disease causation and of the statistical ways of measuring associations between risk factors and diseases. The first section of Chapter 2 contains a review of some basic biologic concepts relating to causation of disease. Although it is impossible to specify concepts that apply to all associations between risk factors and diseases, the intent of this brief review is to present some of the most important issues that should be considered by the epidemiologist when undertaking a study. Then, following a short section on criteria used to test causal hypotheses, the final sections of this chapter cover basic measures that are commonly used to describe disease frequency and to quantify associations between risk factors and diseases. The more complex analyses presented in subsequent chapters build upon the statistical concepts presented here.

BIOLOGIC ASPECTS

Agent-Host-Environment

In classical concepts of infectious disease epidemiology, an agent, or microbe with pathogenic potential, interacts with a host (animal or human) in a particular environment to produce an infection and disease. The concept of an *agent* has since been broadened to include noninfectious agents such as chemical and physical substances as well as infectious agents. Although the concept of host-agent-environment is useful, it is not always clear how a given factor should be categorized. Asbestos, an important risk factor for mesothelioma, may be considered a specific agent for this cancer or an environmental factor that carries the specific agent. Often a complex of two or more factors in combination may be involved in the production of disease.

Almost all diseases have multiple causes. Although an infectious agent may be a *necessary* ingredient in the production of many diseases in susceptible persons, usually the infectious agent is not a *sufficient* cause of the disease. With a few exceptions, such as rabies and measles, cofactors or host characteristics are important in the development and severity of disease. These include age at time of infection and genetic susceptibility, for instance (Evans, 1989). For many diseases of presumed noninfectious etiology, no known necessary or sufficient cause exists, at least in our current state of knowledge; rather, several agents are regarded as risk factors, with no one agent necessary or sufficient. Thus, cigarette smoking is a strong risk factor for lung cancer, but some lung cancer occurs in nonsmokers, and most smokers do not develop lung cancer. A variety of risk factors have been identified for coronary heart disease, including age, gender, cholesterol level, blood pressure, cigarette smoking habits, body build, physical activity, type A behavior, and others, but none of these is a necessary or sufficient factor in the development of coronary artery disease.

The diversity of agents that contribute to disease causation makes generalizations about their characteristics difficult. The intrinsic toxic or pathogenetic properties as well as the duration of exposure needed to induce a disease process are important characteristics of infectious and noninfectious agents. For agents of high infectivity, one exposure may permit the initiation of infection and disease. For other infectious agents and for most noninfectious agents, the dosage may have to be greater or more prolonged to initiate a pathologic process. Once initiated, some noninfectious pathologic or immunologic processes can be self-sustaining or progressive. For example, once a malignant cell has developed it may multiply indefinitely; other cells in which a malignant process has been initiated may require exposure to additional agents, often called promoters, for further multiplication. It should also be emphasized that exposure versus nonexposure is usually not a simple dichotomy and that exposure itself may vary qualitatively and quantitatively and from one point in time to another. Even when all of the dynamic and quantitative aspects of dose and duration of exposure have been established, the response of different hosts to what seem to be identical exposures varies considerably, as discussed below. Usually this outcome is not predictable in advance because of our limited knowledge of the factors controlling host response.

The external *environment* contains biologic, chemical, physical, familial, occupational, and socioeconomic factors, as well as sources of psychological stress and other circumstances that affect the likelihood of disease occurrence. Some of these components are listed in Table 2–1. Much overlap exists in the various categories; for example, the family includes a variety of biologic, social, and other environmental factors. Nevertheless, it is useful to distinguish one component from another because of the different methods used to study them.

Table 2-1. Examples of Environmental Factors Influencing Exposure and Disease

1. *Biologic*: animal, insect vectors; presence of reservoirs; population density; human, animal, bird, insect; food sources; evolutionary process selecting for resistance and susceptibility of the agent or of the host; vegetation
2. *Familial*: number in family; presence of diseases; age distribution; hygienic environment; mobility of members; housing and nutritional environment; cultural and behavioral characteristics
3. *Chemical*: substances in air, water, soil, workplace
4. *Physical*: climate, radiation, vibration
5. *Occupational*: exposure to specific chemical and physical agents; physical and emotional stress
6. *Psychosocial*: stressful life events; social support systems
7. *Socioeconomic*: availability of health services for prevention, diagnosis, control of disease in both the community as a whole and for the individuals within it; poverty and its impact on both disease and nutrition; the need for sanitation; funds to provide clean air, water, milk, food
8. *Special environments*: day-care centers; hospitals, military and recruit camps, nurseries, camps for immigrants and for migrant workers; institutions, prisons
9. *Travel to new environments*: tropical and jungle settings, the Arctic and Antarctic, underseas exploration, outer space

Factors related more to the *host* than to the environment are presented in Table 2–2, which includes both factors that affect the likelihood of exposure and factors that affect the likelihood of clinical disease following exposure. Behavioral, socioeconomic, and hygienic factors influence the probability and nature of exposure to a risk factor. These factors, together with biologic, genetic, immunologic, and psychological characteristics of the host, also influence the nature and the severity of response following exposure. An example of the influence of genetic traits on disease susceptibility is the differences in disease frequency among people of various human leukocyte antigen (HLA) types. In the presence of the HLA antigen B27, the risk of ankylosing spondylitis is more than 100 times greater and of Reiter's disease about 35 times greater than in persons without the B27 antigen (Kaslow and Shaw, 1981). Very limited understanding exists of the mechanisms through which most of these host factors operate. Variation in host response will be discussed further below under Biologic Spectrum.

Routes of Transmission

A broad concept of transmission involves not only the agents that are important in acute infectious diseases but also the transmission or transfer of agents that are important in noninfectious diseases. The following discussion lists common modes of transmission of infectious diseases, with examples of analogous transmission of noninfectious agents where appropriate.

The most frequent pathway for the transmission of common infectious diseases in developed countries is the respiratory, or airborne, route. Transmission may require very close association between the source of infection and a susceptible host, or the agent may be airborne over considerable distances, such as in measles and chicken pox. In a similar way, noninfectious agents may involve close proximity, as in the relation between cigarette smoke and lung cancer, or greater distances, as in the airborne carriage of pollutants over many miles. Whatever the distance and whatever the nature of the agent, the common requirement is that a sufficient dosage be inhaled and reach an appropriate tissue to initiate a pathologic event, whether it be inflammation, irritation, cell death, or malignant change.

The gastrointestinal route is the second most frequent mode of transmission of infectious diseases in developed countries and is probably first in developing countries. Examples are viral diseases caused by rotaviruses; bacterial diseases such as cholera, traveler's diarrhea (mostly due to toxigenic *Escherichia coli*), bacillary dysentery, and the common types of food poisoning; and many intestinal parasites. Various acute and chronic diseases of noninfectious etiology are also the result of ingestion of toxic substances. The ingestion of lead either in drinking water (Jones, 1989) or by eating lead paints, as occurs in children living in houses painted years ago, can lead to both acute and chronic illness depending on the dose

Table 2-2. Examples of Host Factors Influencing Exposure and Disease

1. *Factors influencing exposure and disease occurrence after exposure*
    a. Age
    b. Behavioral patterns: exposure to drugs, alcohol, contraception, life style, eating habits, exercise, sexual activity, smoking
    c. Hygienic habits: personal hygiene, especially hand washing, general cleanliness
    d. Race and ethnic background
    e. Recreational habits: sports, hunting, camping, fishing
    f. Coexisting conditions

2. *Factors influencing occurrence of disease after exposure*
    a. Anatomic defects
    b. Antibiotic resistance
    c. Two or more risk factors operating simultaneously
    d. Dosage and duration of exposure
    e. Exercise of affected part
    f. Genetic makeup
    g. Immune status of host and response to agent
    h. Mechanism of disease production: local versus systemic, direct versus indirect, effect on end organ, functional versus pathologic change
    i. Nutritional status of host
    j. Portal of entry of agents
    k. Psychological and attitudinal factors
    l. Temperature of part of body involved
    m. Trauma

ingested and the duration of exposure. On the other hand, the presence of a substance such as fluoride in drinking water can protect against dental caries (McClure, 1970). Various dietary constituents entering the body through the gastrointestinal route are also believed to play a role in the etiology of many diseases.

The common infections transmitted primarily by the sexual route include gonorrhea, syphilis, chlamydia, and genital herpes. In addition, several important infections are transmitted both sexually and by blood or blood products, including hepatitis B, human immunodeficiency virus type 1 (HIV-1), human T-cell leukemia virus type 1 (HTLV-1), and cytomegalovirus. (Rarely, syphilis is transmitted by transfusions.) Certain malignancies are closely correlated with sexual activity, such as Kaposi's sarcoma in homosexual men infected with HIV-1, and cervical cancer, for which evidence of a causative role for the human papilloma virus, especially types 16 and 18, is strong.

Perinatal exposures to various infectious agents can lead to acute and chronic conditions such as congenital defects, low birthweight, and mental retardation. The routes of infection may differ from one agent to another, and some infectious agents are transmissible by several routes. Congenital abnormalities may result when the fetus is infected through the placenta, as may occur with rubella, cytomegalovirus, HIV-1, syphilis, and toxoplasma infections. Infections may be transmitted to the infant during passage through the birth canal for herpes simplex, varicella, hepatitis B, and HIV-1. Infections just after birth may be transmitted by breast milk, as with HTLV-1 and sometimes cytomegalovirus. Exposures during pregnancy to noninfectious substances may also cause acute and chronic illness in the newborn. For example, thalidomide, a tranquilizer drug taken by pregnant women in Europe, resulted in an epidemic of severe limb defects in the newborn (James and Lamb, 1963). The use of diethylstilbestrol (DES) by pregnant women has been associated years later with the development of vaginal cancer in their daughters (Herbst et al., 1971).

Agents borne by arthropod vectors or by insects include the agents of malaria and the large group of arbovirus infections. At least one chronic disease, Lyme disease, is caused by a tick-borne spirochete-like agent, *Borrelia burgdorferi* (Johnson et al., 1984). As an intermediate host, the snail plays an essential role in the transmission of the various types of schistosomiasis; in Egypt *Schistosoma mansoni* infections are present in a large percentage of the population.

Pathogenic agents present in blood and blood products are transmitted by transfusions and contaminated needles. For instance, the various forms of viral hepatitis, which lead to acute and chronic diseases of the liver, may be transmitted in this way, as well as cytomegalovirus, syphilis, and malaria.

The retroviruses HIV-1, HIV-2, and HTLV-1 are also transmissible by blood and certain blood products, as well as by blood-contaminated needles, and, very rarely, by accidental needle stick of a health worker during care of a patient infected with HIV-1.

The Incubation or Induction Period

The period of time between exposure to a causative agent and the appearance of the first clinical manifestations of the disease is usually termed the *incubation* (or *induction*) *period* by infectious disease epidemiologists and the *induction* (or *latent*) *period* by chronic disease epidemiologists. These periods are often not well defined unless there is a single time of exposure to the causative agent. This period varies with the pathogen, the multiplication time for infectious agents, the place where the major interaction occurs in the affected host, the dosage, and the route taken by the agent in reaching the target organ. For infectious agents, often only a short incubation is necessary for organisms causing effects locally, whereas long incubation periods are common for infections involving spread through the bloodstream or the nervous system. Incubation periods of a few hours are seen for diseases resulting from the direct action of preformed toxins, such as in staphylococcal food poisoning, whereas incubation periods of months or even years are noted for rabies, leprosy, and the slow viral infections. Indeed, in kuru, which is a "slow" viral infection occurring in New Guinea and presumably transmitted by the ingestion of infected human brain tissue, cases were still occurring 27 years after legal cessation of the practice of cannibalism (Prusiner et al., 1982). In addition to all the factors mentioned that affect the incubation period, tremendous variation may occur even when all other factors seem equal. For instance, in an outbreak of hepatitis B resulting from a contaminated yellow fever vaccine given to recruits in the same dose, in the same arm, and on the same day at Camp Polk, the incubation period varied from 40 to 180 days (Paul, 1945).

For diseases with an acute onset, the incubation period can often be estimated, as will be discussed in Chapter 11. For chronic diseases, determination of incubation periods is much more difficult, although under some circumstances the length of the incubation period can be estimated. For Lyme disease, the time of the initial tick bite, the eschar following it, and the demonstration of immunoglobulin M (IgM) type antibodies due to the causative spirochete provide evidence for estimating the incubation period to be an average of 12 days from the tick bite (Steere et al., 1978). The occurrence of bladder cancer following exposure to carcinogenic dyestuffs has varied from under 5 to over 35 years, peaking around 15 to 20 years (Case et al., 1954). For leukemia following exposure to the atomic bomb in

Hiroshima, an average incubation period of some 5 to 10 years was noted (Ichimuru et al., 1978). Available data on the incubation periods between exposure and the appearance of various types of malignant tumors have been reviewed by Armenian and Lilienfeld (1974). The incubation periods for 14 genetic diseases in which the genetic trait has been clearly determined have been summarized by Armenian and Khoury (1981). The age at onset of the disease was taken as the equivalent of the incubation period. In eight biochemical diseases of genetic etiology, the incubation period varied from 2.3 to 27 years. The incubation period for other genetic diseases ranged from 3.0 years for muscular dystrophy to 35 years for Huntington's disease.

In most chronic diseases of infectious or noninfectious etiology, it has not been possible to define or measure the incubation period. Determining the incubation period when the relevant exposures occurred many years previously is difficult. The multiple factors operating in disease pathogenesis, the multiple exposures to each of these factors, and the difficulty in identifying which of the risk factors were essential ones and when exposure to each occurred present further problems. Difficulty in defining the exact onset of the disease also occurs because the onset may be gradual and because characteristic diagnostic features may not be manifest until some time after the pathologic process actually begins. Nevertheless, the above examples show that in a few chronic diseases it is possible to measure the incubation period when a single, predominant causative agent is involved and when the time at which the single exposure to the causative agent took place can be clearly identified.

Biologic Spectrum and Variation in Host Response

One aspect of the way in which human hosts respond to a given causative agent is called the biologic spectrum, which is a measure of the severity of the response, ranging from no response (inapparent or subclinical disease) to varying intensity of the clinical disease from mild to severe to fatal. In some diseases, this spectrum is envisioned as an iceberg, with the part above the water representing the observable, clinical expression of the disease and that below the water line representing subclinical illness detectable only by laboratory or other special tests. The ratio of inapparent, or subclinical, to clinical infection varies greatly with the infecting agent and the age of the host at the time infection occurs. For many viruses, such as those causing poliomyelitis and infectious hepatitis, as well as the Epstein-Barr virus (EBV), infections that occur very early in life are usually inapparent, with inapparent to apparent ratios of 100–1000 to 1. As the age at the time of infection increases to young adulthood, many more infections are clinically expressed. When college students are infected with EBV, about half will develop clinical infectious mononucleosis (Evans and Niederman, 1989). However, a few infectious agents, such as measles and rabies viruses, almost invariably result in clinical illness when infection occurs. There are also susceptible persons who are exposed to various pathogenic agents but who never even become infected because an effective contact between the pathogen and the appropriate cell never occurs.

Many noninfectious diseases are also not apparent unless special tests are applied or unless the disease is detected incidentally. Osteoporosis, or reduced density of bone, is often not diagnosed unless it is revealed by x-rays taken for other reasons or unless a fracture occurs. Moderately elevated blood pressure is often not apparent unless blood pressure happens to be measured as part of a routine medical examination or as part of a screening program.

The clinical expression of recognizable disease may vary considerably. Coronary heart disease may be manifested by angina pectoris, myocardial infarction, or sudden death. Spinal osteoporosis may be manifested by a dowager's hump, back pain, loss of height, or a vertebral fracture. Furthermore, a single agent may affect different organs in the same or different hosts. For example, *Chlamydia trachomatis* infections can result in a variety of genital diseases in both males and females, acute and chronic infections of the eye (including trachoma), arthritis (Reiter's disease), and bronchiolitis and pneumonia in infants. Cigarette smoking can result in an increased risk for lung cancer, bladder cancer, laryngeal cancer, chronic bronchitis and emphysema, back pain, coronary artery disease, low-birthweight infants, and a variety of other conditions.

Markers of the occurrence of an exposure and evidence of its interaction with the host are better developed for diseases of infectious than of noninfectious etiology, mainly because of the ability to detect the occurrence of an immune response in the host. Research is now being undertaken to identify markers of exposure for noninfectious agents as well. The fields of molecular and biochemical epidemiology focus on the use of advanced laboratory methods in combination with analytic epidemiology to identify at the molecular or biochemical level specific environmental and/or host factors that play roles in the causation of disease. This field considers the development of diseases of noninfectious as well as of infectious etiology, and searches for markers that certain exposures have taken place and that the host has reacted to them. When applied to cancer, the laboratory methods include (a) techniques to assess specific characteristics of the host that may affect susceptibility to carcinogens; (b) assays that detect carcinogens in human tissues, cells, or fluids; (c) assays at the cellular level to determine the biologically effective doses of carcinogens; and (d) methods to measure early biologic and biochemical responses to carcinogens (Perera and Weinstein, 1982). Molecular and biochemical epidemiology are discussed further in Chapter 15.

CRITERIA USED TO TEST CAUSAL HYPOTHESES

The earliest efforts to establish the role of a given cause or risk factor in the etiology of a disease began with infectious diseases and focused on the idea that a single agent was both a necessary and sufficient cause of the condition. Among the first attempts to establish guidelines was that of Jacob Henle in 1840, some 40 years before the first bacteria were isolated and cultivated from an infectious disease. These guidelines were further developed by his pupil, Robert Koch, in 1882 in connection with establishing the relation of the tubercle bacillus to tuberculosis. These guidelines of causation constitute what are now called the Koch Postulates, or more properly the Henle-Koch Postulates. They stated three criteria for causation that served as tests of the hypothesis that a specific agent caused a specific disease. These criteria are given here using the original terminology: (a) the parasite occurs in every case of the disease in question and under circumstances that can account for the pathologic changes and clinical course of the disease; (b) it occurs in no other disease as a fortuitous and nonpathogenic parasite; and (c) after being fully isolated from the body and repeatedly grown in pure culture, it can induce the disease anew (Rivers, 1937). The subsequent difficulties in applying these postulates to viral and other infectious agents and to chronic diseases have been reviewed (Evans, 1976, 1993) and their limitations summarized (Evans, 1977). At the time of their enunciation, the concepts of the carrier state, asymptomatic infection, multifactorial causation, and the biologic spectrum of disease were not recognized (Evans, 1977, 1980).

Since the time of Henle and Koch, it has become apparent that most diseases can have several causes, and that one agent can cause several diseases (Evans, 1967, 1991). In other words, rarely is a single agent both necessary and sufficient to produce all cases of a given clinical syndrome. Table 2–3 summarizes some of the criteria used to test causal hypotheses (Evans, 1976). Although it may not be possible to satisfy all the criteria in any given situation, they do provide useful guidelines for the epidemiologist. Also, the criteria do not reflect the complexity and interaction of the various risk factors involved in many chronic diseases, or what has been termed "the web of causation" (MacMahon and Pugh, 1970). For this reason, the term *risk factors* rather than *causative agents* is more commonly used in reference to noninfectious diseases. The term *risk factor* may also be more appropriate for many infectious diseases as we learn that a single

Table 2-3. Criteria Used to Test Causal Hypotheses

1. The hypothesized cause should be distributed in the population in the same manner as the disease.
2. The incidence of the disease should be higher in those exposed to the hypothesized cause than in those not so exposed. (The cause may be present in the external environment or as a defect in host responses.)
3. Exposure to the hypothesized cause should be more frequent among those with the disease than in controls without the disease, when all other risk factors are held constant.
4. Temporally, the disease should follow exposure to the hypothesized causative agent.
5. The greater the dose or length of exposure, the greater the likelihood of occurrence of the disease.
6. For some diseases, a spectrum of host responses should follow exposure to the hypothesized agent along a logical biologic gradient from mild to severe.
7. The association between the hypothesized cause and disease should be found in various populations when different methods of study are used.
8. Other explanations for the association should be ruled out.
9. Elimination or modification of the hypothesized cause or of the vector carrying it should decrease the incidence of the disease (e.g., control of polluted water, removal of tar from cigarettes).
10. Prevention or modification of the host's response on exposure to the hypothesized cause should decrease or eliminate the disease (e.g., immunization, drugs to lower cholesterol, specific lymphocyte transfer factor in cancer).
11. When possible, in experimental settings the disease should occur more frequently in animals or humans appropriately exposed to the hypothesized cause than in those not so exposed; this exposure may be deliberate in volunteers, experimentally induced in the laboratory, or demonstrated in a controlled regulation of natural exposure.
12. All of the relationships and findings should make biologic and epidemiologic sense.

pathogenic agent is but one of many elements involved in the production of clinical illness. Susser has discussed at greater length the complexities of drawing causal inferences from the results of observational epidemiologic studies (Susser, 1977, 1986).

MEASURES OF DISEASE FREQUENCY: RATES AND RISKS

An *incidence rate*, like all quantities meeting the formal definition of a rate (Elandt-Johnson, 1975), is a change per unit time per person at risk (or per 100 or 1000 persons at risk, for instance). Thus, the incidence rate for a first major coronary event in male smokers between the ages of 40 and 64 represents a rate of change from the nondiseased state to the diseased state among persons at risk. The total number of new cases divided by the number of persons at risk per unit time is called the *crude incidence rate*. Often, incidence rates are formed by weighting age-specific rates according to the age distribution of the population to which they are to be generalized or compared. These are referred to as *age-standardized* (or *age-adjusted*) *incidence rates*. *Age-specific incidence rates* are obtained by dividing the number of events within an age group by the number of person-years of observation contributed by persons in that age group. For example, based on 92 events and approximately 10,200 person-years of observation involving men between the ages of 45 and 49 (Pooling Project Research Group, 1978), the incidence rate for a first coronary event among smokers between the ages of 45 and 49 is estimated to be 92/10,200 = 9.0 per 1000 men at risk per year. Person-years of observation are contributed by study participants as long as they have not died, have not been lost to follow-up, and have not had their first coronary event. The incidence rate for a disease is also referred to as the *hazard rate* for developing a disease (Kalbfleish and Prentice, 1980) or as the instantaneous *incidence density* (Miettinen, 1976). When the event under study is death rather than the occurrence of disease, the term *mortality rate* (or *death rate*) is used.

A concept closely related to that of an incidence rate is that of the *risk* or probability of developing a disease over a stated period of time, such as the probability that an individual develops measles during the first 10 years of life or the probability that a person in an occupational group develops respiratory symptoms over a 5-year period of observation. The term risk is also often applied to the average risk for a group of people, even though "average risk" might be a more appropriate term. The average risk is sometimes called the *incidence proportion*. The term *cumulative incidence rate* is also used in this context, but we prefer to avoid use of the term "rate" in reference to a probability or proportion. Because the risk is a probability, its numeric value depends on the length of the period of observation but does not depend on the units in which time is expressed. On the other hand, the numeric value of a rate varies according to the units in which time is expressed. Therefore, an incidence rate of 13.0 per 1000 men at risk per year is equivalent to an incidence rate of 13.0/12 = 1.083 per 1000 men at risk per month.

In many circumstances of practical interest the relationship between rates and risks can be expressed in a simple formula. To describe this relationship, we let $R(t)$ denote the average risk for development of disease among members of a cohort during a specified time period, say from time 0 to time t. Suppose that each cohort member remains at risk and under observation until either the disease occurs or the period of observation ends at time t. It can be shown that when the incidence rate μ in the cohort is constant throughout the period,

$$R(t) = 1 - \exp(-\mu t) = 1 - e^{-\mu t} \qquad (2.1)$$

The symbol e denotes the base of the natural logarithm ($e = 2.71828$), and $\exp(-\mu t)$ denotes e raised to the power $(-\mu t)$. Thus, this equation can be used to relate rates to risks of disease. When the incidence rate varies during the period, equation (2.1) still holds, with μ now representing the average value of the incidence rate during the period.

To use this equation, each incidence rate and length of observation must be expressed in the same units, for example, incidence rate per person per year and length of observation in years. Also, when the incidence rate changes within the time period for which the risk is calculated, the rate must be the *unweighted* average obtained when the total time period is divided into a number of intervals. For instance, in one report (Pooling Project Research Group, 1978), an incidence rate of 13.0 new coronary events per 1000 men at risk per year was obtained by computing the unweighted mean of the age-specific rates for the five age intervals of 40–44, 45–49, 50–54, 55–59, and 60–64. The smaller the intervals into which time is divided, the better will be the estimate of risk obtained in this manner. Nevertheless, fairly wide intervals can be validly used in practice, provided that the incidence does not change markedly within intervals.

Based on an estimated incidence rate of 13.0 per 1000 per year, the mean number of events per man over a 25-year period in a closed cohort (that is, a cohort in which no additions to the cohort take place over time, and persons leave the cohort only through developing the outcome of interest to the study) is $25 \times 0.013 = 0.325$. Assuming that there are no competing risks (that is, events that remove a cohort member from being at risk for the outcome under investigation), the risk that a male smoker will have a first coronary event between the ages of 40 and 64 is therefore estimated as:

$$1 - e^{-0.325} = 0.277$$

Note that conversion of the rate to $0.013/12 = 0.0010833$ events per man at risk per month and conversion of the length of observation to 300 months would yield the same value of 0.277 for the risk.

When the incidence rate is low or the period of observation short, there is a fairly close correspondence between the risk and the product of the mean incidence rate per person and the length of the period of observation. In that instance, the loss of persons at risk because they have developed the disease within the period of observation is small relative to the size of the total group, so that the two quantities correspond quite closely.

When estimating risks from actual data, as when calculating rates, proper account must be taken of persons who die or who are lost to follow-up. If no losses of either type occur over the specified period of observation, then the estimate of risk is simply the proportion of the study group developing the disease over the period of observation. When such losses do occur, however, proper estimation of risks requires special techniques such as those discussed in Chapters 6 and 7.

MEASURES OF ASSOCIATION

As discussed earlier, identification of causal agents usually proceeds only gradually, through the study of what are often referred to as risk factors. Risk factors are in turn identified on the basis of observed variations in disease frequency. If a particular factor is associated with an elevated frequency of occurrence of the disease, and if the association cannot be explained on the basis of confounding or methodological biases, then that factor is regarded as a risk factor for the disease.

An important purpose of observational epidemiologic studies is not only to identify risk factors but also to quantify the magnitude of the effect of risk factors on disease risks or rates. Various measures of the association of a risk factor with disease can be used to quantify this effect. The choice of a measure of association depends in part on one's purposes, on the measurement characteristics of the variables under consideration, on biologic considerations, and on the type of study design employed. In epidemiology, the measures of association used most frequently are those based on incidence rates and on risks of developing disease.

Measures of Association Based on Ratios

One measure of association based directly on incidence or mortality rates is the *rate ratio.* This measure is defined as the ratio of rates for two groups differing in their exposure to a possible risk factor for the disease under study. The rate ratio observed in a study is used to estimate the true rate ratio. For an exposure that is regarded as either present or absent:

$$\text{Rate ratio} = \frac{\text{Incidence rate for exposed}}{\text{Incidence rate for unexposed}}$$

The rate ratio is also sometimes referred to as the *incidence density ratio.* The magnitude of the association between smoking and first coronary event among males between the ages of 40 and 64 may be quantified using the rate ratio. Because the average annual incidence of a first coronary event was observed to be 6.2 per 1000 among male nonsmokers and 13.0 among male smokers between the ages of 40 and 64 (Pooling Project Research Group, 1978), the estimated rate ratio for this association is 13.0/6.2 = 2.1. That is, between ages 40 and 64, male smokers without a previous coronary event have 2.1 times the rate of first coronary events compared with nonsmokers without a previous coronary event.

The *risk ratio,* or *incidence proportion ratio,* is another measure of association that is closely related to the rate ratio. Instead of being based on a comparison of incidence rates, however, the risk ratio is based on a comparison of probabilities of developing the disease. If D denotes the presence of disease, $\bar{D}$ denotes the absence of disease, E denotes the presence of exposure, $\bar{E}$ denotes the absence of exposure, and $Pr(.)$ denotes the probability of an event, then the risk ratio may be expressed in terms of conditional probabilities as:

$$\text{Risk ratio} = \frac{Pr(D|E)}{Pr(D|\bar{E})}$$

For example, because the observed risk of having a first coronary event between the ages of 40 and 64 is 0.277 for men who smoke and 0.144 for those who do not, the estimate of the risk ratio is $0.277/0.144 = 1.9$.

The risk ratio is particularly applicable when the period within which the disease might develop has a fixed duration. Examples include the probability that a newborn is of low birthweight or the risk of illness in the days following a social gathering at which contaminated food was served. For those diseases having lengthy and highly variable incubation or latency periods, the value of the risk ratio depends in part on the length of the period of observation. To take an extreme example, consider mortality from all causes for groups exposed or not exposed to a particular agent. If the mortality rate is twice as high for exposed individuals as for unexposed individuals, then the rate ratio is 2.0. Over a short period of observation, the risk ratio, that is, the ratio of the proportion of each group that has died, will also be close to 2.0, but as the period of observation lengthens, all members of both groups will eventually die. Consequently, even though the rate ratio may remain constant at 2.0 over the entire period of observation, the risk ratio will necessarily approach 1.0 as the individual risks approach 1.0.

A third, frequently used ratio measure of association is the *odds ratio*. For a cohort study, this measure (which is sometimes referred to as the *incidence odds ratio*) is defined as:

$$\begin{aligned}
\text{Odds ratio} &= \frac{Pr(D|E)/[1 - Pr(D|E)]}{Pr(D|\bar{E})/[1 - Pr(D|\bar{E})]} \\
&= \frac{Pr(D|E)/Pr(\bar{D}|E)}{Pr(D|\bar{E})/Pr(\bar{D}|\bar{E})}
\end{aligned}$$

For example, the odds for a first coronary event between the ages of 40 and 64 are $0.277/0.723 = 0.383$ for male smokers and $0.144/0.856 = 0.168$ for male nonsmokers. Consequently, the odds ratio is $0.383/0.168 = 2.3$. For a cross-sectional study an odds ratio can be similarly calculated, but with the symbol D denoting prevalent rather than incident disease.

For a case-control study, the odds ratio is defined as:

$$\text{Odds ratio} = \frac{Pr(E|D)/[1 - Pr(E|D)]}{Pr(E|\bar{D})/[1 - Pr(E|\bar{D})]}$$

$$= \frac{Pr(E|D)/Pr(\bar{E}|D)}{Pr(E|\bar{D})/Pr(\bar{E}|\bar{D})}$$

Because this odds ratio is defined in terms of probabilities of exposure rather than probabilities of disease, it is often referred to as the *exposure odds ratio*. If 40% of cases are exposed and if 25% of controls are exposed, then the estimate of the odds ratio is $(0.400/0.600)/(0.250/0.750) = 2.0$. That is, the odds of exposure are twice as great among cases as among controls. However, the exposure odds ratio and the disease odds ratio are always the same. For example, because $(0.400/0.600)/(0.250/0.750) = (0.400/0.250)/(0.600/0.750) = 2.0$, this odds ratio also indicates that the odds of disease are twice as great in the exposed as in the unexposed.

Although the rate ratio and risk ratio are more readily interpretable as measures of effect (Greenland, 1987), the odds ratio has certain advantages, as will be illustrated in subsequent chapters. First, the odds ratio has certain convenient statistical properties that make it amenable to analysis by means of several important multivariable statistical techniques, including logistic regression and other types of log-linear models (Bishop et al., 1975). Second, when the disease being studied is not common during the period of observation, the odds ratio calculated from a study in a closed cohort or from certain case-control designs (i.e., cumulative incidence case-control studies) approximates the risk ratio (Cornfield, 1951). Finally, in certain other case-control designs (i.e., incidence-density case-control studies), the odds ratio approximates the rate ratio regardless of whether the disease is rare (Sheehe, 1962; Greenland and Thomas, 1982). These specific case-control designs will be discussed in Chapter 8.

When the risk of disease is sufficiently small over the period of observation (under 0.05 in both the exposed and unexposed will usually suffice), the values of the rate ratio, the risk ratio, and the odds ratio are nearly identical. Perhaps for this reason, the logical distinction between these three ratio measures is often not made, and the single term *relative risk* is frequently used to refer to any one of the three. Strictly speaking, however, the term relative risk is most appropriately applied only as a synonym for risk ratio.

So far, ratio measures of association have been discussed only in the context of exposures that are treated as binary (e.g., smokers versus non-smokers). However, the same concepts apply directly to situations in which exposure is treated as a continuous or quantitative variable (e.g., number of cigarettes smoked per day). In that instance, a ratio measure is calculated to describe the relative increase in the rate, risk, or odds associated with an increase of a given magnitude in the quantitative exposure variable. For example, it is estimated that the rate ratio for a first coronary event is 1.15 for each additional ten cigarettes smoked per day, on the average (Pooling Project Research Group, 1978). Specific methods for the estimation of all three ratio measures from actual data will be discussed in subsequent chapters dealing with the design and analysis of specific types of epidemiologic investigations.

Measures of Association Based on Differences

Although ratio measures of association are most frequently employed in epidemiologic research, another important group of measures sometimes used includes those based on the arithmetic difference between rates or risks. The *rate difference* is obtained simply by subtracting the incidence rate for the unexposed group from the corresponding rate for the exposed group. For example, the rate difference for the association between smoking and the incidence of a first coronary event among men between the ages of 40 and 64 is $13.0 - 6.2 = 6.8$ per 1000 men at risk per year. Similarly, the *risk difference* is obtained by subtracting the risk of disease for the unexposed group from the corresponding risk for the exposed group. The risk difference for the association between smoking and first coronary event among men between the ages of 40 and 64 is estimated to be $0.277 - 0.144 = 0.133$.

The choice between ratio measures of association and difference measures is seldom clear-cut. For purposes of public policy decision making, the difference measures may be more useful in that they permit direct calculation of the number of "excess" occurrences of the disease that are associated with the exposure. On the other hand, ratio measures may be preferable when disease etiology is being studied because they contribute to the assessment of the plausibility that an observed association is causal. All other considerations being equal, a rate ratio close to 1.0, even if statistically significant, is more likely than a rate ratio that is much higher (or much lower) than 1.0 to be an artifact of the confounding effects of another risk factor that is correlated with the exposure of interest.

Attributable Fraction

It is sometimes of interest to estimate the proportion of disease occurrence that is attributable to a particular exposure. Provided that the association between the risk factor and disease represents a causal relationship, the *attributable fraction* indicates the proportion of the disease occurrence that potentially would be eliminated if exposure to the risk factor were prevented. The attributable fraction may be calculated either for exposed individuals only or for the population as a whole, and may be based on average risks (incidence proportions) or person-time incidence rates (incidence densities). If the objective is to estimate the proportion of disease that occurred by a certain point in time and that would not have occurred up to that point if the exposure had not occurred ("excess fraction"), then it is usually best to estimate the attributable fraction from the average risks up to that point in time.

The *attributable fraction for the exposed,* or, when expressed as a percent, the *attributable risk percent for the exposed,* is then defined as:

$$\frac{\text{(Risk for exposed)} - \text{(Risk for unexposed)}}{\text{Risk for exposed}}$$

The attributable fraction for the exposed is thus simply the excess disease occurrence associated with the risk factor, expressed as a percentage of the total disease occurrence for those exposed to the risk factor. A mathematically equivalent expression in terms of the risk ratio is

$$\frac{\text{Risk ratio} - 1}{\text{Risk ratio}}$$

In the example involving smoking and first coronary event, the attributable fraction of the exposed is $[(0.277 - 0.144)/0.277] = 0.48$. That is, 48% of the first coronary events occurring among male smokers between the ages of 40 and 64 are attributable to the fact that they smoke. The term "attributable" may be unfortunate in that it often connotes causality. If the association between an exposure and a disease is the result of confounding or other bias, then the apparent excess of disease among the exposed cannot be "attributed" to that exposure.

The *attributable fraction for the population,* or, when expressed as a percent, the *attributable risk percent for the population,* is defined as:

$$\frac{\text{(Risk for the entire population)} - \text{(Risk for the unexposed)}}{\text{Risk for the entire population}}$$

Equivalent expressions in terms of the risk ratio are

$$\text{(Prevalence of exposure among cases)} \times \frac{\text{(Risk ratio} - 1)}{\text{(Risk ratio)}}$$

and

$$\frac{\text{(Prevalence of exposure in the population)} \times \text{(Risk ratio} - 1)}{1 + \text{(Prevalence of exposure in the population)} \times \text{(Risk ratio} - 1)}$$

All of these expressions assume that no confounding of the association between the exposure and the disease is present. For the example, it is convenient to use the latter form. Taking 43% as the estimate of the prevalence of current smoking for men between the ages of 40 and 64 in the general population (National Center for Health Statistics, 1979), the attributable fraction for the population is

$$\frac{0.43 \times 0.90}{1 + (0.43 \times 0.90)} = 0.28$$

That is, it appears that 28% of the first coronary events occurring among all men between the ages of 40 and 64 are attributable to smoking. The attributable fraction for the population is also referred to as the *etiologic fraction* (Miettinen, 1974), although below this term is used in a more specialized sense. Less appropriately perhaps, the etiologic fraction is sometimes called the *attributable risk*, although this term is also sometimes used for the risk difference. Procedures for calculating the attributable fraction for the population when the risk ratio has been adjusted for confounding factors are also available (Greenland and Drescher, 1993; Coughlin et al., 1994; Whittemore, 1983).

The attributable fraction for the population depends not only on the magnitude of the risk ratio but also on the prevalence of exposure in the population. Table 2–4 gives some examples of the value of the attributable fraction for the population as a function of the risk ratio and the prevalence of exposure, assuming no confounding is present. The table indicates that for rare exposures, the attributable fraction for the population is small, even when the exposure is strongly related to the disease. That is, an exposure of low prevalence cannot account for a large proportion of the disease in a population unless it is virtually a necessary condition for the development of the disease.

In addition to the percentage of excess cases occurring during a time interval attributable to a certain cause, one might also wish to estimate the

Table 2–4. Magnitude of the Attributable Fraction in the Population (Expressed as a Percent) as a Function of the Prevalence of Exposure (Expressed as a Proportion) and the Magnitude of the Risk Ratio

Prevalence of Exposure	Risk ratio				
	1.5	2.0	5.0	10.0	50.0
0.01	0.5	1.0	3.8	8.3	32.9
0.05	2.4	4.8	6.0	31.0	71.0
0.10	4.8	9.1	28.6	47.4	83.1
0.20	9.1	16.7	44.4	64.3	90.7
0.50	20.0	33.3	66.7	81.8	96.1
0.80	28.6	44.4	76.2	87.8	97.5

percentage of cases in which the exposure played some etiologic role. Identifying the number of such etiologic cases requires more knowledge of the biology of the exposure-disease relationship than is usually available, but the distinction between "etiologic fraction" and "excess fraction" (Greenland and Robins, 1988) is useful to keep in mind. A more detailed discussion of these issues has been presented by Greenland and Robins (1988).

Correlation Coefficient and Regression Coefficient

Each of the measures of association discussed so far is applicable only when the outcome of interest is either present or absent. Often, however, one is interested in quantifying the magnitude of the association between possible risk factors (also called predictor variables) that are measured on a continuous scale and an outcome that is also measured on a continuous scale (e.g., diet or exercise as they relate to systolic blood pressure). In instances when one wants to examine the association between two continuously distributed variables, a commonly used measure of association is the *product-moment correlation coefficient.* The square of this coefficient indicates the proportion of the variation in the outcome variable that is "explained" or "accounted for" by the predictor variable (Snedecor and Cochran, 1967). Thus, a correlation coefficient of 0.40 between a risk factor and systolic blood pressure would indicate that $(0.40)^2$ or 16% of the variance in systolic blood pressure is accounted for by that risk factor. The correlation coefficient and its multivariable extensions will be discussed in more detail in Chapter 10.

Although the correlation coefficient is commonly used in many fields, more direct information on the quantitative effect that a given increase in one variable has on the level of a second variable can be obtained from a method of analysis called linear regression. Thus, the value of a *regression coefficient* for the relationship between exercise and blood pressure would indicate the decrease (or increase) in the number of millimeters of blood pressure for each increment in exercise (e.g., one hour of tennis per day). On the other hand, the correlation coefficient would indicate only the fraction of a standard deviation by which blood pressure decreases (or increases) for an increment of one standard deviation on the measure of exercise. Since the standard deviation for a particular variable often varies in different population groups, widely different values for the correlation coefficient could be obtained in different groups, even if the underlying biologic relationship remained the same (Greenland et al., 1986, 1991).

REFERENCES

Armenian HK, Khoury MG. 1981. Age of onset of genetic disease. *Am J Epidemiol* 113:596–605.

Armenian HK, Lilienfeld AM. 1974. The distribution of incubation periods of neoplastic diseases. *Am J Epidemiol* 99:92–100.

Bishop YMM, Fienberg SE, Holland PW. 1975. Discrete Multivariate Analysis. Cambridge, MA, M.I.T. Press.

Case RAM, Hosker ME, McDonald DB, Pearson JT. 1954. Tumors of the urinary bladder in workmen engaged in the manufacture and use of certain dye-stuff intermediates in the British chemical industry. *Br J Ind Med* 11:75–104.

Cornfield J. 1951. A method of estimating comparative risks from clinical data. Applications to cancer of the lung, breast and cervix. *J Natl Cancer Inst* 11:1269–1275.

Coughlin SS, Benichou J, Weed DL. 1994. Attributable risk estimation in case-control studies. *Epidemiol Rev* 16:51–64.

Elandt-Johnson RC. 1975. Definitions of rates: some remarks on their use and misuse. *Am J Epidemiol* 102:267–271.

Evans AS. 1967. Clinical syndromes in adults caused by respiratory infection. *Med Clin North Am* 51:803–818.

Evans AS. 1976. Causation and disease: the Henle-Koch postulates revisited. *Yale J Biol Med* 49:175–195.

Evans AS. 1977. Limitations of Koch's postulates. Letter. *Lancet* 2:1277–1278.

Evans AS. 1980. Discussion of paper by Dr. Richmond. In AM Lilienfeld, Editor. Time, Places and Persons: Aspects of the History of Epidemiology. Baltimore, MD, Johns Hopkins University Press, pp 94–98.

Evans AS. 1989. Epidemiological concepts and methods. In AS Evans, Ed. Viral Infections of Humans: Epidemiology and Control. New York, Plenum, pp 3–49.

Evans AS. 1991. Epidemiological concepts. In AS Evans, PS Brachman, Eds. Bacterial Infections of Humans: Epidemiology and Control. New York, Plenum, pp 3–57.

Evans AS. 1993. Causation and Disease. A Chronological Journey. New York, Plenum.

Evans AS, Niederman JC. 1989. Epstein-Barr virus. In AS Evans, Ed. Viral Infections of Humans: Epidemiology and Control. New York, Plenum, pp 265–292.

Greenland S. 1987. Interpretation and choice of effect measures in epidemiologic analyses. *Am J Epidemiol* 125:761–768.

Greenland S, Drescher K. 1993. Maximum likelihood estimation of the attributable fraction from logistic models. *Biometrics* 49:865–72.

Greenland S, Maclure M, Schlesselman JJ, Poole C, Morgenstern H. 1991. Standardized regression coefficients: a further critique and review of some alternatives. *Epidemiology* 2:387–392.

Greenland S, Robins JM. 1988. Conceptual problems in the definition and interpretation of attributable fractions. *Am J Epidemiol* 128:1185–1197.

Greenland S, Schlesselman JJ, Criqui MH, Morgenstern H. 1986. The fallacy of employing standardized regression coefficients and correlations as measures of effect. *Am J Epidemiol* 123:203–208.

Greenland S, Thomas DC. 1982. On the need for the rare disease assumption in case-control studies. *Am J Epidemiol* 116:547–553.

Herbst AL, Ulfelder H, Poskanzer DC. 1971. Adenocarcinoma of the vagina: association of maternal stilbestrol therapy with tumor appearance in young women. *N Engl J Med* 284:878–881.

Ichimuru M, Ichimuru T, Belsky JL. 1978. Incidence of leukemia in atomic bomb survivors belonging to a fixed cohort in Hiroshima and Nagasaki, 1951–71: radiation dose, years after exposure, and type of leukemia. *Jpn J Radiat Res* 19:262–282.

James JIP, Lamb DW. 1963. Congenital abnormalities of the limbs. *Practitioner* 191:159–172.

Johnson RC, Hyde FW, Rumpel CM. 1984. Taxonomy of the Lyme disease spirochetes. *Yale J Biol Med* 57:529–537.

Jones RR. 1989. The continuing hazard of lead in drinking water. *Lancet* 2:669–670.

Kalbfleisch J, Prentice RL. 1980. The Statistical Analysis of Failure Time Data. New York, Wiley.

Kaslow RA, Shaw S. 1981. The role of histocompatibility antigens (HLA) in infection. *Epidemiol Rev* 3:90–114.

MacMahon B, Pugh TF. 1970. Epidemiology: Principles and Methods. Boston, Little, Brown and Company.

McClure FJ. 1970. Water Fluoridation: The Search and the Victory. Washington, DC, U.S. Government Printing Office.

Miettinen OS. 1974. Proportion of disease caused or prevented by a given exposure, trait or intervention. *Am J Epidemiol* 99:325–332.

Miettinen OS. 1976. Estimability and estimation in case-referent studies. *Am J Epidemiol* 103:226–235.

National Center for Health Statistics. 1979. Use Habits Among Adults of Cigarettes, Coffee, Aspirin, and Sleeping Pills: United States, 1976. DHEW Publication no. (PHS) 80–1559. Vital and Health Statistics, Series 10, No. 131.

Paul LW. 1945. Host variation in the manifestation of disease with particular reference to homologous serum jaundice in the Army of the United States. *Dist Columbia Med Assoc* 14:443–449.

Perera FP, Weinstein IB. 1982. Molecular epidemiology and carcinogen-DNA adduct detection: new approaches to studies of human cancer causation. *J Chron Dis* 35:581–600.

Pooling Project Research Group. 1978. Relationship of blood pressure, serum cholesterol, smoking habit, relative weight and ECG abnormalities to incidence of major coronary events: final report of the Pooling Project. *J Chron Dis* 31:201–306.

Prusiner SB, Gajdusek DC, Alpers MP. 1982. Kuru with incubation periods exceeding two decades. *Ann Neurol* 12:1–9.

Rivers TM. 1937. Viruses and Koch's postulates. *J Bacteriol* 33:1–12.

Sheehe PR. 1962. Dynamic risk analysis in retrospective matched pair studies of disease. *Biometrics* 18:323–341.

Snedecor GW, Cochran WG. 1967. Statistical Methods. 6th ed. Ames, IA, Iowa State University Press.

Steere AC, Broderick TF, Malawista SE. 1978. Erythema chronica migrans and

Lyme arthritis: epidemiologic evidence for a tick vector. *Am J Epidemiol* 108:312–321.

Susser M. 1977. Judgment and causal inference: criteria in epidemiologic studies. *Am J Epidemiol* 105:1–15.

Susser M. 1986. The logic of Sir Karl Popper and the practice of epidemiology. *Am J Epidemiol* 124:711–718.

Whittemore AS. 1983. Estimating attributable risk from case-control studies. *Am J Epidemiol* 117:76–85.

Exercises

1. In an observational cohort study of men in the age group 60–69 years, the hypothesis is tested that men who drink cola beverages are at greater risk for stroke than men who do not drink cola beverages. The following fourfold table is obtained:

	Stroke	No Stroke	Total	Proportion with stroke/year
Cola	500	4500	5000	0.10
No cola	20	980	1000	0.02
Total	520	5480	6000	0.09

The *p*-value for the difference in proportions developing strokes is less than 0.01. *In addition to the information that can be obtained from this table,* which of the following pieces of data would help you decide whether the association between drinking cola beverages and stroke is a causal one?

a. The annual incidence rate of stroke in men who drink cola and in those who do not drink cola.

b. The annual incidence rate of stroke in men according to the amount of cola they drink.

c. The annual incidence rate of stroke in men who used to drink cola before the study began.

d. The cost of cola beverages.

e. The relative risk in men who drink cola compared to that in men who do not drink cola.

f. Replication of the findings in other studies.

2. Estimates of 13.0 per 1000 and 6.2 per 1000 have been given in this chapter for the average annual incidence of first coronary events among male smokers and nonsmokers in the age range 40–64. Suppose that the proportion of men who smoke could be reduced through health awareness efforts from 43% to 25%. Assuming that the average amount that smokers smoke remains the same as before, which of the following quantities would you expect to change and if so by how much?

a. Rate ratio

b. Risk ratio

c. Odds ratio

d. Attributable fraction in the exposed

e. Attributable fraction in the population

3. Suppose that in addition to reducing the proportion who smoke to 25%, it is also possible to reduce the average amount that smokers smoke. If the average amount smoked is reduced sufficiently to bring the incidence rate for smokers down to 9.0 per 1000, then what would be the values for each of the five measures listed in Exercise 2?

3

Sources of Routinely Collected
Data on Disease Occurrence

Routinely collected data are often used to provide a rough indication of the frequency of occurrence of diseases and of their descriptive epidemiology. Such data can also serve to provide leads concerning disease etiology. In this chapter, several of the major sources of routinely collected data in the United States are described and their uses and limitations assessed; sources from outside the United States are also briefly discussed where appropriate. Data on international health are described in more detail by Basch (1990) and the National Center for Health Statistics (1988). Although the emphasis in this chapter is on the use of various sources of data for hypothesis generation, many of the strengths and limitations of descriptive studies also apply to analytic studies designed to test hypotheses.

Some data are readily available, in that they are routinely abstracted, tabulated, and published, or can easily be obtained in nonpublished form upon request. Included in this category are mortality and natality data; surveys of the National Center for Health Statistics; data from the Centers for Disease Control and Prevention (CDC) Birth Defects Monitoring Program and the Metropolitan Atlanta Congenital Defects Program; data from the Cancer Surveillance, Epidemiology, and End Results (SEER) program; and data on reportable infectious diseases in the *Morbidity and Mortality Weekly Report* (*MMWR*) from the CDC. Other data can be obtained only by abstracting and tabulating information from records that have been kept primarily for other purposes, such as most hospital records, autopsy reports, physician records, industrial records, insurance records, university student health records, and Armed Forces and Veterans Administration records. Sometimes these records are available in computerized form, but often the investigator has to spend much time and effort abstracting and tabulating the desired information. Finally, no routinely collected source of data exists for some disorders, and the investigator must undertake his or her own study to obtain even basic descriptive information. This chapter will cover only sources of data that are already available in usable form or are available after abstraction and tabulation from records kept primarily for other purposes.

SURVEILLANCE

In most health departments, routinely collected statistics provide the key data for monitoring morbidity and mortality trends and are incorporated under the term *surveillance*. Two recent books are entirely devoted to surveillance (Eylenbosch and Noah, 1988; Teutsch and Churchill, 1994). Epidemiologic surveillance has been defined by the Centers for Disease Control (CDC) (1986) as "the ongoing systematic collection, analysis, and interpretation of health data essential to the planning, implementation, and evaluation of public health practice, closely integrated with the timely dissemination of these data to those who need to know. The final link in the surveillance chain is the application of these data to prevention and control. A surveillance system includes a functional capacity for data collection, analysis, and dissemination linked to public health programs." The sources of data and their application have been described in detail elsewhere (Brachman, 1991; Evans, 1991; Raska, 1983; Thacker and Berkelman, 1988). The World Health Organization (WHO), the Centers for Disease Control (CDC), and many governmental agencies throughout the world use such epidemiologic information as the basis for their operational health policies and immunization programs. Table 3–1 shows the 10 key sources of information that have been designated by WHO for surveillance systems. Most of these are derived from routinely collected reports and have been widely used in the control of communicable diseases. Surveillance data from sources indicated in Table 3–2 as well as other sources of data described in this chapter are also used. Some of these sources fall into the category of routinely collected data, whereas other sources require special efforts on

Table 3–1. Ten Key Sources of Data for Surveillance Systems Designated by the World Health Organization

1. Mortality registration
2. Morbidity reporting
3. Epidemic reporting
4. Laboratory investigations
5. Individual case investigations
6. Epidemic field investigations
7. Surveys
8. Animal-reservoir and vector-distribution studies
9. Biologics and drug utilization
10. Knowledge of the population and environment

Source: Evans (1982).

Table 3-2. Other Sources of Surveillance Data

1. Hospital and medical care statistics
2. Panels of cooperating physicians
3. Public health laboratory reports
4. Absenteeism from work or school
5. Telephone and household surveys
6. Newspaper and news broadcasting reports

Source: Evans (1982).

the part of the investigator. Surveillance techniques are being increasingly applied to chronic diseases, occupational safety and health, health effects of environmental toxic exposures, injuries, personal health practices, and preventive health technologies (Thacker and Berkelman, 1988).

MORTALITY DATA

Over the years, the most commonly used routinely collected source of data has been mortality data. Figure 3-1 shows a copy of the U.S. Standard Certificate of Death, as revised in 1989; it serves as a basic document from which all published mortality statistics arise in the United States. The National Center for Health Statistics, which is the focal agency in the United States for the collection, dissemination, and analysis of vital and health statistics (Israel et al., 1986), prepares Standard Certificates, which serve as models for the states; individual states may make some modifications of the certificates. The funeral director or other person in charge of interment is responsible for completing the parts of the death certificate that require personal information about the deceased and for filing the certificate with the local registrar of the district in which the death occurred. A physician must complete and sign the medical certification section and enter the cause and date of death. In most states, whenever a death is related to accident, suicide, or homicide, or if a physician has not been in attendance, the medical examiner or coroner must sign the certificate. The local registrar, after verifying the completeness of the information, keeps a copy and sends the certificate to the State Registrar. After querying the local registrar for incomplete or inconsistent information, the State Registrar keeps one copy and sends another copy to the National Center for Health Statistics, which in turn prepares and publishes national statistics, mainly in Vital Statistics of the United States.

The middle part of the death certificate shown in Figure 3-1 is concerned with specific causes of death. The immediate cause of death is recorded on line (a) of Part I, and the antecedent conditions, if any, that gave rise to the cause reported on line (a) are listed on lines (b), (c), and

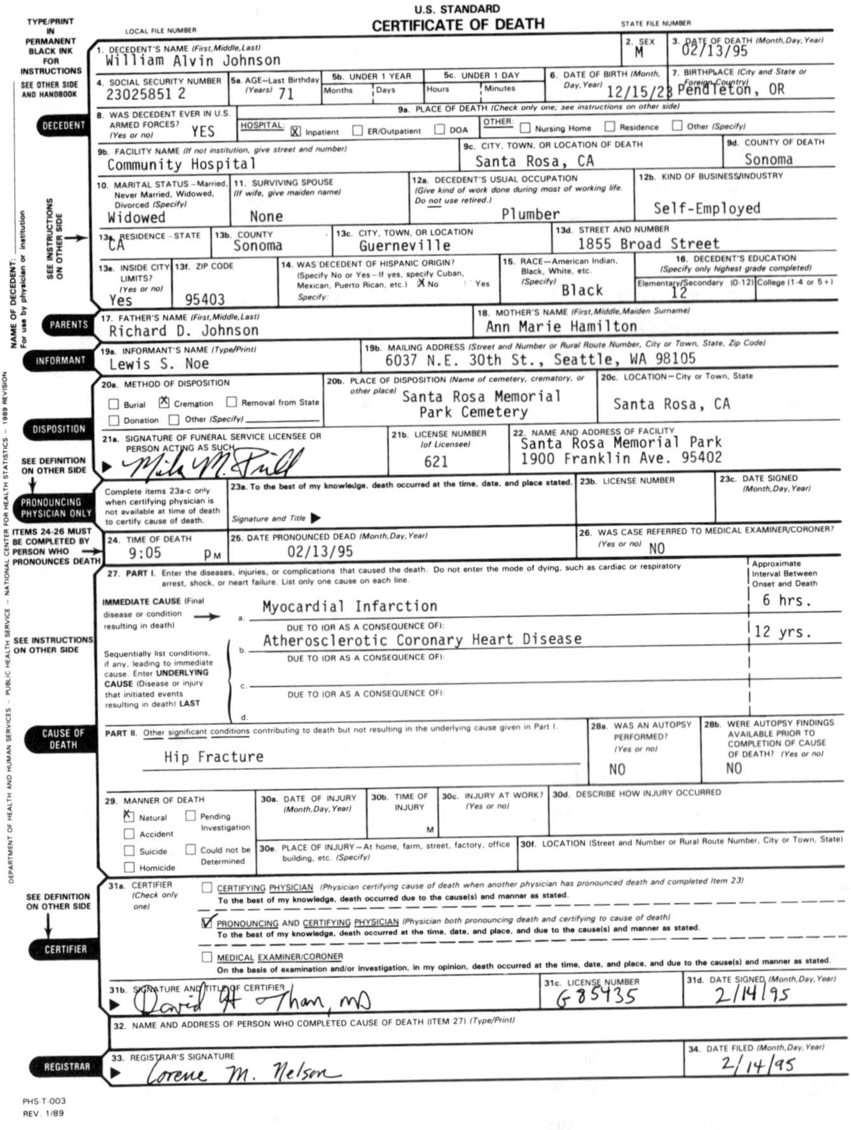
U.S. STANDARD
CERTIFICATE OF DEATH

TYPE/PRINT IN PERMANENT BLACK INK FOR INSTRUCTIONS SEE OTHER SIDE AND HANDBOOK

LOCAL FILE NUMBER

STATE FILE NUMBER

DECEDENT

1. DECEDENT'S NAME (First, Middle, Last): William Alvin Johnson

2. SEX: M

3. DATE OF DEATH (Month, Day, Year): 02/13/95

4. SOCIAL SECURITY NUMBER: 23025851 2

5a. AGE–Last Birthday (Years): 71

5b. UNDER 1 YEAR: Months, Days

5c. UNDER 1 DAY: Hours, Minutes

6. DATE OF BIRTH (Month, Day, Year): 12/15/23

7. BIRTHPLACE (City and State or Foreign Country): Pendleton, OR

8. WAS DECEDENT EVER IN U.S. ARMED FORCES? (Yes or no): YES

9a. PLACE OF DEATH (Check only one; see instructions on other side): HOSPITAL: [X] Inpatient [ ] ER/Outpatient [ ] DOA; OTHER: [ ] Nursing Home [ ] Residence [ ] Other (Specify)

9b. FACILITY NAME (If not institution, give street and number): Community Hospital

9c. CITY, TOWN, OR LOCATION OF DEATH: Santa Rosa, CA

9d. COUNTY OF DEATH: Sonoma

10. MARITAL STATUS – Married, Never Married, Widowed, Divorced (Specify): Widowed

11. SURVIVING SPOUSE (If wife, give maiden name): None

12a. DECEDENT'S USUAL OCCUPATION (Give kind of work done during most of working life. Do not use retired.): Plumber

12b. KIND OF BUSINESS/INDUSTRY: Self-Employed

13a. RESIDENCE – STATE: CA

13b. COUNTY: Sonoma

13c. CITY, TOWN, OR LOCATION: Guerneville

13d. STREET AND NUMBER: 1855 Broad Street

13e. INSIDE CITY LIMITS? (Yes or no): Yes

13f. ZIP CODE: 95403

14. WAS DECEDENT OF HISPANIC ORIGIN? (Specify No or Yes – If yes, specify Cuban, Mexican, Puerto Rican, etc.) [X] No [ ] Yes Specify:

15. RACE – American Indian, Black, White, etc. (Specify): Black

16. DECEDENT'S EDUCATION (Specify only highest grade completed): Elementary/Secondary (0-12): 12; College (1-4 or 5+)

PARENTS

17. FATHER'S NAME (First, Middle, Last): Richard D. Johnson

18. MOTHER'S NAME (First, Middle, Maiden Surname): Ann Marie Hamilton

INFORMANT

19a. INFORMANT'S NAME (Type/Print): Lewis S. Noe

19b. MAILING ADDRESS (Street and Number or Rural Route Number, City or Town, State, Zip Code): 6037 N.E. 30th St., Seattle, WA 98105

DISPOSITION

20a. METHOD OF DISPOSITION: [ ] Burial [X] Cremation [ ] Removal from State [ ] Donation [ ] Other (Specify)

20b. PLACE OF DISPOSITION (Name of cemetery, crematory, or other place): Santa Rosa Memorial Park Cemetery

20c. LOCATION – City or Town, State: Santa Rosa, CA

SEE DEFINITION ON OTHER SIDE

21a. SIGNATURE OF FUNERAL SERVICE LICENSEE OR PERSON ACTING AS SUCH: Mike M. Pull

21b. LICENSE NUMBER (of Licensee): 621

22. NAME AND ADDRESS OF FACILITY: Santa Rosa Memorial Park, 1900 Franklin Ave. 95402

PRONOUNCING PHYSICIAN ONLY

Complete items 23a-c only when certifying physician is not available at time of death to certify cause of death.

23a. To the best of my knowledge, death occurred at the time, date, and place stated. Signature and Title

23b. LICENSE NUMBER

23c. DATE SIGNED (Month, Day, Year)

ITEMS 24-26 MUST BE COMPLETED BY PERSON WHO PRONOUNCES DEATH

24. TIME OF DEATH: 9:05 PM

25. DATE PRONOUNCED DEAD (Month, Day, Year): 02/13/95

26. WAS CASE REFERRED TO MEDICAL EXAMINER/CORONER? (Yes or no): NO

NAME OF DECEDENT: For use by physician or institution — SEE INSTRUCTIONS ON OTHER SIDE

27. PART I. Enter the diseases, injuries, or complications that caused the death. Do not enter the mode of dying, such as cardiac or respiratory arrest, shock, or heart failure. List only one cause on each line.

IMMEDIATE CAUSE (Final disease or condition resulting in death) a. Myocardial Infarction — Approximate Interval Between Onset and Death: 6 hrs.

Sequentially list conditions, if any, leading to immediate cause. Enter UNDERLYING CAUSE (Disease or injury that initiated events resulting in death) LAST

DUE TO (OR AS A CONSEQUENCE OF): b. Atherosclerotic Coronary Heart Disease — 12 yrs.

DUE TO (OR AS A CONSEQUENCE OF): c.

DUE TO (OR AS A CONSEQUENCE OF): d.

CAUSE OF DEATH

PART II. Other significant conditions contributing to death but not resulting in the underlying cause given in Part I: Hip Fracture

28a. WAS AN AUTOPSY PERFORMED? (Yes or no): NO

28b. WERE AUTOPSY FINDINGS AVAILABLE PRIOR TO COMPLETION OF CAUSE OF DEATH? (Yes or no): NO

29. MANNER OF DEATH: [X] Natural [ ] Pending Investigation [ ] Accident [ ] Suicide [ ] Could not be Determined [ ] Homicide

30a. DATE OF INJURY (Month, Day, Year)

30b. TIME OF INJURY: M

30c. INJURY AT WORK? (Yes or no)

30d. DESCRIBE HOW INJURY OCCURRED

30e. PLACE OF INJURY – At home, farm, street, factory, office building, etc. (Specify)

30f. LOCATION (Street and Number or Rural Route Number, City or Town, State)

SEE DEFINITION ON OTHER SIDE

CERTIFIER

31a. CERTIFIER (Check only one)

[ ] CERTIFYING PHYSICIAN (Physician certifying cause of death when another physician has pronounced death and completed Item 23) To the best of my knowledge, death occurred due to the cause(s) and manner as stated.

[X] PRONOUNCING AND CERTIFYING PHYSICIAN (Physician both pronouncing death and certifying to cause of death) To the best of my knowledge, death occurred at the time, date, and place, and due to the cause(s) and manner as stated.

[ ] MEDICAL EXAMINER/CORONER On the basis of examination and/or investigation, in my opinion, death occurred at the time, date, and place, and due to the cause(s) and manner as stated.

31b. SIGNATURE AND TITLE OF CERTIFIER: David H. Than, MD

31c. LICENSE NUMBER: G85435

31d. DATE SIGNED (Month, Day, Year): 2/14/95

32. NAME AND ADDRESS OF PERSON WHO COMPLETED CAUSE OF DEATH (ITEM 27) (Type/Print)

REGISTRAR

33. REGISTRAR'S SIGNATURE: Lorene M. Nelson

34. DATE FILED (Month, Day, Year): 2/14/95

PHS-T-003
REV. 1/89

DEPARTMENT OF HEALTH AND HUMAN SERVICES – PUBLIC HEALTH SERVICE – NATIONAL CENTER FOR HEALTH STATISTICS – 1989 REVISION

Figure 3–1. U.S. Certificate of Death

(d). The underlying cause of death, or the cause that until recently was the only cause recorded in the published vital statistics, is the last cause listed. The underlying cause is the disease or injury that initiated the sequence of morbid events leading directly or indirectly to death, or the circumstances of the accident or violence that produced the fatal injury. Thus, if line (d) is filled in, it is the underlying cause; if line (c) is filled in but not line (d), the cause listed in line (c) is the underlying cause; if line (b) is filled in but not line (c) or (d), the cause listed on line (b) is the underlying cause, and if only line (a) is filled in, then the cause recorded on line (a) is the underlying cause. In Part II, other significant conditions that were present at the time of death and that may have contributed to death, but that were not related to the immediate cause of death as listed on line (a), may be recorded. Thus, in Figure 3–1, atherosclerotic heart disease is the underlying cause because it is the last cause listed in Part I, whereas myocardial infarction is the immediate cause and hip fracture is a contributing cause. Atherosclerotic heart disease is included in the published vital statistics as the underlying cause.

The U.S. Standard Certificate of Death had changed little for several decades, but the 1989 revisions include some changes of note (Freedman et al., 1988). The medical certification section has been changed in an effort to improve accuracy. First, instructions for completing the medical certification section are included on both the front of the certificate, and, in more detail, on the back. Second, additional lines were added to the cause of death section in an effort to enhance completeness of reporting of all of the chronic conditions that may coexist and contribute to death. Third, provision has been made for two physician signatures so that if a physician with little knowledge of the case signs the death certificate to expedite the release of the body to the funeral director, the funeral director can later contact the attending physician to obtain the medical certification. The new death certificate also requests information on the decedent's education as an indicator of socioeconomic status and allows identification of decedents of Hispanic origin. However, recent studies suggest that Hispanic ethnicity and also race are often not accurately recorded on death certificates (Hahn et al., 1992; Sorlie et al., 1992).

Mortality data have been widely used to generate epidemiologic hypotheses for several reasons. First, mortality data are abstracted, tabulated, and published annually in the United States and in many other countries and are therefore inexpensive and convenient to use. Second, because death certificates are required by law when death occurs, they establish the fact of death with virtual certainty. Because everyone eventually dies, the population at risk is known. Finally, because mortality data have been collected on a continuous basis over many years, trends over time can be studied (Riggan et al., 1983), and, because mortality data are collected in many geographic areas, comparisons of rates from one area to another can be made (Pickle et al., 1987). The limitations and potential pitfalls of comparing death rates from one time period or geographic area to another will be discussed later; however, few other data sources permit an investigator to make even rough comparisons over long periods of time or geographic areas. It might also be mentioned that death certificates are useful in studies of survivorship when the main endpoint of interest is whether a person is dead or alive.

The usefulness of mortality data as an indicator of disease frequency in the population depends to a large extent on the particular disease being studied. Diseases that have a high case fatality rate (rate at which persons with a given disease die from that disease within a specified time period), that are rapidly fatal, and that are relatively easily diagnosed are most likely to be recorded accurately on death certificates as underlying causes of death. Lung cancer, for instance, meets these criteria reasonably well, whereas the frequency of chronic bronchitis would not be well represented by mortality data, because by itself it is not usually fatal and it is even less likely to be rapidly fatal. The longer the period between onset and death, the greater the likelihood of occurrence of another disease, which is then (either correctly or incorrectly) recorded on the death certificate as the underlying cause of death. Esophageal cancer, if present, would almost always be listed as the underlying cause of death, since it is generally rapidly fatal. However, persons with chronic leukemia might be listed as having died from pneumonia or some other disease that occurred between the time of diagnosis of leukemia and the time of death, even if leukemia were the underlying cause of the pneumonia. A person with chronic leukemia could die from injuries suffered in an automobile accident completely unrelated to the presence of leukemia, in which case the automobile accident would correctly be listed as the underlying cause of death. Regarding ease of diagnosis, malignant melanoma of the skin would be more likely to be recorded on the death certificate than cancer of the pancreas because the former is more apparent and because simple diagnostic techniques, such as skin biopsy, can be used to confirm the diagnosis. In a study comparing underlying causes of death recorded on death certificates and autopsy reports (Kircher et al., 1985), deaths from neoplasms were most accurately diagnosed, while the highest proportions of disagreement were found for diseases of the respiratory and digestive systems. Diseases most commonly overdiagnosed on death certificates were circulatory disorders, ill-defined conditions, and respiratory diseases. Diseases most commonly underdiagnosed on death certificates were traumatic conditions and gastrointestinal disorders.

A variety of other problems also occur when mortality data are used for epidemiologic purposes. The certification of cause of death may be done carelessly; the physician filling in the cause of death may not be the physician who knows the most about the case (and in fact may be the resident who just happened to be on duty the night the patient died). Physicians in a hurry to fill out the certificate may not take the time to fill it out properly. Diseases to which a stigma is attached, such as suicide, alcohol-related diseases, venereal diseases, or death from abortion, may be underreported. Incorrect codes may be assigned to diseases. The rules regarding assignment of cause of death change periodically. Prior to 1948, for instance, if a person died with both coronary heart disease and diabetes, by rule diabetes was assigned as the underlying cause of death. The 1948 revisions of the International Classification of Diseases (ICD) coding system left it up to the physician to determine the underlying cause. Immediately thereafter, the reported mortality rate from diabetes dropped precipitously, as shown in Figure 3–2. Any time an abrupt change in rates occurs, changes in coding rules should be considered as a possible explanation. Diagnostic fads occur. For instance, during the 1960s, mortality rates from cerebral thrombosis increased, whereas mortality rates for cerebral hemorrhage decreased (Figure 3–3). It has been hypothesized that what was called cerebral hemorrhage at the beginning of the decade was tending to be called cerebral thrombosis at the end of the decade (Acheson, 1966); thrombosis was becoming a popular diagnosis for cardiovascular events during this time period. One diagnostic label may be more popular in one country than in another. Chronic bronchitis was formerly believed to be relatively more common in England and Wales, whereas emphysema was considered more common in the United States, since the ratio of deaths from chronic bronchitis with emphysema to emphysema without mention of bronchitis was at

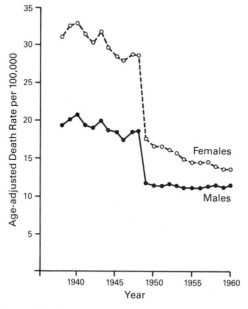

Figure 3–2. Age-adjusted death rates per 100,000 from diabetes mellitus by gender, United States, 1938–1960, whites only.

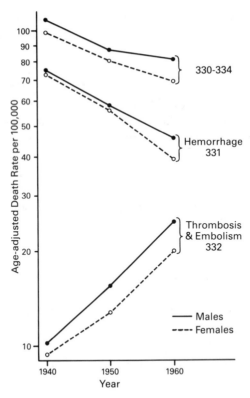

Figure 3–3. Age-adjusted death rates for all cerebrovascular accidents and specific types of cerebrovascular accidents, 1940–1960, by gender, corrected to sixth revision of International Classification of Diseases (from Acheson, 1966).

one time about 1:6 in the United States and 10:1 in England and Wales (Bower, 1961). However, it was subsequently found that the same clinical syndrome was usually called chronic bronchitis in the United Kingdom and emphysema in the United States (Thurlbeck and Angus, 1963). Fletcher et al. (1964) compared 50 patients attending a bronchitis clinic in London with 50 attending an emphysema clinic in Chicago. They noted that the disease was actually similar in most respects, except that the Londoners had a higher frequency of disabling chest infections.

Variations in the quality of medical care among regions or time periods also can make comparisons difficult, since, as diagnostic procedures for a condition improve, mortality rates may appear to increase when in fact the disease is merely being diagnosed more frequently. Finally, many people, especially the elderly, die with several diseases. Selecting any one disease as *the* underlying cause is in many instances unreasonable, and current efforts to publish routinely all causes of death listed on the certificate are helpful in this regard.

In recent years, the National Center for Health Statistics has accumulated data on all causes of death recorded on death certificates. Multiple causes of death are now available on public-use tapes starting with the year 1968 (National Center for Health Statistics, 1984; Israel et al., 1986). These tapes make information readily available from death certificates that could previously be obtained only if an investigator obtained copies of the death certificate and manually coded the causes of death. In 1979, for instance, nearly three quarters of death certificates had more than one condition listed. Nevertheless, frequently not all conditions present at death are reported on the death certificate, particularly if the condition is usually nonfatal, such as obesity, epilepsy, and mental health problems (Israel et al., 1986).

Attention should be drawn to the relatively recent establishment of the National Death Index in the United States. The National Death Index is a central, computerized index of death record information. It includes a standard set of identifying information for each person dying in the United States, Puerto Rico, and the Virgin Islands, starting in 1979 (Patterson and Bilgrad, 1986). Prior to 1979, information on death certificates that could be used to identify individuals was not retained by the National Center for Health Statistics once the annual tabulations had been prepared. In follow-up studies using death as an end point, an investigator had to know that the person had died, the registration area in which the death was recorded, and the approximate date of death in order to obtain a copy of a death certificate (MacMahon, 1983). Now that the National Death Index has been established, approved researchers with some information on name, date of birth, and Social Security number can find out that a death certificate is on file in a given state and can learn the file number. A copy of the death certificate then can be purchased from the state. Data on causes of death are not retained in the National Death Index file; they must be obtained directly from the death certificate (Patterson and Bilgrad, 1986). Details of the various steps involved in using the National Death Index are described by Patterson and Bilgrad (1986) and in a National Center for Health Statistics (1990) publication. In the past, Social Security Administration files have been used to identify deaths among workers. The National Death Index both facilitates determination that a death has occurred and extends coverage to people not in the Social Security system.

In summary, mortality data may help the epidemiologist obtain leads about etiologic agents by identifying demographic subgroups at high risk, facilitating the study of trends in disease occurrence over time, and enabling comparisons of disease occurrence in different geographic regions to be made. However, these data must be interpreted cautiously, and the appropriateness of the disease and the numerous possible pitfalls carefully considered. In most cases, any findings based on mortality data must be regarded strictly as preliminary leads for further investigation.

An annotated bibliography of validation studies of cause of death recorded on death certificates in several countries has been published by the National Center for Health Statistics (National Center for Health Statistics, 1982). In parts of the world in which most deaths are not medically attended, the statistics on causes of death are of very limited value (Moriyama, 1989).

NATALITY DATA

Figure 3–4 shows the U.S. Standard Certificate of Live Birth, 1989 revision. The National Center for Health Statistics recommends the content and format of the birth certificate, but some variation exists among states. As with death certificates, local registrars send copies of birth certificates through state registrars to the National Center for Health Statistics. Birth certificates contain demographic data about the mother, father, and child; in recent years, they have also provided space for recording information on conditions present during the pregnancy, obstetric procedures, types and conditions of labor, method of delivery, congenital malformations, birthweight, length of gestation, Apgar scores, and certain other information. The 1989 revision of the U.S. Standard Certificate of Live Birth contains major changes in the way health-related information is recorded (Freedman et al., 1988). The first change is the replacement of open-ended medical items with items having a checkbox format. (See bottom part of Fig. 3–4.) Also included is a two-part section, "Medical Risk Factors for this Pregnancy" and "Other Risk Factors for this Pregnancy," the latter including tobacco use, alcohol use, and weight gain during the pregnancy, in checkbox format. Information on obstetric procedures, methods of delivery, and abnormal conditions of the newborn is requested in checkbox format. Finally, the revised certificate contains items to identify parents of Hispanic origin, although, as was the case with death certificates, the accuracy of the information on ethnicity and race is questionable (Hahn et al., 1992). Most of the information on birth certificates is confidential, and access requires permission from the appropriate authorities.

The quality of data from birth certificates has been better for some reproductive outcomes than others. Birthweight, for instance, is generally accurately and consistently recorded. Gestational age, on the other hand,

TYPE/PRINT
IN
PERMANENT
BLACK INK
FOR
INSTRUCTIONS
SEE
HANDBOOK

U.S. STANDARD
CERTIFICATE OF LIVE BIRTH

LOCAL FILE NUMBER

BIRTH NUMBER

CHILD

1. CHILD'S NAME *(First, Middle, Last)* | 2. DATE OF BIRTH *(Month, Day, Year)* | 3. TIME OF BIRTH

M

4. SEX | 5. CITY, TOWN, OR LOCATION OF BIRTH | 6. COUNTY OF BIRTH

7. PLACE OF BIRTH: [ ] Hospital [ ] Freestanding Birthing Center
[ ] Clinic/Doctor's Office [ ] Residence
[ ] Other *(Specify)*

8. FACILITY NAME *(If not institution, give street and number)*

CERTIFIER/ ATTENDANT

9. I certify that this child was born alive at the place and time and on the date stated.

Signature ▶

10. DATE SIGNED *(Month, Day, Year)*

11. ATTENDANT'S NAME AND TITLE *(If other than certifier) (Type/Print)*
Name ____
[ ] M.D. [ ] D.O. [ ] C.N.M. [ ] Other Midwife
[ ] Other *(Specify)*

DEATH UNDER ONE YEAR OF AGE
Enter State File Number of death certificate for this child

12. CERTIFIER'S NAME AND TITLE *(Type/Print)*
Name ____
[ ] M.D. [ ] D.O. [ ] Hospital Admin. [ ] C.N.M. [ ] Other Midwife
[ ] Other *(Specify)*

13. ATTENDANT'S MAILING ADDRESS *(Street and Number or Rural Route Number, City or Town, State, Zip Code)*

14. REGISTRAR'S SIGNATURE ▶ | 15. DATE FILED BY REGISTRAR *(Month, Day, Year)*

MOTHER

16a. MOTHER'S NAME *(First, Middle, Last)* | 16b. MAIDEN SURNAME | 17. DATE OF BIRTH *(Month, Day, Year)*

18. BIRTHPLACE *(State or Foreign Country)* | 19a. RESIDENCE—STATE | 19b. COUNTY | 19c. CITY, TOWN, OR LOCATION

19d. STREET AND NUMBER | 19e. INSIDE CITY LIMITS? *(Yes or no)* | 20. MOTHER'S MAILING ADDRESS *(If same as residence, enter Zip Code only)*

FATHER

21. FATHER'S NAME *(First, Middle, Last)* | 22. DATE OF BIRTH *(Month, Day, Year)* | 23. BIRTHPLACE *(State or Foreign Country)*

INFORMANT

24. I certify that the personal information provided on this certificate is correct to the best of my knowledge and belief.

Signature of Parent or Other Informant ▶

INFORMATION FOR MEDICAL AND HEALTH USE ONLY

MOTHER

25. OF HISPANIC ORIGIN? (Specify No or Yes—If yes, specify Cuban, Mexican, Puerto Rican, etc.)

26. RACE—American Indian, Black, White, etc. *(Specify below)*

27. EDUCATION *(Specify only highest grade completed)*
Elementary/Secondary (0-12) | College (1-4 or 5+)

25a. [ ] No [ ] Yes
Specify:

26a.

27a.

FATHER

25b. [ ] No [ ] Yes
Specify:

26b.

27b.

28. PREGNANCY HISTORY *(Complete each section)*

LIVE BIRTHS *(Do not include this child)*		OTHER TERMINATIONS *(Spontaneous and induced at any time after conception)*	29. MOTHER MARRIED? (At birth, conception, or any time between) *(Yes or no)*	30. DATE LAST NORMAL MENSES BEGAN *(Month, Day, Year)*
28a. Now Living	28b. Now Dead	28d.		
Number ____	Number ____	Number ____	31. MONTH OF PREGNANCY PRENATAL CARE BEGAN - First, Second, Third, etc. *(Specify)*	32. PRENATAL VISITS—Total Number *(If none, so state)*
[ ] None	[ ] None	[ ] None	33. BIRTH WEIGHT *(Specify unit)*	34. CLINICAL ESTIMATE OF GESTATION *(Weeks)*
28c. DATE OF LAST LIVE BIRTH *(Month, Year)*		28e. DATE OF LAST OTHER TERMINATION *(Month, Year)*	35a. PLURALITY—Single, Twin, Triplet, etc. *(Specify)*	35b. IF NOT SINGLE BIRTH—Born First, Second, Third, etc. *(Specify)*

MULTIPLE BIRTHS
Enter State File Number for Mate(s)
LIVE BIRTH(S)

FETAL DEATH(S)

36. APGAR SCORE
36a. 1 Minute | 36b. 5 Minutes

37a. MOTHER TRANSFERRED PRIOR TO DELIVERY? [ ] No [ ] Yes If Yes, enter name of facility transferred from:

37b. INFANT TRANSFERRED? [ ] No [ ] Yes If Yes, enter name of facility transferred to:

38a. MEDICAL RISK FACTORS FOR THIS PREGNANCY *(Check all that apply)*

Anemia (Hct. <30/Hgb <10) .... 01 [ ]
Cardiac disease .... 02 [ ]
Acute or chronic lung disease .... 03 [ ]
Diabetes .... 04 [ ]
Genital herpes .... 05 [ ]
Hydramnios/Oligohydramnios .... 06 [ ]
Hemoglobinopathy .... 07 [ ]
Hypertension, chronic .... 08 [ ]
Hypertension, pregnancy-associated .... 09 [ ]
Eclampsia .... 10 [ ]
Incompetent cervix .... 11 [ ]
Previous infant 4000+ grams .... 12 [ ]
Previous preterm or small-for-gestational-age
   infant .... 13 [ ]
Renal disease .... 14 [ ]
Rh sensitization .... 15 [ ]
Uterine bleeding .... 16 [ ]
None .... 00 [ ]
Other ___ 17 [ ]
   (Specify)

38b. OTHER RISK FACTORS FOR THIS PREGNANCY *(Complete all items)*

Tobacco use during pregnancy .... Yes [ ] No [ ]
   Average number cigarettes per day ____
Alcohol use during pregnancy .... Yes [ ] No [ ]
   Average number drinks per week ____
Weight gained during pregnancy ____ lbs.

39. OBSTETRIC PROCEDURES *(Check all that apply)*

Amniocentesis .... 01 [ ]
Electronic fetal monitoring .... 02 [ ]
Induction of labor .... 03 [ ]
Stimulation of labor .... 04 [ ]
Tocolysis .... 05 [ ]
Ultrasound .... 06 [ ]
None .... 00 [ ]
Other ___ 07 [ ]
   (Specify)

40. COMPLICATIONS OF LABOR AND/OR DELIVERY *(Check all that apply)*

Febrile (>100°F. or 38°C.) .... 01 [ ]
Meconium, moderate/heavy .... 02 [ ]
Premature rupture of membrane (>12 hours) ...... 03 [ ]
Abruptio placenta .... 04 [ ]
Placenta previa .... 05 [ ]
Other excessive bleeding .... 06 [ ]
Seizures during labor .... 07 [ ]
Precipitous labor (<3 hours) .... 08 [ ]
Prolonged labor (>20 hours) .... 09 [ ]
Dysfunctional labor .... 10 [ ]
Breech/Malpresentation .... 11 [ ]
Cephalopelvic disproportion .... 12 [ ]
Cord prolapse .... 13 [ ]
Anesthetic complications .... 14 [ ]
Fetal distress .... 15 [ ]
None .... 00 [ ]
Other ___ 16 [ ]
   (Specify)

41. METHOD OF DELIVERY *(Check all that apply)*

Vaginal .... 01 [ ]
Vaginal birth after previous C-section .... 02 [ ]
Primary C-section .... 03 [ ]
Repeat C-section .... 04 [ ]
Forceps .... 05 [ ]
Vacuum .... 06 [ ]

42. ABNORMAL CONDITIONS OF THE NEWBORN *(Check all that apply)*

Anemia (Hct. <39/Hgb. <13) .... 01 [ ]
Birth injury .... 02 [ ]
Fetal alcohol syndrome .... 03 [ ]
Hyaline membrane disease/RDS .... 04 [ ]
Meconium aspiration syndrome .... 05 [ ]
Assisted ventilation <30 min .... 06 [ ]
Assisted ventilation ≥30 min .... 07 [ ]
Seizures .... 08 [ ]
None .... 00 [ ]
Other ___ 09 [ ]
   (Specify)

43. CONGENITAL ANOMALIES OF CHILD *(Check all that apply)*

Anencephalus .... 01 [ ]
Spina bifida/Meningocele .... 02 [ ]
Hydrocephalus .... 03 [ ]
Microcephalus .... 04 [ ]
Other central nervous system anomalies
   (Specify) ___ 05 [ ]
Heart malformations .... 06 [ ]
Other circulatory/respiratory anomalies
   (Specify) ___ 07 [ ]
Rectal atresia/stenosis .... 08 [ ]
Tracheo-esophageal fistula/Esophageal atresia ... 09 [ ]
Omphalocele/Gastroschisis .... 10 [ ]
Other gastrointestinal anomalies
   (Specify) ___ 11 [ ]
Malformed genitalia .... 12 [ ]
Renal agenesis .... 13 [ ]
Other urogenital anomalies
   (Specify) ___ 14 [ ]
Cleft lip/palate .... 15 [ ]
Polydactyly/Syndactyly/Adactyly .... 16 [ ]
Club foot .... 17 [ ]
Diaphragmatic hernia .... 18 [ ]
Other musculoskeletal/integumental anomalies
   (Specify) ___ 19 [ ]
Down's syndrome .... 20 [ ]
Other chromosomal anomalies
   (Specify) ___ 21 [ ]
None ___ 00 [ ]
Other ___ 22 [ ]
   (Specify)

PHS-T-002
REV. 1/89

DEPARTMENT OF HEALTH AND HUMAN SERVICES – PUBLIC HEALTH SERVICE – NATIONAL CENTER FOR HEALTH STATISTICS – 1989 REVISION

Figure 3–4. U.S. Certificate of Live Birth

usually depends on recall of the date of the last menstrual period, is frequently subject to rounding error, and is consequently less accurate. Tests to determine Apgar scores may not be uniformly performed at exactly the appropriate time, and conditions occurring during pregnancy may not be known by the physician filling out the certificate. Many congenital malformations are not recorded on the birth certificate. The only ones that have been recorded with a fairly high degree of consistency are those that are very severe and easily diagnosed at birth, such as anencephaly and spina bifida cystica. Most other malformations have been recorded in such a small proportion of cases that examining their frequency by means of birth certificates is of very limited value. Thus, low birthweight and perhaps neural tube defects are about the only relatively common events that have been recorded reasonably reliably. It is hoped that the new checkbox format will improve recording of at least the listed conditions. However, unlike the death certificates, in which a cause of death has to be listed, it is easy to fail to check a box even where medical conditions do exist.

FETAL DEATHS

The 1989 revision of the U.S. Standard Report on Fetal Death is shown in Figure 3–5. Fetal death certificates have not been particularly useful for epidemiologic purposes (Kirby, 1993). While most states require certification of all fetal losses after 20 weeks of gestation, some require that *all* fetal losses be reported. In many very early fetal deaths, the pregnancy is not even recognized, and many known pregnancies that terminate very early go unreported because the mother did not seek medical care. Late fetal deaths (that is, those occurring after 28 weeks) are reported fairly reliably, but intermediate fetal deaths (at 20–27 weeks of gestation) are inconsistently reported. Reporting of specific fetal malformations is very unreliable, both because they are usually of less clinical concern than abnormalities among the live-born and because many abnormalities are difficult or impossible to diagnose in an early fetus. The 1989 revisions of the medical section of the U.S. Standard Report of Fetal Death are for the most part similar to those for the U.S. Standard Certificate of Live Birth described above. In addition, the fetal death certificate also requests information on maternal and paternal occupation (Freedman et al., 1988).

OTHER DATA FROM THE NATIONAL CENTER FOR HEALTH STATISTICS

The National Center for Health Statistics conducts a variety of surveys and studies of interest to epidemiologists. A summary of the data collected has

U.S. STANDARD
REPORT OF FETAL DEATH

STATE FILE NUMBER

1. FACILITY NAME *(If not institution, give street and number)*

2. CITY, TOWN, OR LOCATION OF DELIVERY | 3. COUNTY OF DELIVERY | 4. DATE OF DELIVERY *(Month, Day, Year)* | 5. SEX OF FETUS

PARENTS

6a. MOTHER'S NAME *(First, Middle, Last)* | 6b. MAIDEN SURNAME | 7. DATE OF BIRTH *(Month, Day, Year)*

8a. RESIDENCE-STATE | 8b. COUNTY | 8c. CITY, TOWN, OR LOCATION | 8d. STREET AND NUMBER

8e. INSIDE CITY LIMITS? *(Yes or no)* | 8f. ZIP CODE | 9. FATHER'S NAME *(First, Middle, Last)* | 10. DATE OF BIRTH *(Month, Day, Year)*

11. OF HISPANIC ORIGIN? (Specify No or Yes—If yes, specify Cuban, Mexican, Puerto Rican, etc.) | 12. RACE—American Indian, Black, White, etc. *(Specify below)* | 13. EDUCATION *(Specify only highest grade completed)* | | 14. OCCUPATION AND BUSINESS/INDUSTRY *(Worked during last year)*

| | | Elementary/Secondary (0-12) | College (1-4 or 5 +) | Occupation | Business/Industry |

MOTHER

11a. ☐ No ☐ Yes Specify: | 12a. | 13a. | | 14a. | 14b.

FATHER

11b. ☐ No ☐ Yes Specify: | 12b. | 13b. | | 14c. | 14d.

15. PREGNANCY HISTORY *(Complete each section)*

LIVE BIRTHS		OTHER TERMINATIONS *(Spontaneous and induced at any time after conception)*
15a. Now Living Number ____ ☐ None	15b. Now Dead Number ____ ☐ None	15d. *(Do not include this fetus)* Number ____ ☐ None
15c. DATE OF LAST LIVE BIRTH *(Month, Year)*		15e. DATE OF LAST OTHER TERMINATION *(Month, Year)*

16. MOTHER MARRIED? (At delivery, conception, or any time between) *(Yes or no)* | 17. DATE LAST NORMAL MENSES BEGAN *(Month, Day, Year)*

18. MONTH OF PREGNANCY PRENATAL CARE BEGAN—First, Second, Third, etc. *(Specify)* | 19. PRENATAL VISITS—Total Number *(If none, so state)*

20. WEIGHT OF FETUS *(Specify Unit)* | 21. CLINICAL ESTIMATE OF GESTATION *(Weeks)*

22a. PLURALITY—Single, Twin, Triplet, etc. *(Specify)* | 22b. IF NOT SINGLE BIRTH—Born First, Second, Third, etc. *(Specify)*

23a. MEDICAL RISK FACTORS FOR THIS PREGNANCY *(Check all that apply)*

Anemia (Hct. < 30/Hgb. < 10) .... 01 ☐
Cardiac disease .... 02 ☐
Acute or chronic lung disease .... 03 ☐
Diabetes .... 04 ☐
Genital herpes .... 05 ☐
Hydramnios/Oligohydramnios .... 06 ☐
Hemoglobinopathy .... 07 ☐
Hypertension, chronic .... 08 ☐
Hypertension, pregnancy-associated .... 09 ☐
Eclampsia .... 10 ☐
Incompetent cervix .... 11 ☐
Previous infant 4000 + grams .... 12 ☐
Previous preterm or small-for-gestational-age infant .... 13 ☐
Renal disease .... 14 ☐
Rh sensitization .... 15 ☐
Uterine bleeding .... 16 ☐
None .... 00 ☐
Other .... 17 ☐
(Specify)

23b. OTHER RISK FACTORS FOR THIS PREGNANCY *(Complete all items)*

Tobacco use during pregnancy .... Yes ☐ No ☐
Average number cigarettes per day ____
Alcohol use during pregnancy .... Yes ☐ No ☐
Average number drinks per week ____
Weight gained during pregnancy ____ lbs.

24. OBSTETRIC PROCEDURES *(Check all that apply)*

Amniocentesis .... 01 ☐
Electronic fetal monitoring .... 02 ☐
Induction of labor .... 03 ☐
Stimulation of labor .... 04 ☐
Tocolysis .... 05 ☐
Ultrasound .... 06 ☐
None .... 06 ☐
Other .... 07 ☐
(Specify)

25. COMPLICATIONS OF LABOR AND/OR DELIVERY *(Check all that apply)*

Febrile (>100°F. or 38°C.) .... 01 ☐
Meconium, moderate/heavy .... 02 ☐
Premature rupture of membrane (>12 hours) .... 03 ☐
Abruptio placenta .... 04 ☐
Placenta previa .... 05 ☐
Other excessive bleeding .... 06 ☐
Seizures during labor .... 07 ☐
Precipitous labor (< 3 hours) .... 08 ☐
Prolonged labor (>20 hours) .... 09 ☐
Dysfunctional labor .... 10 ☐
Breech/Malpresentation .... 11 ☐
Cephalopelvic disproportion .... 12 ☐
Cord prolapse .... 13 ☐
Anesthetic complications .... 14 ☐
Fetal distress .... 15 ☐
None .... 00 ☐
Other .... 16 ☐
(Specify)

26. METHOD OF DELIVERY *(Check all that apply)*

Vaginal .... 01 ☐
Vaginal birth after previous C section .... 02 ☐
Primary C-section .... 03 ☐
Repeat C-section .... 04 ☐
Forceps .... 05 ☐
Vacuum .... 06 ☐
Hysterotomy/Hysterectomy .... 07 ☐

27. CONGENITAL ANOMALIES OF FETUS *(Check all that apply)*

Anencephalus .... 01 ☐
Spina bifida/Meningocele .... 02 ☐
Hydrocephalus .... 03 ☐
Microcephalus .... 04 ☐
Other central nervous system anomalies *(Specify)* .... 05 ☐
Heart malformations .... 06 ☐
Other circulatory/respiratory anomalies *(Specify)* .... 07 ☐
Rectal atresia/stenosis .... 08 ☐
Tracheo esophageal fistula/Esophageal atresia ... 09 ☐
Omphalocele/Gastroschisis .... 10 ☐
Other gastrointestinal anomalies *(Specify)* .... 11 ☐
Malformed genitalia .... 12 ☐
Renal agenesis .... 13 ☐
Other urogenital anomalies *(Specify)* .... 14 ☐
Cleft lip/palate .... 15 ☐
Polydactyly/Syndactyly/Adactyly .... 16 ☐
Club foot .... 17 ☐
Diaphragmatic hernia .... 18 ☐
Other musculoskeletal/integumental anomalies *(Specify)* .... 19 ☐
Down's syndrome .... 20 ☐
Other chromosomal anomalies *(Specify)* .... 21 ☐
None .... 00 ☐
Other .... 22 ☐
(Specify)

28.

PART I. Fetal or maternal condition directly causing fetal death. — IMMEDIATE CAUSE

Enter only one cause per line for a, b, and c.

a. | Specify Fetal or Maternal

Fetal and/or maternal conditions, if any, giving rise to the immediate cause(s), stating the underlying cause last.

DUE TO (OR AS A CONSEQUENCE OF):
b. | Specify Fetal or Maternal

DUE TO (OR AS A CONSEQUENCE OF):
c. | Specify Fetal or Maternal

PART II. Other significant conditions of fetus or mother contributing to fetal death but not resulting in the underlying cause given in Part I. | 29. FETUS DIED BEFORE LABOR, DURING LABOR OR DELIVERY, UNKNOWN *(Specify)*

30. ATTENDANT'S NAME AND TITLE *(Type/Print)*
Name _____
☐ M.D. ☐ D.O. ☐ C.N.M. ☐ Other Midwife
☐ Other *(Specify)* _____

31. NAME AND TITLE OF PERSON COMPLETING REPORT *(Type/Print)*
Name _____
Title _____

PHS-T-007
REV. 1/89

DEPARTMENT OF HEALTH AND HUMAN SERVICES — PUBLIC HEALTH SERVICE — NATIONAL CENTER FOR HEALTH STATISTICS — 1989 REVISION

Figure 3–5. U.S. Report of Fetal Death

been provided by Kovar (1989). Most of the reports from the National Center for Health Statistics are part of the Vital and Health Statistics series, which includes several hundred publications. Advance Data from Vital and Health Statistics was started in 1976 to permit early release of certain findings. These advance reports are generally followed by detailed publications in the Vital and Health Statistics series. The National Center for Health Statistics publishes the Vital Statistics of the United States and Monthly Vital Statistics Report. In addition to the mortality and natality data described above, marriage and divorce statistics are included in these series.

Table 3–3 lists the recent Vital and Health Statistics series. In addition to the publications on methodology, several ongoing surveys are of considerable interest to epidemiologists. In the National Health Interview Survey, at present about 128,000 people in about 49,000 households throughout the United States are included each year. Information is collected on demographic characteristics, the incidence of acute illnesses and injuries, the prevalence of chronic conditions and impairments, the extent of disability, the utilization of health care services, and other health-related topics. The questionnaires used in this survey consist of (a) a set of basic health and demographic items, and (b) one or more sets of questions on current health topics. Only episodes of illness that resulted in a visit to a physician or in restricted activity are included in the publications from the National Health Interview Survey. The target population is the civilian noninstitutionalized population of the United States. Perhaps the parts of this survey most valuable for epidemiologists are the incidence data by age, gender, and other demographic characteristics for acute conditions, and the measures of associated days of restricted activity, days lost from work, and days lost from school. Because it does not include institutionalized persons, this data source is less valuable as an indicator of the prevalence of chronic conditions. Members of the armed forces are also not included.

A major limitation of the National Health Interview Survey is that it accepts answers from proxy respondents when household members are not at home at the time of interview. This practice undoubtedly reduces the accuracy of the data. Also, information provided by the respondents is not subject to verification by physician. Less underreporting would be expected to occur for diseases included on the checklist of illnesses than for diseases that respondents have to bring up themselves, but even with checklists most diseases are underreported in household interview surveys. Nevertheless, for conditions that result in activity restriction, that are significant to the affected individual, that occurred close to the time of the interview, and for which lay individuals understand the diagnosis, this survey undoubtedly provides useful information. Compared to surveys that require actual physical examination, it includes larger numbers of people, has higher response rates, and can be administered by a nontechnical staff.

Table 3–3. Vital and Health Statistics Series of the National Centers for Health Statistics

Series No.	Title	Description
1.	Programs and collection procedures	Reports describing programs and data collection methods
2.	Data evaluation and methods research	Studies of new statistical methodology and analytic techniques, and evaluation of reliability of collected data
3.	Analytic and epidemiological studies	Reports presenting analytical or interpretive studies based on vital and health statistics
4.	Documents and committee reports	Findings of major committees concerned with vital and health statistics, and recommended vital statistics certificates
5.	Comparative international vital and health statistics reports	Reports comparing U.S. vital and health statistics with those of other countries
6.	Cognitive and survey measurement	Reports using methods of cognitive science to design, evaluate, and test survey instruments
10.	Data from the National Health Interview Survey	Reports based on data collected in a continuing national household interview survey of the civilian non-institutionalized U.S. population
11.	Data from the National Health Examination Survey and the National Health and Nutrition Examination Survey, including the Hispanic Health and Nutrition Examination Survey	Reports on data collected through direct examination, testing, and measurement of national samples of the civilian noninstitutionalized U.S. population
13.	Data on health resources utilization	Statistics on the utilization of health professionals and facilities providing long-term care, ambulatory care, hospital care, and family planning services
14.	Data on health resources: manpower facilities	Professional and facilities statistics on the number, geographic distribution, and characteristics of health professionals
15.	Data from special surveys	Statistics on health and health-related topics collected in special surveys that are not a part of the continuing data systems of the National Center for Health Statistics
16.	Computations of advance data from health and demographic surveys	Reports providing early release of data from the National Center for Health Statistics health and demographic surveys

(*continued*)

Table 3-3. (*Continued*)

Series No.	Title	Description
20.	Data on mortality	Various statistics on mortality other than as included in the annual or monthly reports
21.	Data on natality, marriage, and divorce	Various statistics on natality, marriage, and divorce other than as included in the annual or monthly reports
23.	Data from the National Survey of Family Growth	Reports based on data collected in periodic surveys of a nationwide probability sample of women 15–44 years of age
24.	Compilation of data on natality, mortality, marriage, divorce, and induced termination of pregnancy	Advanced reports based on data from the National and Vital Statistics system and reports on induced termination of pregnancy based on data from the National and Health Statistics system

Source: Kovar (1989).

In the National Hospital Discharge Survey, included under Data on Health Resources Utilization in Table 3–3, data are obtained by sampling records of short-term general and specialty hospitals in the United States. Military and Veterans Administration hospitals and hospital units in institutions such as prisons are excluded. The universe of the survey consists of about 7500 short-stay non-Federal hospitals in the United States. In 1991, 247,000 patients discharged from 484 of these hospitals were included. Within each sampled hospital, discharges are randomly sampled from the daily listing sheets. For each selected discharge, information from the face sheet is abstracted on diagnoses, surgical procedures, and length of stay. Up to seven diagnoses and four procedures are coded for each discharge. For common diseases for which the treatment generally requires hospitalization, these data may give a good indication of frequency of occurrence. For uncommon conditions, however, the sample size is not large enough for meaningful statistics, although combining data over several years can improve precision. Also, multiple discharges for the same medical problem are not distinguished.

The National Ambulatory Medical Care Survey is also included under Data on Health Resources Utilization. In 1991 this survey included 1,354 nonfederally employed physicians in office-based patient-care practice. Physicians in the specialties of anesthesiology, pathology, and radiology are excluded. A sample is taken from master files of the American Medical Association and the American Osteopathic Association. In general, about three quarters of the randomly selected physicians agree to participate. A random week of the year is selected for each physician, and patient visits are sampled during that week. Information about the visits includes diagnoses, treatment, disposition, and length of time the visit lasted. About 34,000 patient visits were included in 1991.

In view of the numerous changes in ways of providing health care over the past decade, the National Center for Health Statistics is integrating the provider-based surveys such as the National Hospital Discharge Survey and the National Ambulatory Medical Care Survey and expanding them into the National Health Care Survey. Data collection is being extended into other health care settings, such as hospital outpatient clinics, emergency rooms, ambulatory acute care facilities, outpatient surgical units, free-standing surgicenters, health agencies, hospices, and community-based long-term care facilities (McCaig, 1994). A Patient Follow-up Component will be included in the National Health Care Survey; this component will provide information on outcomes of patient care and subsequent use of care through periodic contacts with patients or patients' families.

The National Health and Nutrition Examination Surveys (NHANES I and NHANES II) have provided data from physical examinations, clinical and laboratory tests, and questionnaires on a sample of the noninstitutionalized civilian population of the United States. NHANES I was a prevalence study undertaken during 1971–1975, and included about 20,000 individuals in the age range 1–74 years. It was designed to measure overall health status, with particular emphasis on nutritional status, dental health, skin problems, and eye conditions. A more detailed health examination was given to a subsample of 6913 adults aged 25–74 years, with emphasis on chronic lung disease; disabling arthritis of the hip, knee, and lower spine; cardiovascular disease; hearing level; health-care needs; and general well-being.

NHANES II, also a prevalence survey, included 20,000 individuals from six months to 74 years of age and was carried out during 1976–80. It was designed to permit some assessment of changes in the population's nutritional status and certain other variables over time, compared with NHANES I. In NHANES II, measurement of nutritional status involved a physician's examination, medical history information, body measurements, laboratory assessments on blood and serum, and a dietary interview. Also included were assessments of diabetes, kidney disease, heart disease, hypertension, certain allergies, disc degeneration, pulmonary function, hearing and speech problems, and exposure to certain potentially toxic substances. The Hispanic Health and Nutrition Examination Survey (HHANES) was carried out in 1982–1984 to obtain data on the health and nutritional status of three Hispanic groups: Mexican Americans in certain areas of the southwestern United States, Cuban Americans residing in Dade County, Florida, and Puerto Ricans residing in the New York area. The specific data collected depended in part on the age of the participant. In general, a variety of information on demographic characteristics, health status, health insurance coverage, health services utilization, smoking, alcohol consumption, drug abuse, depression, reproductive history, and diet was obtained by means of questionnaire. A physician performed a medical examination, a dentist performed a dental examination, various tests and procedures were undertaken, and several body measurements were made. Previous surveys of this type, which were called the Health Examination Surveys and which involved physical examinations, were undertaken in 6700 adults aged 18–79 in 1960–1962, 7100 children aged 6–11 in 1963–1965, and 6700 children aged 12–17 in 1966–1970. All of these surveys that involve physical examination have the disadvantage of smaller sample size than the surveys based on interview, but nevertheless they provide valuable information on the more common diseases surveyed, especially those that require physical examination and special tests and procedures for diagnosis.

NHANES III began in September 1988 and will continue for about 6 years. This survey includes persons aged 2 months and older, with no upper age limit. All participants undergo physical examination, body measurements, and a dietary interview. Depending on the age of the participant, other components of the examination include a dental examination, health interview, cognitive and neurological tests, blood and urine tests, hearing tests, vision examination, allergy skin test, spirometry, electrocardiogram, x-rays, ultrasound examination of the gallbladder, and measurements of bone density. Data are being collected in two 3-year segments, so that statistical analysis can take place at the end of each of the segments as well as for the full survey.

The NHANES I Epidemiologic Follow-up Study of 1982–1984 was undertaken to permit investigation of the relationships between the physiological, nutritional, behavioral, and demographic characteristics collected in the NHANES I survey of 1971–1975 and subsequent morbidity and mortality from specific diseases and conditions. Personal interviews, abstraction of hospital records, nursing home records, and death certificates were used to determine the subsequent health experience of 93% of the original cohort of 14,407 persons aged 25–74 years. In 1985–1986, a Continued Follow-up of the Elderly NHANES I Cohort was conducted. Persons who had been 55 years and older at NHANES I were contacted, and computer-assisted telephone interviews administered. Abstracts from health care facilities and death certificates were also used. In 1986–1987, attempts were made to contact the entire NHANES I cohort again. Data on health status were obtained through telephone interviews, hospital and nursing home records, and death certificates.

The Longitudinal Study of Aging is a group of surveys based on the Supplement on Aging to the 1984 National Health Interview Survey. The Supplement on Aging obtained data on family structure and frequency of contacts with children, housing, use of community and social supports, occupation and retirement, ability to perform work-related functions, conditions and impairments, functional limitations, and providers of help for those activities. Information was obtained for about 16,000 people aged 55 years and older. These data are being linked to cause-of-death information from the National Death Index. Subsamples of the participants have been interviewed in subsequent years, mainly in order to measure changes in various social and health-related variables over time.

Finally, the National Mortality Followback Survey and the National Maternal and Infant Health Survey supplement the vital registration systems by providing more detailed information about events surrounding death and birth, respectively, for samples of death and birth certificates. The National Mortality Followback Survey of 1986, for instance, interviewed next-of-kin or other knowledgeable informants to obtain information on socioeconomic status, assets, education, use of health care resources in the last year of life, disability prior to death, and health habits such as smoking and drinking alcoholic beverages. This survey also examined the reliability of items reported on death certificates by comparing these items with the same items reported by the survey respondent. The 1988 National Maternal and Infant Health Survey consisted of a natality survey based on 10,000 certificates of live birth, a fetal mortality survey based on 4000 reports of fetal death, and an infant mortality survey based on 6000 death certificates. Information was obtained from mothers named on the vital records, and from the mothers' health care providers. Areas of interest in this survey included causes of low birthweight and infant death; barriers and facilitators to prenatal care; the effects on pregnancy outcome of maternal smoking, marijuana and cocaine use, and alcohol consumption; the effects of sexually transmitted diseases on pregnancy outcome; and use and evaluation of public programs. Medical data on the mothers and infants during the 6 months following delivery were also obtained from hospital records.

Any single source of data from the National Center for Health Statistics presents an incomplete picture of the frequency and impact of disease, but taken as a whole, the surveys provide a wealth of information on the health status of the population of the United States. Although information obtained from interviews is necessary to find out about a person's symptoms and to learn how a person feels he or she is affected by a disease, such data are of course dependent on the ability and willingness of individuals to answer the questions posed, and it is known that the frequency of occurrence of most conditions is underestimated in interview surveys, although some overreporting may also occur (Sanders, 1962; Edwards et al., 1994). Diagnoses made by such means as physical examination or x-ray do not rely on the subjective reporting of symptoms. However, many people with "objective" evidence of disease do not feel any adverse effects, whereas some people with symptoms show no evidence of disease on examination or x-ray. Data based on records of visits to physicians or hospitals exclude people who did not seek medical care. Nevertheless, by using each of these sources when appropriate, much can be learned about the descriptive epidemiology of diseases. In addition, the recent addition of longitudinal components such as the NHANES I Epidemiologic Follow-up Study and the Longitudinal Study of Aging greatly facilitate the conduct of analytic epidemiologic studies that could be done only to a limited extent with the cross-sectional data previously available.

A few other countries have also conducted major morbidity surveys. Canada, for instance, has undertaken the Canada Health Survey of 1978–1979 and Canada's Health Promotion Survey of 1985. In Finland, the Social Insurance Institution's Mini-Finland Health Survey was conducted during 1977–1980 and the Mobile Clinic Health Examination Survey during 1966–1972.

HCIA

HCIA (Baltimore, Maryland), a successor to the former Commission on Professional and Hospital Activities (CPHA), compiles data from a variety of public and private sources in the United States on characteristics of hospital inpatients and outpatients and their care. Of particular interest to epidemiologists, the National Inpatient Profile is based on information abstracted from about 1.6 million patient discharge records from participating short-term general hospitals and then extrapolated to the United States as a whole. It provides estimates, by ICD-9 code, of the annual number of discharge diagnoses and procedures performed in hospitals in the United States, together with demographic, clinical, and reimbursement characteristics of the patients. A comparison of characteristics of inpatients included in the 1991 National Hospital Discharge Survey of the National Center for Health Statistics with characteristics of the inpatients included in the 1992 HCIA discharge statistics show them to be similar in most respects (HCIA, 1993). Thus, the HCIA inpatient database provides an alternative to the National Hospital Discharge Survey that is based on larger numbers of discharges and more recent data, but is not from a scientifically selected sample of hospitals. HCIA is currently developing a similar source of data on outpatient visits.

CENTERS FOR DISEASE CONTROL CONGENITAL MALFORMATIONS SURVEILLANCE PROGRAMS

The Centers for Disease Control and Prevention (CDC) has two major programs that collect data on congenital malformations, the Metropolitan Atlanta Congenital Defects Program and the Birth Defects Monitoring Program. The Metropolitan Atlanta Congenital Defects Program (MACDP), which covers about 27,000 births per year, is directed by the CDC, the Georgia Mental Health Institute, and the Emory University School of Medicine. Its purposes are to monitor intensively the occurrence of malformations in a defined geographic area and to maintain a case registry for epidemiologic and genetic studies. It collects data on any liveborn or still-born infant who has a structural, chromosomal, or biochemical abnormality present at birth and diagnosed before the infant is one year of age and whose parents resided in Metropolitan Atlanta at the time of birth. Staff of MACDP review and abstract records of hospitals and physicians in Metropolitan Atlanta. The states of Florida and Nebraska also have registries of congenital defects, but these rely on reporting by participating hospitals; this reporting is mandatory in Nebraska and voluntary in Florida.

The Birth Defects Monitoring Program (BDMP) is sponsored by the CDC, the National Institute of Child Health and Development, the March of Dimes, and previously the Commission on Professional and Hospital Activities (Edmonds et al., 1981). The primary purpose of the BDMP is to monitor the frequency of birth defects and other conditions in the newborn. The BDMP monitors 161 diagnoses, including structural, chromosomal, biochemical, and genetic disorders. During 1981–1986, approximately 1236 hospitals voluntarily participated in the BDMP, including about 21% of all births in the United States (Centers for Disease Control, 1988). Data are abstracted from the medical records in these hospitals for all liveborn and stillborn infants delivered. Although these data are not population-based and are not a representative sample of births in the United States, they are the largest single source of uniformly collected discharge data on birth defects in newborn infants. Data from both of the CDC surveillance programs are routinely published. An example of data

Table 3–4. Prevalence Rates Per 10,000 Births of Major Congenital Malformations, by Race/Ethnicity, United States, 1981–1986

Malformation	Blacks	Hispanics	American Indians	Asians	Whites
Anencephaly	2.1	4.4	3.6	4.4	3.0
Spina bifida without anen-cephaly	3.3	5.9	4.1	1.8	5.1
Hydrocephalus without spina bifida	8.1	4.6	10.8	4.8	5.4
Microcephalus	4.8	2.8	2.6	1.9	2.1
Ventricular septal defect	14.4	13.8	19.1	21.0	17.4
Atrial septal defect	2.1	1.2	4.1	2.5	2.1
Valve stenosis and atresia	5.9	1.9	8.2	2.8	3.2
Patent ductus arteriosus	49.9	20.7	33.5	25.1	26.5
Pulmonary artery stenosis	5.4	1.4	0	1.8	1.5
Cleft palate without cleft lip	3.7	3.7	9.8	4.6	5.9
Cleft lip with or without cleft palate	4.4	8.6	17.5	12.9	9.7
Clubfoot without central nervous system defects	19.9	19.1	15.5	14.4	27.5
Hip dislocation without cen-tral nervous system defects	13.8	24.0	31.4	25.0	32.3
Hypospadias	24.6	14.9	17.5	16.5	32.7
Rectal atresia and stenosis	2.8	3.0	4.6	3.8	3.7
Fetal alcohol syndrome	6.0	0.8	29.9	0.3	0.9
Down's syndrome	6.5	11.6	6.7	11.3	8.5
Autosomal abnormalities, ex-cluding Down's syndrome	2.1	2.1	3.1	2.9	2.2
Total	179.9	144.4	222.0	157.8	189.8

Source: Centers for Disease Control (1988).

from the BDMP is given in Table 3–4, which shows rates of congenital malformations by race/ethnicity in the United States for the years 1981–1986.

CANCER SURVEILLANCE, EPIDEMIOLOGY, AND END RESULTS (SEER) PROGRAM

The SEER program of the National Cancer Institute at present includes nine population-based cancer registries in the United States. Although individual registries such as the Connecticut Tumor Registry have been in existence since 1935, the SEER network includes cases diagnosed from 1973 to the present. The goals of the SEER program (Young et al., 1981) are to:

1. Determine the incidence of cancer in selected geographic areas of the United States with respect to demographic and social characteristics of the population.
2. Estimate cancer incidence for the United States on an annual basis.
3. Monitor trends over time in incidence of specific forms of cancer with respect to geographic area and demographic and social characteristics of the population.
4. Determine survival experience for cancer patients diagnosed among residents of selected geographic areas of the United States.
5. Monitor trends over time in cancer patient survival with respect to form of cancer, extent of disease, therapy, and demographic, socioeconomic, and other parameters of prognostic importance.
6. Identify cancer etiologic factors by conducting special studies that disclose groups of the population at high or low risk for cancers. These groups may be defined by social, occupational, environmental, dietary, or other characteristics, and by drug history.
7. Identify factors related to patient survival through special studies of referral patterns, diagnostic procedures, treatment methods, and other aspects of medical care.
8. Promote specialty training in epidemiology, biostatistics, and tumor registry methodology, operation, and management.

The geographic areas included in the SEER network were selected to provide representation from various regions and ethnic groups in the United States. All incident cancers except certain skin cancers occurring in residents of these defined geographic areas are reported to the registries from the hospitals within and near these registry areas. A person's residence is determined primarily by the address on the hospital record; thus, if a nonresident is staying with a resident relative, the nonresident may mistakenly be included. Second and subsequent admissions for the same cancer are identified and excluded from incidence data so that actual incidence rates of newly diagnosed cancers can be obtained. Information is collected on demographic characteristics of the patient, anatomic site, histologic cell type, extent of disease at the time of diagnosis, treatment given, and subsequent vital status of the patient. The reports from the individual SEER registries are sent to the National Cancer Institute, where they are compiled and published. Because almost all cancers except skin cancer are seen in a hospital at some time during the course of diagnosis and treatment, such a registry system works well for cancers. Incidence and survivorship data are published periodically (Young et al., 1981; Horn et al., 1984) and provide information on demographic characteristics of people at high risk, on time trends, on geographic variation within the United States, and on factors related to survivorship. Data on treatment is generally of better quality for radiation therapy, which takes place in a hospital, than for chemotherapy, which is frequently administered on an outpatient basis. Cases reported to SEER registries have also served as a source of cases for case-control studies, although rapid reporting systems may have to be implemented for case identification in such studies.

INTERNATIONAL CANCER STATISTICS

The International Agency for Research on Cancer (IARC) has published cancer statistics in six volumes of *Cancer Incidence in Five Continents* over a 25-year period (International Agency for Research on Cancer, 1992). Recent volumes include incidence rates reported from registries covering 137 populations in 36 countries on five continents. Data from several registries have appeared in all six volumes over the 25-year period, so that trends over time can be examined in some geographic areas. In general, only those registries that have a reliable system for identifying and registering new cases of cancer are included. In some instances, data from registries covering areas where incidence data are of particular interest but where some degree of incompleteness is suspected are also included; such data are clearly differentiated from the data considered reliable. Another publication of the International Agency for Research on Cancer, Cancer Occurrence in Developing Countries (International Agency for Research on Cancer, 1986), covers developing countries in which high quality registration is not possible.

THE REPORTING OF NOTIFIABLE DISEASES

At present, cases of only six diseases are required to be reported to the World Health Organization (WHO) because of their epidemic potential and the possibility of their transmission from one country to another: cholera, plague, louse-borne relapsing fever, smallpox, louse-borne typhus fever, and yellow fever. These notifiable diseases must be reported by telex to the WHO from any country in the world in which the cases are diagnosed.

WHO reports the occurrence of notifiable diseases from most of the countries of the world in the *WHO Weekly Epidemiological Record.* This publication includes editorial comment on the significance of disease trends and on developments in the Expanded Immunization Program of WHO. There is also a monthly report (the *WHO Epidemiological and Vital Statistics Report*), and a *WHO Annual Report.* Although these data may enable overall trends to be observed, the variability in the reporting of cases in many parts of the world, especially in developing countries, and the questionable validity of the denominator data on which disease incidence rates are based, markedly limit the use of these data for accurate descriptive studies. Similar surveillance information is published by many countries of the world and by the Pan American Health Organization (PAHO), which summarizes data for the Americas on a weekly, monthly, and annual basis.

In the United States, the Centers for Disease Control and Prevention (CDC), formerly called the Centers for Disease Control and before that the Communicable Disease Center, has had responsibility since 1960 for receiving morbidity reports on notifiable diseases from the states and larger cities and for issuing the *Morbidity and Mortality Weekly Report* (*MMWR*). The number of notifiable diseases is considerably larger than the six required to be reported by WHO, and varies somewhat from one year to another. The decision as to what diseases should be declared notifiable is made through the Association of State and Territorial Epidemiologists. This decision is based mainly on the ability to control the disease. Thus, streptococcal infections, chickenpox (varicella), and infectious mononucleosis are not reportable in most states and are not recorded in *MMWR*. Exceptions to this are diseases of major and worldwide importance such as cholera, plague, and AIDS. New infectious diseases may be identified that require notification, such as when the Hanta virus recently appeared in humans in the United States. The weekly *MMWR* provides tables summarizing the number of cases of the common notifiable diseases for that week compared to the number that occurred during the same week in the previous year, as well as cumulative totals for the current year compared to the past year. A brief summary table of notifiable diseases of low frequency is also included. Most of these conditions are also listed in the tabular form by region, state, New York City, and four trust areas (Guam, Puerto Rico, Virgin Islands, and Pacific Trust Territories). A fourth table lists the number of deaths by age groups for these geographic areas as well as deaths from pneumonia and influenza. Many issues contain a section called "Current Trends," in which morbidity, mortality, and other data are reported in narrative and graphic form, and a section called "Epidemiologic Notes and Reports," in which other health conditions of interest are delineated. Sections on "Perspectives in Disease Prevention and Health Promotion," "Progress in Chronic Disease Prevention," and "Topics in Minority Health" are included in some issues.

In recent years *MMWR* has also provided descriptive information on such topics as congenital malformations, injuries, chronic diseases, behaviors that affect health such as cigarette smoking, and health promotion and disease prevention activities such as screening. Beginning in 1989, *MMWR* has published monthly Chronic Disease Reports to provide basic information on chronic disease mortality, associated risk factors, and preventive measures (Centers for Disease Control, 1989a). Recommendations for immunization practices have been published from time to time (Centers for Disease Control, 1991), including guidelines for immunocompromised persons (Centers for Disease Control, 1993).

One issue each year of *MMWR* is published as the "Annual Summary"; this issue reviews in detail statistical data for the year before (e.g., the October 21, 1994, issue is the Summary of Notifiable Diseases, United States, 1993). In the 1993 Summary (Centers for Disease Control, 1994), for instance, Part I gives summaries of 49 currently notifiable conditions in the United States, as well as the distribution of cases by month, geographic location, patient's age, and race/ethnicity. Part II provides graphs and maps of the summary data for many of the notifiable conditions included in tabular form in Part I. Part III contains tables of the number of cases of notifiable diseases reported over the past 50 years. Table 3–5 shows the number of cases of notifiable diseases for the period 1989–1993. Part III also gives tables of the number of deaths associated with specific notifiable diseases reported for the period 1982–1991.

As with any data collected over time, changes in case definition can have a significant effect on apparent trends over time. For instance, in September 1987 the CDC case definition of AIDS was revised to include a broader spectrum of diseases characteristically found in persons with human immunodeficiency virus (HIV) infection. This change in case definition had a large effect on the number and epidemiologic characteristics of reported cases (Centers for Disease Control, 1989b). Twenty-nine percent of the 40,836 cases reported between September 1987 and December 1988 would not have been included without the revisions. A higher proportion of cases meeting only the revised criteria than cases meeting the previously used criteria were female (15% vs. 9%), black or Hispanic (34% vs. 26% black, 21% vs. 14% Hispanic), or heterosexual intravenous drug users (35% vs. 18%). A lower proportion of those meeting only the 1987 case definition had a history of male homosexual or bisexual activity without intravenous drug use (41% vs. 63%). Figure 3–6 shows the effect of this changed case definition on the number of reported cases of AIDS. The definition of AIDS was further extended on January 1, 1993, to include all human immunodeficiency virus–infected persons with severe immunodepression, pulmonary tuberculosis, recurrent pneumonia, or invasive cervical cancer (Centers for Disease Control, 1992). Using this new definition, 103,500 cases of AIDS were reported in 1993 among persons aged 13 years and older. This represented an increase of 111% over the 49,016 cases reported in 1992. If the old definition had been used, a 2% decrease compared to the 1992 figure would have been seen.

Table 3–5. Number of Cases of Notifiable Diseases Reported for Period 1989–1993

Disease	1993	1992	1991	1990	1989
U.S. total resident population (in thousands) 1990 census; July 1 estimate 1989 and 1991–1993	257,908	255,082	252,177	248,710	248,239
Acquired immunodeficiency syndrome (AIDS)	103,533	45,472	43,672	41,595	33,722
Amebiasis	2,970	2,942	2,989	3,328	3,217
Anthrax	—	1	—	—	—
Aseptic meningitis	12,848	12,223	14,526	11,852	10,274
Botulism, total (including wound and unspecified)	97	91	114	92	89
Food-borne	27	21	27	23	23
Infant	65	66	81	65	60
Brucellosis	120	105	104	85	95
Chancroid	1,399	1,886	3,476	4,212	4,692
Cholera	18	103	26	6	—
Diphtheria	—	4	5	4	3
Encephalitis: primary	919	774	1,021	1,341	981
Post-infectious	170	129	82	105	88
Gonorrhea	439,673	501,409	620,478	690,169	733,151
Granuloma inguinale	19	6	29	97	7
Haemophilus influenzae[a]	1,419	1,412	2,764	. . . .	
Hansen disease	187	172	154	198	163
Hepatitis A	24,238	23,112	24,378	31,441	35,821
Hepatitis B	13,361	16,126	18,003	21,102	23,419
Hepatitis non-A, non-B	4,786	6,010	3,582	2,553	2,529
Hepatitis, unspecified	627	884	1,260	1,671	2,306
Legionellosis	1,280	1,339	1,317	1,370	1,190
Leptospirosis	51	54	58	77	93
Lyme disease	8,257	9,895	9,465	. . . .	
Lymphogranuloma venereum	285	302	471	277	189
Malaria	1,411	1,087	1,278	1,292	1,277
Measles (rubeola)	312	2,237	9,643	27,786	18,193
Meningococcal infections	2,637	2,134	2,130	2,451	2,727
Mumps	1,692	2,572	4,264	5,292	5,712
Murine typhus fever	25	28	43	50	41
Pertussis (whooping cough)	6,586	4,083	2,719	4,570	4,157
Plague	10	13	11	2	4

(continued)

Table 3–5. (*Continued*)

Disease	1993	1992	1991	1990	1989
Poliomyelitis, paralytic	3	6	6	7	5
Psittacosis	60	92	94	113	116
Rabies, animal	9,377	8,589	6,910	4,826	4,724
Rabies, human	3	1	3	1	1
Rheumatic fever, acute	112	75	127	108	144
Rocky Mountain spotted fever	456	502	628	651	623
Rubella (German measles)	192	160	1,401	1,125	396
Rubella congenital syndrome	5	11	47	11	3
Salmonellosis (excluding typhoid fever)	41,641	40,912	48,154	48,603	47,812
Shigellosis	32,198	23,931	23,548	27,077	25,010
Small pox	. . . . . . Last documented case occurred in 1949.				
Syphilis (primary and secondary)	26,498	33,973	42,935	50,223	44,540
Total all stages	101,259	112,581	128,569	134,255	110,797
Tetanus	48	45	57	64	53
Toxic-shock syndrome	212	244	280	322	400
Trichinosis	16	41	62	129	30
Tuberculosis	25,313	26,673	26,283	25,701	23,495
Tularemia	132	159	193	152	152
Typhoid fever	440	414	501	552	460
Varicella (chickenpox)	134,722	158,364	147,076	173,099	185,441
Yellow fever	Last indigenous case reported 1911; last imported, 1924				

aNot notifiable nationally prior to 1991.

Source: Centers for Disease Control (1994).

The reports of the notifiable diseases in the United States in the *MMWR* and in the Annual Summary represent an important source of morbidity information for a variety of diseases, but the limitations of the data should be recognized. Some of the limitations are that (a) not all infectious and communicable diseases are on the notifiable list, including many common viral and other diseases for which there are presently no effective control measures; (b) the diagnosis may not be supported by confirmatory laboratory tests, a major problem for many viral diseases; and (c) the reporting system depends on a chain of events, including the occurrence of a clinical disease of sufficient severity to warrant medical care, the

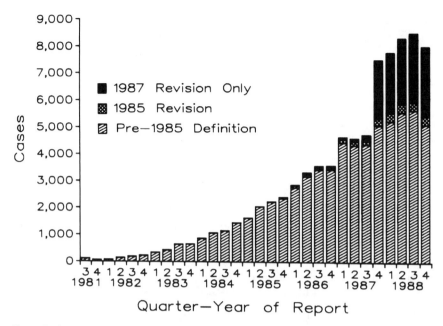

Figure 3–6. AIDS cases, by quarter of report and case definition—United States, 1981–1988 (from Centers for Disease Control, 1989b).

availability of medical and diagnostic services, the ability of the medical care provider to diagnose the illness correctly, and the reporting of the disease to the health department. Once reported to the local authority, the information is forwarded to the state health department and from there to the CDC. The most serious weakness in this chain in the United States is the failure of the physician or other health care provider to report the illness to the local health authority. One study of 570 cases of notifiable communicable diseases from 11 hospitals in Washington, D.C., revealed that only 35% of all notifiable diseases were in fact reported. This included 11% of viral hepatitis cases, 50% of meningococcal meningitis cases, and 11% of tuberculosis cases (Marier, 1977). To increase the completeness of these reporting systems, active surveillance methods such as community household surveys, telephone reporting, hospital record abstraction, and special surveys have been used.

DATA ABSTRACTED FROM HOSPITAL RECORDS

In many hospitals, obtaining information on disease occurrence involves abstracting the desired information from various records kept in the hospitals. Computerized systems, which are being developed with increasing frequency, will be discussed briefly at the end of this section. In contrast to mortality data, the population at risk to be admitted to a given hospital for a given disease is usually not known. (An exception to this is prepaid health care plans, which will be discussed later.) Within the hospital records, however, good diagnostic information may be available, so that the quality of medical information is, in general, much higher than for mortality data. In addition, just as mortality data are most useful for studying the occurrence of rapidly fatal diseases, hospital data are most appropriate for the study of diseases that are traditionally treated in hospitals, preferably at an early stage.

Many of the uses and limitations of hospital data described by Masi (1962) several years ago still pertain. Sometimes hospital data are used for the purpose of generalizing only to hospitalized patients. Studies of hospital-acquired infections, adverse drug effects, and delayed effects of medical treatment may fall into this category. More often, however, hospital data are used with the intent of applying results to the community as a whole. This may involve estimating disease incidence, as is done by cancer registries receiving reports of cancer from hospitals, or obtaining information on disease etiology by means of case-control studies, to be discussed in Chapters 8 and 9. As pointed out by Masi (1962), in considering whether hospital data should be used, the appropriateness of the disease and the appropriateness of the hospitals and their catchment area need to be considered.

Regarding the appropriateness of the disease, first, the condition should be conventionally treated in a hospital. For instance, most cancers are at some time treated in a hospital, coronary heart disease sometimes is, and mental illness frequently is not. Second, the condition should be adequately defined. Thus, "chronic brain syndrome" would not meet this criterion, whereas a fracture, diagnosed by x-ray, would. Third, no selection for hospitalization should occur. Males, for instance, are more likely than females to have surgery for prolapsed lumbar intervertebral disc, whereas the latter are more likely to undergo prolonged bed rest, usually at home, for similar symptoms (Kelsey and Ostfeld, 1975). Unmarried persons are more likely to be treated in hospital for peptic ulcers than married individuals (Schwartz and Anguera, 1957). Fourth, for a rare disease that usually requires hospitalization, identification of patients through hospitals may be necessary; otherwise a prohibitively large sample would have to be taken of some other source of data. Cancer of the breast in males, for instance, is so rare that finding cases through physicians or in a community survey would be impractical and unwieldy.

The appropriateness of the hospitals and their catchment area must also be considered. Ideally, a defined population with available census data should exist. To achieve this it may be necessary to include several hospitals within a defined area and to survey hospitals from neighboring areas as well; patients who are not residents of the geographic area will, of course, have to be excluded when incidence rates are calculated. The hospitals should serve most people from the geographic area. Hospitals in southwestern Connecticut or northeastern New Jersey, for instance, do not serve all the individuals in these areas, since some residents seek care at hospitals in New York City. No significant migration to hospitals in other areas should occur; if such migration does take place, these hospitals would have to be checked for residents of the area of interest. Such migration is especially likely to occur if specialized procedures or equipment are needed. Specialized hospitals should be analyzed separately because they will draw cases from a very wide geographic area.

The investigator should have access to all hospitals in the geographic area. If some hospitals will not permit research to be undertaken, then cases will be missed. Finally, when trying to identify all cases of a disease seen at a particular hospital, it is important to use multiple sources within the hospital. Although sources in hospital record departments should in theory be able to identify all patients seen with a given disease over a certain time period by means of the code number assigned to the disease, cases are missed for a variety of reasons. Therefore, if one is obtaining information on incidence cases of hip fracture, x-ray log books and operating room log books should also be searched. For cases of cancer, pathology and operating room log books should be examined. Many investigators who have initially relied only on record room sources have been surprised by the number of cases missed there that are identified from other sources.

Other problems that occur when information from hospital records is used are, first, that the cases seen at hospital differ from cases not seen at hospital according to personal characteristics (age, sex, marital status, socioeconomic class, occupation, race), severity of disease, presence of associated conditions, administrative admissions policies, the particular facilities available within a hospital, and the practice of the physician treating the case. Second, in deciding whether to admit patients, physicians are influenced by their own education, the current medical literature, and the occurrence of epidemics. The medical records themselves are often incomplete and the information unstandardized from hospital to hospital or from physician to physician within a hospital. Likewise, diagnostic variability exists among different hospitals and physicians. In the United States hospitals are generally reimbursed according to the Diagnostic Related Group (DRG) system, which is based on discharge diagnosis rather than any standard diagnostic criteria; thus, what is listed as a discharge diagnosis may be influenced by reimbursement considerations. When hospital records are used, all these factors must be kept in mind, and every effort made to apply standard diagnostic criteria.

Over the next several years it is likely that in many countries an increasing amount of information from hospital records will be computerized. In the past it has been possible in many hospitals for authorized persons to obtain, by means of a computer, identification numbers of persons with discharge diagnoses of interest. The discharge diagnoses and their code numbers are taken from the hospital record face sheet for each admission. Then, the hospital records themselves can be requested and abstracted. More recently, some hospital computing systems make it possible to obtain readily, through a convenient computer terminal, clinical and laboratory information for a given patient. If only specific subsets of patients are of interest, assistance from programming staff is generally needed. One computerized system called Clin Query, recently developed at the Beth Israel Hospital in Boston, permits the researcher or clinician himself/herself to search the database to identify specific subsets of patients of interest (Safran et al., 1989). Each night, data from the approximately 70 discharged patients are transferred to the Clin Query system. The data include 42 types of administrative information, the results of up to 300 laboratory and diagnostic tests, all medications and blood products received, admitting and discharge diagnoses, and procedures performed. Several hundred video display terminals are available from which to access the data. Within a few minutes, the user can identify all patients with various combinations of attributes, and the associated clinical and laboratory data are displayed. When information from the medical record not included in the Clin Query system is needed, the medical record itself can be requested and the desired information abstracted. The HELP system developed at the University of Utah (Pryor et al., 1983) is another computerized system that allows retrieval of information from subpopulations of hospitalized patients and facilitates comparisons of characteristics of the subpopulations; associated statistical programs assist the user in analyzing the data.

AUTOPSY RECORDS

Autopsy reports contain detailed and usually accurate information about what a pathologist observed at autopsy and in the histologic examination that followed. The pathologist's findings may or may not be correlated with clinical observation, but the autopsy is generally regarded as the final court of diagnosis. Persons seen at autopsy tend to be a highly select group of hospitalized patients who, as noted above, are themselves select; furthermore, the proportion of deaths that are autopsied has been decreasing in recent years. This proportion was estimated to be less than 14% in the United States in 1985 (Carter, 1985). Interesting cases and undiagnosed diseases are likely to be seen at autopsy. Males are more likely to be autopsied than females, and young people are more likely to be autopsied than older people (McMahon, 1962), probably because more interest exists in their cause of death. If a physician on the staff of the hospital is particularly interested in a specific disease, autopsies may frequently be requested on patients with that disease. Accordingly, autopsy information has somewhat limited usefulness in epidemiologic studies and is mainly used as a source of information on the diagnostic accuracy of cases collected from another source. Another use of autopsy data (MacMahon and Pugh, 1970) is in determining the prevalence of a nonfatal disease, because the proportion of persons in whom the disease is found at autopsy gives an indication of the prevalence of that disease at the age at which the patient died, as long as cases with the nonfatal disease of interest are no more or less likely to be autopsied than other individuals. Autopsy data have shown, for instance, that the majority of women have fibrocystic breast disease at the time of death (Frantz et al., 1951), even though it is diagnosed in life in a much smaller percentage of women.

PHYSICIAN RECORDS

Records of physicians in office-based practice might appear to be a valuable source of data on diseases usually treated in a physician's office. However, obtaining permission to use these records is frequently difficult because of concerns about privacy and confidentiality. Also, most physicians' records are extremely brief, providing such limited information as primary symptoms, basic laboratory data, primary diagnosis, method of payment, and perhaps demographic characteristics. Often the handwriting and abbreviations are in the physician's own special shorthand, since the record is primarily for his or her own use.

INDUSTRIAL RECORDS

Industrial records can provide valuable epidemiologic information, if permission can be obtained to use them. Such records were the source of data for studies concerned with absence due to chronic bronchitis in postmen exposed to varying levels of air pollution in England and Wales (Reid and Fairbairn, 1958), and studies of coronary heart disease in London bus drivers and conductors (Morris et al., 1953). Employees in many industries must undergo preemployment and periodic examinations. Although some questions may be raised about the thoroughness of these examinations, in many instances workers receive the same routine tests year after year for many years; the records therefore can be used to obtain data on the incidence of disease and on changes in various measurements over time. Information will usually be available on reasons for sickness absence and disability. If the occupational environment is suspected of contributing to the disease, studies in industry can evaluate this possibility. Using industrial records is more convenient and less expensive than undertaking one's own study to measure exposures and diseases and is therefore relatively inexpensive. The population is defined; it consists of all workers in a given industry or component of an industry over a defined period of time. Finally, industrial populations are relatively stable compared with the general population.

One of the main disadvantages of using data from industrial populations is the potential lack of generalizability. Working people are systematically different from the general population. Comparisons with the general population are often invalid because of the "healthy-worker effect;" that is, workers are on the average healthier than the general population and would be expected to have lower disease rates. Administrative policies affect sickness absence and disability benefits, and these may not be comparable from one industry or plan to another. People may report ill health who are not really sick. People may leave a job because of a disease, and the investigator may not know this. Data may not be standardized among plants. Information in individual records has not been collected for research purposes, and the information desired may not have been recorded. For studies of specific exposures, it may be difficult to find an appropriate comparison group. Finally, workers may choose to seek medical care outside of the plant.

PREPAID INSURANCE GROUPS

Records of participants in prepaid health insurance plans, such as Kaiser-Permanente or the Health Insurance Plan of Greater New York, are useful for epidemiologic studies. To a large extent, the population of prepaid health plans can be defined, although of course some movement of people in and out of these plans occurs. Records of earlier illnesses, prescriptions, and other forms of treatment can be linked with records of later illnesses, because people enrolled in these plans have a financial incentive to obtain all of their care through the plan. Records are available over time, and in some instances they are computerized. Disadvantages, in addition to the select nature of these populations, include the difficulty of gaining access to these records and the fact that the data were collected and recorded for purposes other than research. A health plan member may also be covered under a different health care plan to which another family member subscribes, so that in some instances care may be sought elsewhere. Finally, concern often arises among the personnel of the plan that the research will in some way interfere with patient care.

An example of the use of such records for both descriptive and analytic epidemiologic purposes comes from the Kaiser-Permanente Medical Care Program of Northern California, where records were used to determine the incidence of clinically manifest cryptococcosis in a defined population over the period 1971–1980 and to learn about other characteristics of those affected (Friedman, 1983). It was found that almost all the cases had predisposing immunosuppressive disorders, a view not widely accepted at the time.

DATA ON PSYCHIATRIC DISORDERS

Two major sources exist on the prevalence of psychiatric disorders in the general population of the United States. First, the National Institute of Mental Health Epidemiologic Catchment Area (ECA) Program has provided data on the incidence, prevalence, and other characteristics of several psychiatric disorders in about 18,000 community residents in the Baltimore, New Haven, North Carolina, St. Louis, and Los Angeles areas based on a structured interview, the Diagnostic Interview Schedule (DIS) (Regier et al., 1984; Regier et al., 1988; Eaton et al., 1989). Second, Dohrenwend et al. (1980) extrapolated from previously undertaken community studies in various defined geographic locations to provide estimates of prevalence rates of psychiatric disorders in the United States as a whole.

Otherwise, most data on the frequency of mental illness in the United States are based on records of patients admitted to mental hospitals and other treatment facilities. For instance, the Division of Biometry of the National Institute of Mental Health collects hospital admissions statistics from throughout the country and issues reports. However, because many psychiatric disorders are not treated by physicians, these sources give underestimates of true frequencies of occurrence. The one exception to this may be schizophrenia, which has been found to come to medical attention in over 80% of cases (Dohrenwend et al., 1980).

OTHER SOURCES OF DATA

Other special populations occasionally used for epidemiologic study are school populations, university students, people enrolled in life insurance plans, and members of the Armed Forces. All three branches of the military, as well as the Veterans Administration, maintain computer records of patients based on information on the cover sheets of hospital records (IPES system). These records are kept in different places for each service. None keeps computerized records of outpatient visits. Permission for use of these data should be obtained from the Surgeon General of the military service responsible for the data or from the Medical Director of the Veterans Administration. It may also be possible to obtain permission through the office of the Research and Development Command of each service.

The record system of the Mayo Clinic (Kurland and Molgaard, 1981) has provided a large amount of data on disease incidence in the population of a defined geographic area, Olmsted County, Minnesota. The Mayo Clinic and the associated medical facilities in Rochester, Minnesota, attract a worldwide clientele, yet at the same time serve virtually the entire population of Olmsted County, where the Mayo Clinic is located. The ability to separate these two patient populations and the excellent clinical records that have been kept over many years have facilitated many population-based studies. This system has permitted the linking of disease occurrence, therapeutic agents, and other medically related exposures at one point in time with disease incidence at a later time. Use of these records has enhanced our understanding of the epidemiology and clinical course of epilepsy, for instance. Incidence and prevalence rates have been determined, underlying or antecedent neurological diseases identified as causes, certain factors predictive of remission described, and survivorship following various types of seizures studied (Hauser and Kurland, 1975). Determination of incidence rates of rheumatoid arthritis in males and females over a 25-year period (Fig. 3–7) in Olmsted County led to the suggestion that oral

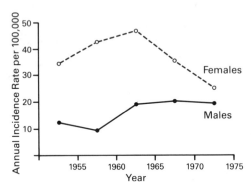

Figure 3–7. Annual incidence rate per 100,000 of rheumatoid arthritis in Rochester, Minnesota, 1950–1974, based on initial diagnosis of rheumatoid arthritis, age-adjusted to the 1960 U.S. white population (from Linos et al., 1980).

contraceptives might be protective against rheumatoid arthritis (Linos et al., 1978, 1980), a hypothesis still being investigated.

The National Institute of Occupational Safety and Health (NIOSH) publishes documents on the frequency of diseases of presumed occupational etiology in a variety of industries and on a variety of etiologic agents found in the occupational environment.

Computerized data files from Medicaid and Medicare programs are sometimes used for descriptive and analytic epidemiologic studies (Ray and Griffin, 1989; Bright et al., 1989; Fisher et al., 1990). Large numbers of people are included in both programs. Medicaid is a joint federal-state program for financing medical care for qualifying poor people in the United States. Medicare provides financing for medical care for persons aged 65 years and older. Medicaid files, for instance, generally include diagnostic information from hospitalizations and outpatient visits, demographic characteristics, prescriptions filled, surgical procedures performed, and fiscal and other information. The exact information received and the availability of data vary somewhat from state to state. The uses and limitations of using Medicaid data for epidemiologic studies, particularly studies to monitor unanticipated effects of marketed pharmaceutical agents, have been reviewed (Ray and Griffin, 1989; Bright et al., 1989). One recent example of a contribution to epidemiologic knowledge from Medicaid files was a Michigan-based study that identified an association between use of long half-life psychotropic drugs and incidence of hip fracture (Ray et al., 1987). The advantages and disadvantages of a variety of automated sources of data for pharmacoepidemiologic research have been discussed by Strom and Carson (1990).

REFERENCES

Acheson RM. 1966. Mortality from cerebrovascular disease in the United States. In Cerebrovascular Disease Epidemiology, A Workshop. Washington, D.C., U.S. Government Printing Office, Public Health Service Publication No. 1441.

Basch PF. 1990. Textbook of International Health. New York, Oxford University Press.

Bower G. 1961. Deaths and illness from bronchitis, emphysema, and asthma. *Am Rev Respir Dis* 83:684–689.

Brachman PS. 1991. Surveillance. In: AS Evans, PS Brachman, Eds. Bacterial Infections of Humans. New York, Plenum, pp 59–72.

Bright RA, Avorn J, Everitt PE. 1989. Medicaid data as a resource for epidemiologic studies: strengths and limitations. *J Clin Epidemiol* 42:937–945.

Carter JR. 1985. The problematic death certificate. *N Engl J Med* 313:1285–1286.

Centers for Disease Control. 1986. Comprehensive plan for epidemiologic surveillance: Centers for Disease Control, August 1986. Atlanta, GA, CDC.

Centers for Disease Control. 1988. Leading major congenital malformations among minority groups in the United States, 1981–1986. *MMWR* 37 (No. SS–3):17–24.

Centers for Disease Control. 1989a. Chronic disease reports in the *Morbidity and Mortality Weekly Report*. *MMWR* 38 (No. S–1):1–8.

Centers for Disease Control. 1989b. Update: Acquired immunodeficiency syndrome —United States, 1981–1988. *MMWR* 38:229–235.

Centers for Disease Control. 1991. Update on adult immunization. Recommendations of the Immunization Practices Advisory Committee (ACIP). *MMWR* 40 (No. RR–12):1–94.

Centers for Disease Control. 1992. Revised classification system for HIV infection and expanded surveillance case definition for AIDS among adolescents and adults. *MMWR* 41 (No. RR–17):1–19.

Centers for Disease Control. 1993. Recommendations of the Advisory Committee on Immunization Practices (ACIP): Use of vaccines and immune globulins in persons with altered immunocompetence. *MMWR* 42 (No. RR–4):1–18.

Centers for Disease Control. 1994. Summary of notifiable diseases, United States, 1993. *MMWR* 42:1–73.

Dohrenwend BP, Dohrenwend BS, Gould MS, Link B, Neugebauer R, Wunsch-Hitzig R. 1980. Mental Illness in the United States. New York, Prager.

Eaton WW, Kramer M, Anthony JC, Dryman A, Shapiro S, Locke BZ. 1989. The incidence of specific DIS/DSM-III mental disorders: data from the NIMH Epidemiologic Catchment Area Program. *Acta Psychiatr Scand* 79:163–178.

Edmonds LD, Layde PM, Levy MJ, Flynt JW, Erickson JD, Oakley GP Jr. 1981. Congenital malformations surveillance: two American systems. *Int J Epidemiol* 10:247–252.

Edwards WS, Winn DM, Kurlantgick V, Sheridon S, Retchin S, Collins JG. 1994. Evaluation of National Health Survey Diagnostic Reporting. National Center for Health Statistics Vital and Health Statistics. Series 2, Number 120.

Evans AS. 1989. Surveillance and seroepidemiology. In: AS Evans, Ed. Viral Infections of Humans. New York, Plenum, pp 51–73.

Eylenbosch WJ, Noah ND, Eds. 1988. Surveillance in Health and Disease. New York, Oxford University Press.

Fisher ES, Baron JA, Malenka DJ, Barrett J, Bubolz TA. 1990. Overcoming potential pitfalls in the use of Medicare data for epidemiologic research. *Am J Public Health* 80:1487–1490.

Fletcher CM, Jones NL, Burrows B, Nidess AH. 1964. American emphysema and British bronchitis. *Am Rev Respir Dis* 90:1–13.

Frantz VIC, Pickren JW, Melcher GW, Auchincloss H Jr. 1951. Incidence of chronic cystic disease in so-called normal breasts: study based on 225 postmortem examinations. *Cancer* 4:762–783.

Freedman MA, Gay GA, Brockert JE, Potrzebowski PW, Rothwell CJ. 1988. The 1989 revisions of the U.S. Standard Certificates of Live Birth and Death and the U.S. Standard Report of Fetal Death. *Am J Public Health* 78:168–172.

Friedman GD. 1983. The rarity of cryptococcosis in Northern California: the 10-year experience of a large defined population. *Am J Epidemiol* 117:230–234.

Hahn RA, Mulinare J, Teutsch SM. 1992. Inconsistencies in coding of race and ethnicity between birth and death in US infants. *JAMA* 267:259–263.

Hauser WA, Kurland LT. 1975. The epidemiology of epilepsy in Rochester, Minnesota, 1935 through 1967. *Epilepsia* 16:1–66.

HCIA, Baltimore, MD. 1993. Unpublished data.

Horn JW, Asire AJ, Young JL Jr, Pollack EJ. 1984. SEER Program: Cancer Incidence and Mortality in the United States 1973–81. Bethesda, MD, U.S. Department of Health and Human Services, National Institutes of Health. NIH Publication No. 85–1837.

International Agency for Research on Cancer. 1986. Cancer Occurrence in Developing Countries. DM Parkin, Ed. IARC Scientific Publications No. 75. Lyon, France.

International Agency for Research on Cancer. 1992. Cancer Incidence in Five Continents. Vol. VI. IARC Publication No. 120. Lyon, France, IARC Scientific Publications.

Israel RA, Rosenberg HM, Curtin LR. 1986. Analytical potential for multiple cause-of-death data. *Am J Epidemiol* 124:161–179.

Kelsey JL, Ostfeld AM. 1975. Demographic characteristics of persons with acute herniated lumbar intervertebral disc. *J Chron Dis* 28:37–50.

Kirby RS. 1993. The coding of underlying cause of death from fetal death certificates: Issues and policy considerations. *Am J Public Health* 83:1088–1091.

Kircher T, Nelson J, Burdo H. 1985. The autopsy as a measure of the accuracy of the death certificate. *N Engl J Med* 313:1263–1269.

Kovar MG. 1989. Data systems of the National Center for Health Statistics. National Center for Health Statistics. Vital and Health Statistics Series 1, No. 23. DHHS Publication No. (PHS) 89–1325.

Kurland LT, Molgaard CA. 1981. The patient record in epidemiology. *Sci Am* 245:54–63.

Linos A, Worthington JW, O'Fallon WM, Kurland LT. 1978. Rheumatoid arthritis and oral contraceptives. *Lancet* 1:871.

Linos A, Worthington JW, O'Fallon WM, Kurland LT. 1980. The epidemiology of rheumatoid arthritis: a study of incidence, prevalence and mortality. *Am J Epidemiol* 111:87–98.

MacMahon B. 1983. The National Death Index. *Am J Public Health* 73:1247–1248.

MacMahon B, Pugh TF. 1970. Epidemiology, Principles and Methods. Boston, Little Brown and Company.

Marier R. 1977. The reporting of communicable diseases. *Am J Epidemiol* 105:587–590.

Masi AT. 1962. Potential uses and limitations of hospital data in epidemiologic research. *Am J Public Health* 55:658–667.

McCaig LF. 1994. National Hospital Ambulatory Medical Care Survey: 1992 emergency department summary. Advance data from vital and health statistics; No. 245. Hyattsville, MD, National Center for Health Statistics.

McMahon CA. 1962. Age-sex distributions of selected groups of human autopsied cases. *Arch Pathol* 73:40–47.

Moriyama IM. 1989. Problems in measurement of accuracy of cause-of-death statistics. *Am J Public Health* 79:1349–1350.

Morris JN, Heady JA, Raffle PAB, Roberts CG, Parks JW. 1953. Coronary heart disease and physical activity at work. *Lancet* 2:1053–1057.

National Center for Health Statistics. 1982. Annotated bibliography of cause of death validation studies, 1958–80. Vital and Health Statistics, Series 2, No. 89. DHHS Pub. No. (PHS) 82–1363.

National Center for Health Statistics. 1984. Multiple causes of death in the United States. Monthly Vital Statistics Report, Vol. 32, No. 10, Suppl. 2.

National Center for Health Statistics. 1988. International Health Data Reference Guide 1987. DHHS Publication No. (PHS) 88–1007.

National Center for Health Statistics. 1990. National Death Index User's Manual. DHHS Publication No. (PHS) 90–1148.

Patterson BM, Bilgrad R. 1986. Use of the National Death Index in cancer studies. *J Natl Cancer Inst* 77:877–881.

Pickle LW, Mason TJ, Howard N, Hoover R, Fraumeni JF Jr. 1987. Atlas of U.S. Cancer Mortality Among Whites: 1950–1980. Washington, D.C., U.S. Department of Health and Human Services. DHHS Publication No. (NIH) 87–2900.

Pryor TA, Gardner RM, Clayton PD, Warner HR. 1983. The HELP system. *J Med Systems* 7:87–102.

Raska K. 1983. Epidemiologic surveillance in the control of infectious diseases. *Rev Infect Dis* 5:1112–1117.

Ray WA, Griffin MR. 1989. Use of Medicaid data for pharmacoepidemiology. *Am J Epidemiol* 129:837–849.

Ray WA, Griffin MR, Schaffner W, Baugh PK, Melton LJ. 1987. Psychotropic drug use and the risk of hip fracture. *N Engl J Med* 316:363–369.

Regier DA, Boyd JH, Burke JD Jr, Rae DS, Myers JK, Kramer M, Robins LN, George LK, Karno M, Locke BZ. 1988. One-month prevalence of mental disorders in the United States based on five Epidemiologic Catchment Area sites. *Arch Gen Psychiatry* 45:977–986.

Regier DA, Myers JA, Kramer M, Robins LN, Blazer DG, Hough RL, Eaton WW, Locke BZ. 1984. The NIMH Epidemiologic Catchment Area Program. *Arch Gen Psychiatry* 41:934–941.

Reid DD, Fairbairn AJ. 1958. The natural history of chronic bronchitis. *Lancet* 2:1147–1152.

Riggan WB, Van Bruggen JW, Acquavella JF, Beaubier J, Mason TJ. 1983. U.S. Cancer Mortality Rates and Trends, 1950–1979. Washington, D.C., U.S. Environmental Protection Agency, National Cancer Institute. EPA-600/1–83–015a.

Safran C, Porter D, Lightfoot J, Rury CD, Underhill LH, Bleich HL, Slack WV. 1989. Clin Query: A system for online searching of data in a teaching hospital. *Ann Intern Med* 111:751–756.

Sanders BS. 1962. Have morbidity surveys been oversold? *Am J Public Health* 52:1648–1659.

Schwartz D, Anguera G. 1957. Une cause de biais dans certaines enquêtes médicales: le temps de sejour des malades. *Communication à L'Institute International de Statistique*. 30ème session. Stockholm.

Sorlie PD, Rogot E, Johnson NJ. 1992. Validity of demographic characteristics on the death certificate. *Epidemiology* 3:181–184.

Strom BL, Carson JL. 1990. Use of automated databases for pharmacoepidemiology research. *Epidemiol Rev* 12:87–107.

Teutsch SM, Churchill RE. 1994. Principles and Practice of Public Health Surveillance. New York, Oxford University Press.

Thacker SB, Berkelman RL. 1988. Public health surveillance in the United States. *Epidemiol Rev* 10:164–190.

Thurlbeck WM, Angus GE. 1963. The relationship between emphysema and chronic bronchitis as assessed morphologically. *Am Rev Respir Dis* 87:815–819.

Young JL Jr, Percy CL, Asire AJ, Berg JW, Cusano MM, Gloeckler LA, Horm JW, Lourie WI Jr, Pollack ES, Shambaugh EM. 1981. Surveillance, epidemiology, and end results: incidence and mortality data, 1973–77. National Cancer Institute Monograph 57. Washington, D.C.: U.S. Government Printing Office. NIH Publication No. 81–2330.

Exercises

How would you go about obtaining the following information? Give reasons for your choice, and discuss the strengths and weaknesses of the method you choose.

1. Incidence rates of breast cancer in Connecticut residents by age and gender

2. The incidence rate of acute appendicitis in residents of _____ (nearest large city)

3. The incidence rate of anencephaly in _____ (your state)

4. The distribution of hearing levels among adults in the United States

5. The prevalence rate of hay fever in adult residents of New Hampshire

6. Geographic differences, within the United States, in the frequency of strokes (cerebral vascular accidents)

7. Changes in blood pressure levels over time (i.e., as people get older)

8. The incidence rate of coronary heart disease among bus drivers in _____ (nearest large city)

9. The most frequent causes of death among elderly residents of _____ (nearest large city) with hip fractures in the three years following the fracture

4

Prospective Cohort Studies: Planning and Execution

NATURE OF PROSPECTIVE COHORT STUDIES

In a cohort study concerned with disease etiology, the investigator starts with a group of individuals apparently free of the disease(s) of interest. This group of individuals, or cohort, is divided into those exposed to a possible risk factor and those not exposed, and is then followed through time in order to determine the incidence rate (or mortality rate) among the exposed and the incidence rate (or mortality rate) among the unexposed. In a *prospective* cohort study, the investigator collects information on the exposure status of the cohort members at the time the study begins, and identifies new cases of disease (or deaths) from that time forward. This contrasts with the *retrospective* cohort study, to be discussed in Chapter 5, in which exposure status is established from information recorded at some time in the past, and disease incidence (or mortality) is determined from then until the present.

Prospective cohort studies are sometimes started at the time of first exposure to a suspected risk factor, such as when employees first start working at a plant or at the time people first start using a drug. Perhaps more often, the exposure has already been occurring for some time when it is measured at the beginning of a study. When previous exposure has taken place, it is desirable to estimate by means of questionnaires or records the duration and intensity of such exposure, thus adding a retrospective element to many prospective cohort studies.

In many instances, however, it is impossible to know how long exposure has occurred. For example, when a substance such as serum cholesterol is measured at the beginning of a study, it is not generally known how long the cholesterol has been at that particular level and what previous levels have been, unless such information happens to have been recorded on medical records. Also, a cohort initially should include only individuals free of the disease(s) of interest, but the disease process may already have begun in some cohort members, even though it cannot be detected by available means. It is important to remember when interpreting results that the cohort members have often had unrecorded exposures of interest or sub-clinical disease before entry into the cohort.

This book focuses on observational cohort studies. However, many aspects of measurement, follow-up, analysis, and, to a certain extent, con-trol of confounding pertain to experimental studies as well. One particular type of cohort study, the panel study, will be deferred to Chapter 10 be-cause the design and analysis of panel studies differ in some respects from the more traditional cohort studies to be discussed here.

Strengths and weaknesses of observational prospective cohort studies will not be enumerated here, as they have been extensively discussed else-where (Friedman, 1994; Lilienfeld and Stolley, 1994; Hennekens and Bur-ing, 1987; Mausner and Kramer, 1985). Because of the large sample size and high cost almost always associated with prospective cohort studies of all but the commonest of outcomes, they are usually initiated under two cir-cumstances: first, when sufficient evidence has been obtained from less expensive case-control, cross-sectional, or retrospective cohort studies to indicate that a prospective cohort study is warranted, and second, when a new agent that requires monitoring for its possible association with several diseases has been introduced into the environment, such as oral contracep-tives or hormone replacement therapy.

ESTIMATES MADE FROM COHORT STUDIES

Before discussing specific issues in study design, it will be useful to review briefly the estimates that the investigator usually wants to make from the data collected in a cohort study, because the nature of these estimates to a large extent dictates the information to be collected. The statistical proce-dures for making these estimates will be covered in Chapters 6 and 7, but it is useful to keep in mind from the outset the need to collect certain relevant information. First, the investigator wants to estimate the incidence rates of disease in those exposed and those not exposed to the possible risk factors of major interest, in those exposed to various levels and for various lengths of time, and in those exposed to certain combinations of risk factors. The investigator may also want to determine whether changes in exposure levels are related to occurrence of disease.

It is important to take any confounding variables into account when making estimates of the incidence rates or mortality rates associated with a given factor; otherwise, as in any type of study, misleading conclusions may be reached about the role of that factor. Determining whether exposure to one factor modifies the effect of exposure to another is also an integral part of the data analysis.

Another estimate usually made is the rate ratio (or risk ratio). In order to obtain a measure of the magnitude of an association between a risk factor and a disease and in order to help determine the likelihood that an association between a risk factor and a disease is causal (see Chapter 2), the investigator usually wants to estimate (a) the rate (or risk) in the exposed persons relative to the rate (or risk) in the unexposed persons, (b) the rate (or risk) in persons exposed to each of several levels of a risk factor relative to that in the unexposed, and (c) the rate (or risk) in persons exposed to various combinations of risk factors relative to those not exposed to any risk factors. Again, confounding variables should be controlled for when these rate ratios (or risk ratios) are computed.

Finally, the investigator or health planner may want to estimate the attributable fraction, or the proportion of cases of a disease that result from a given cause or given combination of causes.

ASSEMBLING THE COHORT

Before beginning a study, those who are susceptible and those who are immune or who for other reasons are not at risk for the disease(s) under study should be identified. With infectious agents, susceptibility is generally determined by measuring serum antibody levels so that the incidence or attack rate can be determined among susceptibles only. Distinguishing susceptible and immune persons at the start of the study is of such importance and the cost of tests for the presence or absence of antibody is sufficiently low that routine application of such tests to potential cohort members is almost mandatory. However, such definitive separation into susceptible and immune cannot be done in certain situations, including diseases for which reinfection is common in the presence of antibody (such as respiratory syncytial virus), diseases that result from reactivation of a latent infection (herpes viruses, tuberculosis, toxoplasmosis), and certain malignancies of presumed viral etiology (African Burkitt's lymphoma due to Epstein-Barr virus) in which it is the *height* of the antibody level, not its mere presence, that is associated with the disease.

In diseases of presumed noninfectious etiology, such relatively definitive markers of susceptibility are at present usually not available, although people without an organ at risk should be removed from the cohort, such as women who had a hysterectomy in a study concerned with the etiology of cancer of the endometrium. People with a known or suspected history of the disease(s) under study generally should be eliminated unless recurrences are of interest. If disease recurrence and first occurrence are both of interest, then those with a history of the disease should be noted and considered as a separate group in the analysis. Identifying those not at risk for a disease and those who have already had the disease may involve conducting a prevalence study at the beginning of a cohort study.

As mentioned previously, the identification of persons with current or past asymptomatic or subclinical disease sometimes presents difficulties. The use of laboratory tests, electrocardiograms, x-rays, cytological examinations, and other special procedures may help to identify persons who should be excluded from the study or placed in a special category, but in general, these procedures must be simple, harmless, and inexpensive if they are to be applied to the entire cohort.

Cohorts are sometimes chosen because they are representative of the general population, as in the Framingham Heart Study (Dawber et al., 1951) or the Tecumseh Community Health Study (Epstein et al., 1970). Although the ability to generalize from such studies makes them highly desirable, they are usually very expensive and tend to be associated with relatively large loss to follow-up. Also, an exposure of interest may be uncommon in the general population, so that it may sometimes be more efficient to select a cohort with a higher proportion exposed. For these reasons, cohorts representing limited population subgroups are often selected.

In many instances, unless the cohort under study is limited to a group at high risk for the disease, prohibitively large sample sizes would be needed for enough new cases of disease to develop. For instance, the Framingham Heart Study did not include individuals under 30 years of age (Dawber et al., 1951), because their risk of coronary heart disease was known to be very low over the next decade or so. If one wanted to learn more about the epidemiology of idiopathic adolescent scoliosis (abnormal lateral curvature of the spine), a cohort study would be needed because many of the suggested etiologic agents (e.g., muscle imbalance, ocular-motor disturbances) could be consequences rather than causes of the disease. Scoliotic curves of 10 degrees or more will develop in about 2% of children between the ages of 6 and 16 years. If an unselected group of 6-year-olds were to be followed for 11 years, a sample size of about 2900 would be needed to detect a relative risk of 3 for an exposure present in 10% of the population (assuming no loss to follow-up, $\alpha = 0.05$, $\beta = 0.20$, and a two-sided test of significance; see Chapter 12). However, if the study were limited to siblings of children with scoliosis, a sample size of only about 700 would be needed, as the risk is about 3.5 times greater for scoliosis among siblings of cases than in the general population. (In reality, somewhat larger sample sizes would be needed because of the inevitable dropouts during the period of the study.) Such a study would, of course, assume that the same risk factors pertain to the population as a whole as to siblings of children with scoliosis. This assumption is not unreasonable, given the probable polygenic mode of inheritance of adolescent scoliosis, with strong influence from environmental factors. If risk factors were identified in this somewhat select population, a next step might be to try to confirm these findings in a cohort from a more general population. Such a study would require a large sample size, as indicated above, and would therefore be considerably more expensive, but might be worth carrying out, once a less expensive study had provided justification.

One commonly used cohort is people working in a particular industry or occupation. Such individuals often have exposures of particular interest, are less likely to be lost to follow-up because of their lower mobility than the general population, have a certain amount of relevant information recorded in their medical and employment records, and in many instances undergo initial and then periodic medical examinations. Morris et al. (1966), for instance, assembled a cohort from an occupational group, London busmen, in order to identify and confirm risk factors for coronary heart disease. Because most of these men tended to stay at their jobs for many years, follow-up was greatly facilitated. Also, the possibly protective effect of physical activity was of considerable interest, and the conductors had a great deal of physical activity on their jobs. Paffenbarger and Hale (1975) used a cohort of longshoremen to study the relationship between physical activity and coronary heart disease for much the same reasons, that is, a relatively high proportion with the exposure of primary interest and the ease of follow-up. Studies of the relationship between type A behavior and coronary heart disease have been undertaken in employed populations because of ease of follow-up and because the scale used to measure type A behavior is in part based on work-related behavior (Rosenman et al., 1975). Thus, studies of occupational cohorts not only may lead to the identification of etiologic agents in the workplace, but in addition may provide an efficient means of identifying risk factors operating in the general population.

A cohort that has provided a great deal of information about several exposure-disease relationships in women is the Nurses' Health Study cohort (Hennekens et al., 1979; Stampfer et al., 1991; Stampfer et al., 1993). Nurses were selected for the cohort not because of any particular occupational exposure, but because it was believed that their cooperation would be at a high level and that they could report disease occurrence with a high degree of accuracy. This cohort was established in 1976, when questionnaires were sent to all married female registered nurses born between 1921 and 1946 and living in 11 states of the United States. Of the 172,413 women who were sent a questionnaire, 121,700 responded. The questionnaire sought data on known or suspected risk factors for cancer and coronary heart disease such as height, weight, smoking habits, use of estrogen replacement therapy and use of oral contraceptives. A follow-up questionnaire is mailed to the cohort members every 2 years to update information on possible risk factor exposure and to determine whether major medical events have occurred. Subsequently, new areas of interest, such as a dietary history, have been added to the questionnaire. Numerous publications have resulted from this study concerning such exposures as oral contraceptives, estrogen replacement therapy, cigarette smoking, alcohol consumption, diet, and use of hair dyes, and such conditions as cancers, coronary heart disease, and hip fracture. Following such a large cohort over so many years might be prohibitively expensive, except that most of the information is collected through a questionnaire sent through the mail. Studies of the validity and reliability of selected items of information have in general shown the quality of the data to be good (Colditz et al., 1986). Nurses are one of the few groups that can be expected to provide medical information in a relatively accurate manner. A cohort study of a new group of nurses has now begun.

Cohorts from prepaid health plans also offer several advantages. Like occupational cohorts, they can be more easily identified and followed than the general population. Thus, if a subgroup of their membership is sampled and invited to participate in a prospective cohort study, follow-up is likely to be considerably easier than in the general population. For instance, the Oakland Unit of the Kaiser Permanente Medical Care Program of Northern California contributes participants to the cohort being followed in the Coronary Artery Risk Development in Young Adults (CARDIA) prospective study (Sidney et al., 1991).

Prepaid health care plans have the additional advantage that records are routinely kept of medications and drugs prescribed, surgical procedures undertaken, and the results of laboratory tests performed as well as of diseases that the cohort members develop. Therefore, prepaid health plans are a valuable resource for studies of medically related exposures and diseases for which care usually is sought. A prospective cohort study in the Walnut Creek facility of the Kaiser Permanente Medical Care Program examined through medical records the possible associations between the use of oral contraceptives and a large number of diseases (The Walnut Creek Contraceptive Study, 1976). As with cohort studies in industry, access to these records by investigators not employed at these facilities is limited, but, when such investigations are undertaken, they can provide a great deal of information.

Prospective seroepidemiologic studies of infectious diseases have been carried out in school, college, university, and military populations. They have contributed to knowledge of disease incidence, etiology, ratio of inapparent to apparent infection, biologic spectrum of clinical illness associated with a given infectious agent, contribution of various agents to a given clinical syndrome, level of antibody needed to protect against reinfection or recurrent clinical disease, and duration of immunity. Prospective studies of the Epstein-Barr virus (EBV), for instance, established that this agent is causally related to infectious mononucleosis. The studies of EBV and infectious mononucleosis involved cohorts of students at Yale University (Evans et. al., 1968), at the West Point Military Academy (Hallee et al., 1974), and at five English colleges and universities (University Health Physicians and P.H.L.S., 1971).

Other reasons for selecting a restricted cohort are that determining exposure status may require a method of measurement that is most easily applied in a special setting and that enrolling and making measurements on cohort members when they happen to be visiting a medical facility reduces cost. In seroepidemiologic studies, the ability to obtain a portion of each blood sample drawn at the time of entry physical exam or for routine diagnostic testing has greatly facilitated these investigations. Women having their first antenatal visits have been enrolled in cohort studies of outcomes of pregnancy because this is a convenient time to approach the women and to make measurements. The relationship between alcohol consumption and spontaneous abortions, for instance, has been studied by determining drinking habits through a questionnaire administered at the time of prenatal visits and linking the information to subsequent pregnancy outcomes (Harlap and Shiono, 1980). Hatch et al. (1993) studied the relationship between exercise during pregnancy and pregnancy outcome by forming a cohort of women identified at the time of the first prenatal visit. Cohort members were then queried about their physical activity (and other attributes) during each trimester of pregnancy, and this information was related to pregnancy outcomes as determined from physicians and hospital records. Cohort studies of perinatal events have the additional advantage of requiring only a relatively short period of follow-up.

A variety of other cohorts too numerous to be listed here have been used for prospective cohort studies. It is hoped that these examples provide an idea of the types of cohorts that may be used and of some of the reasons for selecting a particular cohort. When cohorts not strictly representative of the general population are selected, caution should be exercised in applying the results to the population as a whole. Careful consideration must be given to whether there is some reason that risk factors identified in the selected cohort may or may not apply to the general population. However, advantages of reduced sample size, ease of identifying exposures, ease of follow-up, and the associated reduced cost frequently tip the scales in favor of a more restricted cohort.

Finally, the large sample size often needed in prospective cohort studies sometimes necessitates collaborative studies involving several geograph-ically separated cohorts. One example of such a collaborative effort is the Study of Osteoporotic Fractures (Cummings et al., 1990), which is relating a variety of potential risk factors for low bone mass and falls to the risk of fracture in various bones; the cohort began with 9704 women from four geographic areas in the United States.

DETERMINING EXPOSURE STATUS

The techniques used to measure the possible risk factor(s) of interest vary considerably from one study to another and from one risk factor to another. In a study based on the general population, such as the Framingham study (Dawber et al., 1951), the cohort is assembled and measurements of the possible risk factors of interest are made by means of questionnaires (e.g., age, smoking habits), laboratory tests (e.g., serum cholesterol, hemo-globin), physical measurements (e.g., blood pressure, height), and various special procedures (e.g., electrocardiograms, x-rays). In these studies, the investigators make the measurements and then classify the cohort members into various exposure categories. The questionnaire can include items on the length of previous exposure to variables such as cigarette smoking, as well as questions on current exposure status.

Exposures may be identified from existing records, as in studies aimed at identifying occupational exposures and medications as risk factors. For instance, in a study by the Royal College of General Practitioners (1974; Kay and Hannaford, 1988) in England, women obtaining their first pre-scription for oral contraceptives were identified through physicians' re-cords. Information on oral contraceptive use was then updated by the participating physicians every 6 months so that changes in oral contracep-tive use through the course of follow-up could be determined. Sometimes more detailed information can be obtained about the extent, nature, and length of exposure by supplementing data from records with information obtained from personal interview. In their study of physical activity and coronary heart disease in longshoremen, Paffenbarger and Hale (1975) estimated the energy output required in 49 types of longshoring jobs, and classified longshoremen each year into three categories according to the energy output of the job. Table 4–1 shows the main finding of this study: The longshoremen in the high-physical-activity category had substantially

Table 4-1. Age-Adjusted Mortality Rates Per 10,000 Man-Years from Coronary Heart Disease (CHD) according to Physical Activity Level at Work

Work Activity Level (kcal/min)	CHD Death Rate
Heavy (5.2–7.5)	26.9
Moderate (2.4–5.0)	46.3
Light (1.5–2.0)	49.0

Source: Paffenbarger and Hale (1975).

lower mortality rates from coronary heart disease than did those in the medium and low categories. Controlling in the analysis for other risk factors for coronary heart disease did not change this association.

Prospective cohort studies of infectious diseases raise other issues. The presence, duration, and intensity of exposure to an infectious agent depend on the source of the infection and the means of transmission. When the source of infection and means of transmission are well defined and of one type, or are unique, then division into exposed or not exposed groups may be quite simple. For instance, in the famous outbreak of cholera from the Broad Street well, Snow could identify those drinking or not drinking water from this source (Snow, 1855). For many infections in which multiple sources of exposure or multiple means of transmission occur, separation of the exposed and unexposed groups may be impossible. Indeed, many investigations of infectious diseases are carried out in order to establish the nature of the exposure and/or means of transmission. This is done by classifying the various specific times of exposure and then determining the incidence of disease in those exposed in various ways. The investigation of a food-borne outbreak is a good example (see Chapter 11); if the highest rates of illness occur among persons eating a specific food at a particular time and place, then the probable source of infection and mode of transmission are suggested.

A rapidly growing area in the study of the epidemiology of noninfectious diseases is the attempt to develop biologic markers of exposure and of biologically effective exposures. Biomarkers of exposure refer to biological measurements of internal dose or body burden, such as blood lead levels as a marker of environmental lead exposure (Stein and Hatch, 1987). For infectious diseases, such markers of exposure (i.e., antibodies) have long existed; for example, in a prospective cohort study of chronic hepatitis B as a cause of primary liver cancer, serum markers of hepatitis B were used to define exposure, since hepatitis B is often asymptomatic (Beasley et al., 1981). For noninfectious agents, it is hoped that biomarkers of exposure will be more precise or accurate than measurements made by questionnaire; with questionnaires a person may not know exactly what he/she was exposed to, may forget exposures, or may deliberately misinform the investigator. Biomarkers also may be useful when environmental data are poor approximations of individual dose (because of individual variation in uptake and pharmacokinetics, for instance), when it is desired to document exposure in target tissue, and when one wishes to quantify the biological load from an exposure. Finally, biomarkers can be used to validate in small samples of individuals information obtained from less expensive and more feasible sources such as questionnaires.

Changes in exposure to putative risk factors during the course of follow-up often occur. People decide to change jobs or to use a different method of contraception. Male homosexuals may start using condoms or stop frequenting gay bars because of fear of AIDS. The participants may even change their behavior because of the study, a situation often referred to as the "Hawthorne effect." For instance, if every year people are asked about their diets, they may begin to eat different foods. A hypertensive cohort member may hear about blood pressure so much that he or she starts to take hypertensive medication during the course of a study in which blood pressure is being considered as a possible risk factor for other diseases. The investigator can do little about these changes, because the participants are free to choose and because many of the changes are in fact desirable. Nevertheless, it is important to note such changes and the reasons for them so that in the analysis, length of exposure and the reasons for changes in exposure can be considered. Exposure levels may also change as a result of actions outside the control of either the study subjects or the investigator. For instance, air pollution control equipment may be installed in a plant. Again, such changes should be noted, and may provide additional insight into what changes in risk occur as a result of intervention.

SELECTION OF COMPARISON GROUPS OF UNEXPOSED INDIVIDUALS

Choice of a comparison, or referent, group sometimes follows naturally from the choice of the exposed group. If a population is sampled and participants are classified on exposure status as measured by the investigator, then the natural comparison group is an *internal comparison group* of those from the same sample who do not have the exposure. Use of an internal comparison group not only increases the likelihood that the exposed and unexposed cohort members come from a similar subgroup of the population, but generally means that they will be subject to the same follow-up procedures and will therefore have the same chance of having disease detected. In the Framingham study, for instance, cohort members were classified according to cholesterol level, blood pressure, and many other variables. When cholesterol level is considered, those with high levels would be the exposed group and those without high levels the comparison group; when blood pressure level is considered, those with high blood pressure would be the exposed group and those without high levels the nonexposed group. When several variables are being considered simultaneously, the unexposed group would be those with exposure to none of the risk factors.

In some studies there is no obvious referent group. This can occur, for instance, if everyone has at least some exposure or if the number of persons in the group with no exposure or a low level of exposure is small. Methods of analyzing and interpreting data with no specific referent group are described in Chapters 6 and 7. However, if it is deemed useful to consider one group as the referent group, the investigator can select whatever group he/she thinks appropriate, but it is a good idea to select a referent group with relatively large numbers, in order to have adequate precision when disease rates in groups with other levels of exposure are compared to the disease rate in the referent group.

In some studies, exposed individuals are selected on the basis of a particular exposure, and in many such instances, no internal comparison groups exists, so an *external comparison group* must be sought. Often the comparison group is the general population of the area from which the exposed group is obtained. In a study of the possible relationship between exposure to carbon disulfide and coronary heart disease, for instance, death rates among workers exposed to carbon disulfide in a viscose rayon plant were compared to death rates in two other groups, one of which was the general Finnish population (Hernberg et al., 1973). General population comparison groups are usually not ideal in studies evaluating risks from occupational exposures, however. Not only are persons selected for employment on the average healthier than the general population, but once they became employed, they tend to have better economic circumstances and better access to medical care than the general population; they also may make changes in their lifestyle that are conducive to better health (Wen et al., 1983). Therefore, an external comparison group is often used that is believed to be susceptible to the same selective factors as the exposed group, provided the comparison group does not have exposures that might also increase the risk for disease(s) of interest. In the study of carbon disulfide exposure and coronary heart disease, the mortality experience of the exposed cohort of workers in the viscose rayon industry was compared to workers in the paper industry from the same town as well as to the general population. The workers with carbon disulfide exposure did in fact have the highest mortality rates from coronary heart disease, but, as would be expected from the healthy worker effect, the rates in the paper workers were lower than those in the general population.

Sometimes both external and internal comparison groups are used. In a study of cancer mortality among white underground uranium miners in the Colorado Plateau area (Wagoner et al., 1965), one comparison group was white males in the four-state area in which most of the miners lived. Compared to this control group, the miners had almost four times the risk of dying from respiratory cancer. An internal comparison was also made by using records of occupational histories and measurements of radiation levels within the mines to categorize the men according to their estimated cumulative radiation exposure. The results of this internal comparison are shown in Table 4–2.

Concern that persons selected because of exposure status may be more or less healthy than the general population extends to etiologic agents other than occupational exposures. For instance, if the exposure of interest is use of oral contraceptives, the question arises as to whether the comparison group should consist of women not using oral contraceptives or be limited to women using another method of contraception. Women using no method of contraception may differ from women using some other method of contraception with respect to sexual practices, desire to become pregnant, and fertility status. On the other hand, women choosing various methods of contraception differ according to such characteristics as religion, ethnic group, and overall health status. As in many situations, no single comparison group is obviously best. Fortunately, in England two prospective cohort studies have been undertaken of long-term effects of oral contraceptives, one using as a comparison group women not taking oral contraceptives (Royal College of General Practitioners, 1974; Kay and Hannaford, 1988), the other, which identified oral contraceptive users at a family planning

Table 4–2. Age-Adjusted Incidence Rates Per 10,000 Man-Years of Respiratory Cancer According to Estimated Cumulative Exposure to Airborne Radiation

Cumulative Radiation Exposure (Working-Level Months)	Incidence Rate
<120	3.10
120–839	6.55
840–1799	15.46
1800–3719	37.06
≥3720	116.12

Source: Wagoner et al. (1965).

clinic, employing as a comparison group women using a diaphragm or an intrauterine device (Vessey et al., 1976, 1989). With a few exceptions, results from the two cohort studies have been consistent, thus allowing one to have increased confidence in the validity of findings. Should the comparison groups give different results, then the investigator must try to find out why the results are different. Also, there is generally less certainly about the results when such inconsistencies occur.

No matter what type of comparison group is decided upon, comparability to the exposed group with respect to other characteristics that might affect the likelihood of disease must be evaluated carefully before conclusions are reached. The possibility of self-selection into the initial exposed and unexposed groups always needs to be considered. For instance, people selecting jobs with high levels of physical activity may be more healthy to begin with, and this initial state of health, rather than the physical activity on the job, could be the reason for their reduced incidence of coronary heart disease. In an early study to test the hypothesis that physical exercise protects against coronary heart disease, London bus conductors, who had a great deal of exercise while working, were compared with bus drivers, who were sitting almost all the time (Morris et al., 1953). Coronary heart disease incidence rates were in fact observed to be higher in the bus drivers than in the conductors. This finding might be construed as evidence that physical activity protects against coronary heart disease, but the drivers and conductors were not completely alike in other characteristics that could affect their risk for coronary heart disease. It was noted that the waist size of the uniforms of the drivers was on the average larger than that of the conductors at the time of initial employment, so that the heavier body weight of the drivers could be another reason for their increased risk for coronary heart disease. Also, the stress of driving through the streets of London might have put the drivers at higher risk than the conductors.

If the relevant exposures have been measured, the methods of multivariable analysis to be described in Chapters 6 and 7 can be used to help sort out which of these variables are predictive of coronary heart disease independent of the effects of other variables. However, other explanations sometimes cannot be ruled out because the appropriate measurements have not been or cannot be made, and the investigator is left with inconclusive results. Careful thought must enter into the choice of the comparison group and of the measurements to be made on all cohort members so that either (a) the unexposed cohort members are firmly believed to be comparable to exposed cohort members, except for the exposure, in their likelihood of developing the disease, or (b) ways in which the two groups differ in risk can be taken into account in the analysis.

MEASUREMENT OF DISEASE

Determining which cohort members develop the disease(s) of interest varies a great deal, depending upon the particular diseases being studied and the resources available. No matter what method is being used, under most circumstances procedures for disease identification should be comparable for exposed and unexposed; whenever possible, disease ascertainment should be done by persons unaware of the exposure status of the cohort members.

In some studies, the outcome of interest is whether the cohort member has died, and, if so, what were the specific causes of death. Methods of determining whether a person has died will be covered in a subsequent section of this chapter. Obviously, using mortality as the outcome is reasonable only if the diseases of interest are frequently fatal. In many studies, the causes of death as recorded on the death certificate are accepted, despite the various limitations discussed in Chapter 3. In other studies the death certificate is only a starting point, and additional information on causes of death is collected from medical records, physicians, autopsy reports, and next of kin. For most diseases, obtaining this more complete information is highly desirable in order to increase accuracy.

For diseases that usually require hospitalization, records of the hospitals at which cohort members are likely to seek care can be monitored. For instance, the cohort in a study of long-term effects of oral contraceptives consisted of large numbers of women living in the Boston, Massachusetts, area who had been identified through Massachusetts town books and whose oral contraceptive use was determined by a postal questionnaire (Ory et al., 1976). Hospitals in the Boston area were then monitored for admissions of cohort members. This method of follow-up, which has the advantage of being relatively inexpensive, is probably of value for diseases that are generally treated at hospitals, such as cancers, whereas for conditions such as benign breast diseases or gallbladder disease, a relatively large number of disease occurrences would be missed. In addition, over the course of time a certain proportion of women moved out of the area. Thus, this method works best when the diseases of interest require hospitalization and when the follow-up time is no more than a few years. In a similar manner, population-based disease registries can provide a means of case identification in areas where such registries exist.

For diseases generally seen by physicians, use of physician records can provide a means of determining the occurrence of disease, if physicians are willing to make them available. In the study of the Royal College of General Practitioners (1974) on long-term effects of oral contraceptives, information on disease occurrence was obtained from physicians' records. Because in England a person almost always sees his or her general practitioner before care from a specialist is sought, this method of identification of disease occurrence works well in England. In the United States, prepaid health plans offer similar advantages.

When the investigator depends on existing records for ascertainment of disease occurrence, however, the information collected by different hospitals or physicians may not be standardized, diagnostic criteria may vary from one physician to another, and some records will be more complete than others. Not all people will seek care from the monitored hospitals or physicians. If exposed cohort members are more or less likely to seek care at these facilities than unexposed cohort members, then disease occurrence may be overestimated or underestimated in those exposed relative to those not exposed. People may not even know that they have a disease and may therefore have no reason to seek care.

For these reasons, it is necessary in many studies actually to examine the cohort members periodically after they have entered the study cohort, despite the expense. In the Framingham Heart Study, for instance, cohort members were given biennial physical examinations and questionnaires and underwent special diagnostic procedures such as electrocardiograms and chest x-rays. When cohort members have moved from the area, information on disease occurrence may have to be obtained through postal questionnaires, queries to their physicians and hospitals, and surveillance of death certificates.

For infectious diseases, several methods of ascertaining disease occurrence are available, but often correct diagnosis depends on laboratory tests and on appropriate recording and/or reporting of the diagnosis. Mortality data are of limited value because most infections are not fatal; in addition, the investigator must determine whether the infection was the underlying cause of death or, as often occurs with pneumonia, represented a terminal event in a person dying from some other disease. Other means of active ascertainment of the occurrence of infectious diseases that do not involve actual contact of cohort members include review of hospital and clinic records, acquisition of data from hospitals and public health laboratories, and surveys of practicing physicians.

More active ascertainment must be employed for less severe infections for which medical care is not usually sought, such as many respiratory diseases, intestinal diseases, or the common childhood diseases. Ascertainment may involve determining absenteeism from school or industry, periodic household surveys, telephone surveys, postal card self-reporting, or the use of daily calendar sheets of symptoms. These techniques are explained and illustrated in studies carried out in Tecumseh, Michigan (Monto and Ullman, 1974), in the Cleveland Family Study (Dingle et al., 1964), and in the special "Virus Watch" as well as other family studies summarized by Fox (1974), in which intensive correlation of minor illness with viral excretion was made. For subclinical or asymptomatic infections, ascertainment depends on periodic serologic tests and/or isolation of the infectious agent. Because infection without clinical disease is common for many infectious agents, the measurement of disease patterns without serologic testing or isolation of the organism would give a very inadequate measure of the infection rate in many instances.

DIAGNOSTIC CRITERIA

It is important that determination of presence or absence of disease be made in a uniform manner for exposed and unexposed cohort members. Accordingly, diagnostic criteria should be established before the study begins. The nature of the diagnostic criteria varies considerably, depending on the particular disease and the method used to identify disease.

On the one hand, if only information from death certificates is used to determine disease occurrence, then the investigator merely accepts the diagnoses recorded on the death certificates, keeping in mind the inevitability of inaccuracies. Errors in assignment of causes of death will usually result in dilution of any association between a risk factor and a disease if the errors are of approximately equal magnitude in exposed and unexposed (see Chapter 13). However, in some instances, the exposure may influence what is recorded on the death certificate, thus creating false associations or exaggerating real associations. For instance, in studies concerned with the relationship between occupational exposure to asbestos and mortality from mesothelioma, it has been found that mesothelioma is more likely to be recorded as the cause of death if it is known that the worker had been exposed to asbestos than if it is not known that the worker had this exposure (Enterline, 1976).

If information on cause of death from death certificates is supplemented by information from other sources such as medical records, autopsy reports, and next of kin, then clear criteria must be established a priori as to which sources of data have precedence in assigning cause of death. If this is not done, the chances of subjective bias entering into the decision are increased. Also, the cause of death should be assigned without knowledge of the exposure.

When hospital records are used to determine disease occurrence, some studies accept the discharge diagnoses listed on the face sheet of the medical record. Although this is the quickest and therefore least expensive way of using the records, the accuracy and completeness of the recorded diagnoses cannot be assumed. Therefore, in many studies, all or parts of medical records are searched for relevant information. For some diseases, one relatively definitive diagnostic criterion exists, such as the pathology report for cancers and appendicitis or an x-ray report for a fracture; the abstraction from the record can then be limited to just this piece of information. In other instances, a variety of sources may be needed, and again, it is important to establish a priori how all this information will be combined to reach a decision. The attending physician may be queried for more information if needed, and this information can be added to the recorded data according to preexisting rules.

If physicians' office records are being used to determine disease occurrence, it is often necessary to accept his or her diagnosis without qualification because office records are usually much briefer than hospital records.

When physical examination and special tests are needed to identify new cases of disease, as in many studies of cardiovascular diseases, either new diagnostic criteria must be established or existing criteria applied. Committees are usually assembled to develop criteria, and the criteria decided upon must be evaluated carefully and sometimes revised. The Cardiovascular Health Study, for instance, has established diagnostic criteria for various cardiovascular events, including subtypes of stroke (National Heart, Lung, and Blood Institute, unpublished). First, stroke is defined as the rapid onset of a persistent brain deficit thought to be due to obstruction or rupture in the arterial system and not secondary to brain trauma, tumor, or infection. The deficit must last more than 24 hours unless death intervenes or there is a persistently demonstrable lesion that is consistent with deficit (by CT scan). The diagnosis of stroke will be made by the Toxicity and Endpoint Committee, based on the suspicion of the consulting neurologist that a stroke has occurred and the satisfaction of the appropriate criteria. It will include strokes occurring during surgery. Cases who satisfy these criteria for stroke are subdivided into those with hemorrhagic, ischemic, and unknown type stroke. As an example, the criteria for hemorrhagic stroke are given in Table 4–3.

Subdivision by certainty of diagnosis is useful in many situations in which definitive criteria cannot be applied to all cases. The Cardiovascular Health Study, for instance, uses criteria for hospitalized myocardial infarction that categorize potential cases as definite, probable, suspect, and no myocardial infarction; fatal events are classified as definite fatal myocardial infarction, definite fatal coronary heart disease, possible fatal coronary heart disease, and noncoronary heart disease death.

The clinical diagnosis of an infectious disease is usually confirmed by the isolation of the agent and/or the detection of a rise of a certain magni-

Table 4–3. Hemorrhagic Stroke Subtype Classification in the Cardiovascular Health Study

1. Definition

   Blood in subarachnoid space or intraparenchymal hemorrhage by CT Scan. (Intraparenchymal blood must be dense and not mottled—mixed hyperdensity or hypodensity.);   OR

   Bloody spinal fluid by lumbar puncture;   OR

   Death from stroke within 24 hours of onset and no lumbar puncture or CT or autopsy;   OR

   Surgical or autopsy evidence of hemorrhage as cause of clinical syndrome.

2. Subtype

   A. Subarachnoid Hemorrhage

      Headache or coma or combination with possibly some focal deficit and CT shows subarachnoid blood in basal cistern, tissues or convexity or blood clots in these locations. May also see aneurysm or arteriovenous malformation with enhancement;   OR

      Similar clinical picture with bloody cerebrospinal fluid. Headaches, stiffness and coma outweighs focal deficit. May have subhyloid hemorrhage, third nerve palsy.

   B. Intraparenchymal Hemorrhage

      CT shows intraparenchymal increased density (not mottled). Location is compatible with deficit;   OR

      Bloody cerebrospinal fluid with a progressive focal deficit;   OR

      Autopsy evidence for intraparenchymal hemorrhage.

   C. Indeterminate Type Hemorrhagic Stroke

      Death within 24 hours of onset without evidence by CT, surgery or autopsy location of blood;   OR

      Bloody lumbar puncture but no definite clinical picture compatible with either subarachnoid hemorrhage or intraparenchymal hemorrhage.

Source: National Heart, Lung, and Blood Institute (unpublished)

tude in antibody titer. However, false positives and false negatives may occur because of variations in laboratory techniques, the presence of two infectious agents, the occurrence of nonspecific inhibitors, or the occurrence of cross-reacting antigens in serologic tests (Evans, 1989). IgM-specific antibody is usually a reflection of a primary infection but also occurs in some reactivated infections. The specific laboratory tests to be used and the criteria for diagnosis should be established in advance. Sera should be coded and tested blindly.

If data are collected by questionnaire, participants may be asked if they have had a given condition, or they may be asked about the presence or absence of a variety of symptoms and then be classified by standard criteria on the basis of their symptoms. Another approach is to ask the participants if they have seen a doctor for certain symptoms or for a certain disease, and then query the physician as to the nature of the illness.

In some studies, criteria are based on data from several of these sources. In a study of hepatitis in university students in Taiwan (Beasley et al., 1983), criteria were based on serologic evidence of conversion and a history of various signs and symptoms as indicated in interview and medical records. Accordingly, serologic evidence for the development of hepatitis among previously susceptible individuals was defined as follows:

> *Infection:* Infection with hepatitis A virus (HAV) was considered to have occurred if a student had a positive test for anti-HAV. Infection with hepatitis B was considered to have occurred if a student had a positive test for hepatitis B surface antigen (HBsAg), or for antibodies to hepatitis B core protein or surface antigen (anti-HBc or anti-HBs).
>
> *HBsAg carrier:* A student was considered a carrier if he or she was HBsAg positive for six months or more.

The additional information on medical history from interview and records was used to classify the cases into clinical and subclinical cases and to identify cases of non-A, non-B hepatitis.

Another problem occurs when an exposure being considered as a possible risk factor is also part of the established diagnostic criteria. For instance, the presence of hyperuricemia is usually considered an integral part of the diagnostic criteria for gout, but if one wants to quantify the relationship between serum uric acid levels and risk for gout, then hyperuricemia must be omitted from the diagnostic criteria (Brauer and Prior, 1978).

SPECTRUM OF DISEASE

Although investigators often think of diseases as being present or absent depending upon whether certain criteria are met, it is important to keep in mind that conditions such as blood pressure or density of bone are in actuality continuously distributed in the population. Some arbitrary cutoff point of blood pressure level or density of bone must be used to place a person in the category of having or not having hypertension or osteoporosis, respectively.

Some diseases may be composed of different subtypes that are etiologically distinct. When this occurs, combining all cases into one overall group may make it difficult to identify risk factors for any one subtype. What was once called "juvenile rheumatoid arthritis," for instance, is in reality composed of several subtypes, each with its own etiology (Masi and Medsger, 1979). Fibrocystic breast disease may be subdivided according to the presence or absence of certain histopathologic characteristics; research is ongoing to determine whether the various subtypes have different etiologies.

In addition, a considerable amount of disease is undetected clinically. For many infectious diseases, such as hepatitis and poliomyelitis, subclinical disease is a well-known phenomenon. There is undoubtedly also a great deal of undetected disease of noninfectious etiology. A person may have undetected coronary atherosclerosis and therefore not be classified as having coronary artery disease. A person may have a slowly growing tumor that is undetected for some time. Risk factors for clinical and subclinical disease may to a certain extent be different, a possibility that should be considered in data analysis. For instance, the psychological profiles of persons having clinically apparent myocardial infarction (determined by symptom history and electrocardiogram) and "silent" myocardial infarctions (determined only by electrocardiogram with no reported symptoms) have been found to be different.

CONFOUNDING VARIABLES

As in any epidemiologic study, failure to take into account confounding variables can cause the investigator to conclude that a factor increases the risk for disease when in fact it does not, or the investigator may fail to detect a causal association that does exist. Methods of measuring confounding variables are the same as methods of measuring exposures of primary interest, that is, through questionnaires, physical measurements, laboratory tests, and measures of the physical environment. The same limitations of these methods of measurement apply to confounding variables. It is also important to keep in mind that if confounding variables are not accurately measured, they cannot be adequately taken into account in the study design or in the analysis; hence, all criteria for good measurement of exposures of primary interest also apply to measurement of confounding variables. Ways of taking confounding variables into account in the analysis will be described in subsequent chapters.

EFFECTS OF NONPARTICIPATION

Unless all information on exposure status is obtained from existing records, some potential participants will almost inevitably be unavailable for inclusion, and the nonparticipants will almost always differ in some way from participants. For instance, at the time most studies begin, a higher proportion of nonparticipants than participants are smokers (Criqui et al., 1978;

Doll and Hill, 1964). In the Framingham study (Gordon et al., 1959), a higher proportion of nonparticipants than participants died in the 5 years after the initiation of the study, suggesting that the nonrespondents were on the average more likely to be seriously ill than the respondents. It is generally recognized that nonparticipation by persons invited to be in a study may affect generalizability of results. Less frequently discussed is the effect that nonparticipation may have on rate ratios, risk ratios, and odds ratios.

The effect of nonparticipation on measures of association depends on both the size of the group omitted from the study and its specific characteristics. Bias is likely to be greatest when the proportion of nonparticipants is high and when the participants differ greatly from nonparticipants in likelihood of developing the disease. The effects also vary according to the particular measure of association used to quantify the exposure-disease relationship.

If the proportions participating differ according to likelihood of exposure but not disease, then the values of the rate ratio, risk ratio, and odds ratio are all unbiased. For instance, if in a study of the association between cigarette smoking and coronary heart disease, a higher proportion of nonsmokers participated than of smokers, but participants and nonparticipants were otherwise equally likely to develop coronary heart disease, then these measures of association would not be biased. If the proportions participating differ with respect to disease but not exposure, then the rate ratio and risk ratio are biased but the odds ratio is not. For diseases affecting only a small proportion of the population, however, the magnitude of the bias for the rate ratio and risk ratio is likely to be small. If, for instance, the risk of coronary heart disease is 10% in smokers and 5% in nonsmokers over several years, and if 0.80 of people who will develop coronary heart disease but only 0.40 of people who will not develop it participate, then the odds ratio will remain at 2.00, while the risk ratio will change, but only from 2.00 to 1.91.

In a prospective cohort study, it is more likely that the proportions participating will differ with respect to exposure than with respect to disease. In prospective cohort studies the disease has not yet occurred at the time that the sample is selected, and it is unlikely that future events can affect the selection process. If, however, proportions participating differ according to the presence or absence of other risk factors for the disease, then it is quite possible that bias can be introduced for the estimation of the rate ratio or risk ratio, a situation that resembles confounding and that can be controlled in much the same way (Miettenen and Cook, 1981).

The most serious impact of nonparticipation on study results occurs when the proportions participating do not vary only with respect to exposure or only with respect to disease, but instead vary according to specific combinations of exposure and disease. For example, if individuals who both have the exposure and develop the disease are less (or more) likely to participate in a study than is the remainder of the cohort, then the value of the rate ratio, risk ratio, and odds ratio can be quite different from the population values one hopes to estimate. For instance, if only 0.50 of smokers who were going to develop coronary heart disease participated, but 0.90 of smokers who were not going to develop coronary heart disease participated and also 0.90 of nonsmokers regardless of whether they were going to develop coronary heart disease participated, then the risk ratio in the above example would be estimated as 1.16 instead of 2.00, and the odds ratio as 1.17 instead of 2.11.

In evaluating study results, it is thus important to consider whether persons with any particular exposure-disease combination are more or less likely to be selected than would be expected on the basis of selection factors that depend on exposure status only and selection factors that depend on disease status only. One way in which selection bias of this type can occur is when participants are aware of the details of the hypotheses under investigation. Suppose, for example, that participants are told that the purpose of a prospective cohort study is to examine the relationship between smoking cigarettes and the incidence of coronary heart disease. Persons who both smoke and who have been told by their physicians that they have major risk factors for coronary heart disease (e.g., high blood pressure, family history, obesity) may view the study as particularly relevant (or threatening), and therefore the participation fraction for persons who are both exposed and destined to develop the disease may be substantially different from the selection fraction for the three other groups.

The extent to which the results of a particular study may be affected by selection biases of the type that can seriously distort measures of association is a judgmental issue. Empirical data relevant to making such a judgment are seldom available. Therefore, the most satisfactory way of dealing with selection bias is to do everything possible to ensure that very nearly all persons selected for inclusion do in fact participate. In prospective cohort studies, obtaining high participation rates is especially challenging in light of the long-term commitment that is typically asked of participants.

FOLLOW-UP OF COHORT MEMBERS

Keeping track of large numbers of cohort members over a period of many years is a major challenge in highly mobile populations such as that of the United States. Therefore, a major portion of the efforts of study staff must be devoted to follow-up.

A number of procedures can be employed to facilitate follow-up. One procedure is to ask that each study participant provide the name and address of one or more individuals who do not live with the participant but who are likely to know his or her whereabouts. The investigator is then able to contact these people in the event that the study participant cannot be located. Another useful means of tracing participants is through state departments of motor vehicles. Because these records are computerized and contain names, birthdates, and often Social Security numbers, computer linkage is feasible even for large numbers of cohort members. Record linkage for epidemiologic research is also possible through birth records and through credit bureaus. The Postal Service can be requested to provide information on changes of address. Multiple sources of information must often be employed before the participant can be located.

When the outcome of primary interest is mortality, death certificates generally constitute the major source of data. As discussed in Chapter 3, a National Death Index (NDI) has been established by the National Center for Health Statistics. The NDI is a computer index of all deaths occurring in the United States since 1979. The file includes name, birthdate, and Social Security number (if available), so that computer linkage with data on cohort members can readily be performed. Qualified investigators can have access to the NDI for a fee. The NDI provides the investigator with the date of death, the state in which the death occurred, and the death certificate number of any death that matches a cohort member within specified criteria. The investigator can then request copies of individual death certificates from the states. A detailed description of how one uses the NDI has been written by Patterson and Bilgrad (1986).

The quality of the results provided by the NDI has been evaluated in several studies (Boyle and Decouflé, 1990; Calle and Terrell, 1993; Stampfer et al., 1984; Wentworth et al., 1983), and has been found to be very good, especially if a Social Security number is available (Calle and Terrell, 1993). For instance, 98.4% of known deaths in a cohort of men were successfully matched by NDI (Wentworth et al., 1983), as were 96.5% of known deaths in a cohort of women (Stampfer et al., 1984). In the absence of a social security number, whites and males are more likely to be successfully identified than nonwhites and females. Also, availability of a middle initial has been found to be helpful, and use of a nickname to be problematic, emphasizing the importance of the ascertainment of full names of cohort members. A number of false-positive matches are likely to occur, but these can often be identified by computer algorithms and by manual review of other information on the record (Calle and Terrell, 1993). One epidemiologist has remarked that the impressive performance of the NDI should satisfy "all but the most compulsive" (MacMahon,

1983). The vast majority of those not matched by the NDI can safely be regarded as alive as of the most recent date for which the NDI has been updated.

When disease incidence rather than mortality is of interest, whatever types of individual follow-up that are needed to hold losses to follow-up to an absolute minimum should be used. Losses to follow-up tend to produce the same sorts of biases in the risk and rate ratios or odds ratio as do losses due to nonparticipation (Critqui et al., 1978; Greenland, 1977; Kleinbaum et al., 1981). Because losses to follow-up can occur at any time, there may be a greater potential for these losses being related to diseases status than are losses due to nonparticipation, which by definition occur early in the study.

One way in which the investigator may be alerted to bias as a result of loss to follow-up is through discovering that the exposed and unexposed groups differ in terms of the proportion lost to follow-up. However, such a difference does not *necessarily* imply a bias, nor does lack of such a difference necessarily imply the absence of bias. Consequently, the only way to ensure that bias stemming from loss to follow-up does not distort the study results is to minimize losses through intensive efforts to locate each cohort member. Additional methods for the follow-up of cohort members are discussed in the next chapter under retrospective cohort studies.

REFERENCES

Beasley, RP, Hwang L-Y, Lin C-C, Chen C-S. 1981. Hepatocellular carcinoma and hepatitis B virus: a prospective study of 22,707 men in Taiwan. *Lancet* 2:1129–1132.

Beasley RP, Hwang, L-Y, Linn C-C, Ko, Y-O, Twu S-J. 1983. Incidence of hepatitis among students at a university in Taiwan. *Am J Epidemiol* 117:213–222.

Boyle CA, Decoufflé P. 1990. National sources of vital status information: extent of coverage and possible selectivity in reporting. *Am J Epidemiol* 131:160–168.

Brauer GW, Prior IAM. 1978. A prospective study of gout in New Zealand and Maoris. *Ann Rheum Dis* 37:466–472.

Calle EE, Terrell DD. 1993. Utility of the national death index for ascertainment of mortality among Cancer Prevention Study II participants. *Am J Epidemiol* 137:235–241.

Colditz GA, Martin P, Stampfer MJ, Willett WC, Sampson L, Rosner B, Hennekens CH, Speizer FE. 1986. Validation of Questionnaire information on risk factors and disease outcomes in a prospective cohort study of women. *Am J Epidemiol* 123:894–900.

Criqui MH, Barrett-Connor E, Austin M. 1978. Differences between respondents and non-respondents in a population-based cardiovascular disease study. *Am J Epidemiol* 108:367–372.

Cummings SR, Black DM, Nevitt MC, Browner WS, Canley JA, Genant HK,

Mascioli SR, Scott JC, Seeley DG, Steiger P. 1990. Appendicular bone density and age predict hip fracture in women. The Study of Osteoporotic Fractures Research Group. *JAMA* 263:665–668.

Dawber TR, Meadors GF, Moore FE Jr. 1951. Epidemiological approaches to heart disease: the Framingham Study. *Am J Public Health* 41:279–286.

Dingle JH, Badger GF, Jordan WS Jr. 1964. Illness in the Home: A Study of 25,000 Illnesses in Groups in Cleveland. Cleveland, Press of Western Reserve.

Doll R, Hill AB. 1964. Mortality in relation to smoking: ten years' observations of British doctors. *Br Med J* 1:1399–1410, 1466–1467.

Enterline PE. 1976. Pitfalls in epidemiological research: an examination of the asbestos literature. *J Occup Med* 18:150–156.

Epstein FH, Napier JA, Block WD, Hayner NS, Higgins MP, Johnson BC, Keller JB, Metzner HL, Montoye HJ, Ostrander LP Jr, Ullman BM. 1970. The Tecumseh Study. *Arch Environ Health* 21:402–407.

Evans AS. 1989. Epidemiological concepts and methods. In: AS Evans, Ed. Viral Infections of Humans. New York, Plenum, pp 3–49.

Evans AS, Niederman JC, McCollum RW. 1968. Seroepidemiologic studies of infectious mononucleosis with EB virus. *N Engl J Med* 279:1121–1127.

Fox JP. 1974. Family-based epidemiologic studies. The second Wade Hampton Frost lecture. *Am J Epidemiol* 99:165–179.

Friedman GD. 1994. Primer of Epidemiology. New York, McGraw-Hill.

Gordon T, Moore FE Jr, Shurtleff D, Dawber TR. 1959. Some epidemiologic problems in the long-term study of cardiovascular disease. Observations on the Framingham study. *J Chron Dis* 10:186–206.

Greenland S. 1977. Response and follow-up bias in cohort studies. *Am J Epidemiol* 106:184–187.

Hallee TJ, Evans AS, Niederman JC, Brooks CM, Voegtly JH. 1974. Infectious mononucleosis at the United States Military Academy. A prospective study of a single class over four years. *Yale J Biol Med* 47:182–195.

Harlap S, Shiono PH. 1980. Alcohol, smoking, and incidence of spontaneous abortions in the first and second trimesters. *Lancet* 2:173–176.

Hatch MC, Shu X-O, McLean DE, Levin B, Begg M, Reuss L, Susser M. 1993. Maternal exercise during pregnancy, physical fitness, and fetal growth. *Am J Epidemiol* 137:1105–1114.

Hennekens CH, Buring JE. 1987. Epidemiology in Medicine. Boston, Little Brown and Company.

Hennekens CH, Speizer FE, Rosner B, Bain CJ, Belanger C, Peto R. 1979. Use of permanent hair dyes and cancer among registered nurses. *Lancet* 1:1390–1393.

Hernberg S, Nurminen M, Tolonen M. 1973. Excess mortality from coronary heart disease in viscose rayon workers. *Work Environ Health* 10:93–98.

Kay CR, Hannaford PC. 1988. Breast cancer and the pill—a further report from the Royal College of General Practitioners' oral contraceptive study. *Br J Cancer* 58:675–680.

Kleinbaum DG, Morgenstern H, Kupper LL. 1981. Selection in epidemiologic studies. *Am J Epidemiol* 113:452–463.

Lilienfeld DE, Stolley PD. 1994. Foundations of Epidemiology. New York, Oxford University Press.

MacMahon B. 1983. The National Death Index. *Am J Public Health* 73:1247–1258.

Masi AT, Medsger TA Jr. 1979. Epidemiology of rheumatic disease. In: DJ McCarty, Editor. Arthritis and Allied Conditions. Philadelphia, Lea & Febiger, pp 11–35.

Mausner JS, Kramer S. 1985. Mausner and Bahn Epidemiology. An Introductory Text. Philadelphia, W. B. Saunders.

Miettenen OS, Cook EF. 1981. Confounding: essence and detection. *Am J Epidemiol* 114:593–603.

Monto AS, Ullman BM. 1974. Acute respiratory illness in an American community. *JAMA* 227:164–169.

Morris, JN, Heady JA, Raffle PSD, Roberts CG, Parks JW. 1953. Coronary heart disease and physical activity of work. *Lancet* 2:1053–1057.

Morris JN, Kagan A, Pattison DC, Gardner JM, Raffle PAB. 1966. Incidence and prediction of ischaemic heart disease in London busmen. *Lancet* 2:553–559.

National Heart, Lung, and Blood Institute. Cardiovascular Health Study, Unpublished document.

Ory H, Cole P, MacMahon B, Hoover R. 1976. Oral contraceptives and reduced risk of benign breast diseases. *N Engl J Med* 294:419–422.

Paffenbarger RS Jr, Hale W. 1975. Work activity and coronary heart mortality. *N Engl J Med* 292:545–50.

Patterson BM, Bilgrad R. 1986. Use of the National Death Index in cancer studies, *J Natl Cancer Inst* 79:877–881.

Rosenman RH, Brand RJ, Jenkins CD, Friedman M, Straus R, Wurm M. 1975. Coronary heart disease in the Western Collaborative Study. Final follow-up experience of 8½ years. *JAMA* 233:872–877.

Royal College of General Practitioners. 1974. Oral Contraceptives and Health. London, Pitman.

Sidney S, Jacobs DR, Haskell WL, Armstrong MA, Dimicco A, Oberman A, Savage PJ, Slattery ML, Sternfeld B, Van Horn L. 1991. Comparison of two methods of assessing physical activity in the Coronary Artery Risk Development in Young Adults (CARDIA) Study. *Am J Epidemiol* 133:1231–1245.

Snow J. 1855. On the mode of communication of cholera. London; reprinted in Snow on Cholera. WH Frost, Editor. New York: The Commonwealth Fund, 1936.

Stampfer MJ, Colditz GA, Willett WC, Manson JE, Rosner B, Speizer FE, Hennekens CH. 1991. Postmenopausal estrogen therapy and cardiovascular disease. Ten-year follow-up from the Nurses' Health Study. *N Engl J Med* 325:756–762.

Stampfer MJ, Hennekens CH, Manson JE, Colditz GA, Rosner B, Willett WC. 1993. Vitamin E consumption and the risk of coronary heart disease in women. *N Engl J Med* 328:1444–1449.

Stampfer MJ, Willett WC, Speizer FE, Dysert DC, Lipnick R, Rosner B, Hennekens CH. 1984. Test of the national death index. *Am J Epidemiol* 119:837–839.

Stein Z, Hatch M. 1987. Biological markers in reproductive epidemiology: prospects and precautions. *Environ Health Perspect* 74:67–75.

University Health Physicians and P.H.L.S. 1971. Infectious mononucleosis and its relationship to EB virus antibody. *Br Med J* 4:643–646.

Vessey MP, Doll R, Peto R, Johnson B, Wiggins P. 1976. A long-term follow-up study of women using different methods of contraception—an interim report. *J Biosoc Sci* 8:373–427.

Vessey MP, McPherson K, Villard-Mackintosh L, Yeates D. 1989. Oral contraceptives and breast cancer: latest findings in a large cohort study. *Br J Cancer* 59:613–617.

Wagoner JK, Archer VE, Lundin FE Jr, Holaday DA, Lloyd JW. 1965. Radiation as the cause of lung cancer among uranium miners. *N Engl J Med* 273:181–188.

Walnut Creek Contraceptive Study. 1976. A Prospective Study of the Side Effects of Oral Contraceptives. Volume II. Additional Findings in Oral Contraceptive Users and Nonusers. S. Ramcharan, Ed. Washington D.C., U.S. Government Printing Office, DHEW Publication No. (NIH) 76–563.

Wen CP, Tsai SP, Gibson RL. 1983. Anatomy of the healthy worker effect: a critical review. *J Occup Med* 25:283–289.

Wentworth DN, Neaton JD, Rasmussen WL. 1983. An evaluation of the Social Security Administration Master Beneficiary Record File and the National Death Index in the ascertainment of vital status. *Am J Public Health* 73:1270–1274.

Exercises

1. Design a prospective cohort study to test one of the following hypotheses. Discuss the strengths and weaknesses of your proposed study. Describe in general terms what you would want to do in the statistical analysis, but do not be concerned with details of the analysis until after Chapters 6 and 7 have been read.

    a. Alcohol consumption during pregnancy affects the risk of preterm delivery.

    b. Kissing among teenagers affects the risk of infectious mononucleosis.

    c. Physical activity affects the risk of breast cancer among women.

    d. Use of oral contraceptives affects the risk of coronary heart disease.

2. In a hypothetical prospective cohort study to determine whether low calcium intake among older women affects their risk of hip fracture, there is concern that initial participation rates are higher in women with high calcium intake than in women with low calcium intake. (It is estimated that initial participation rates are 90% in those with calcium intake above the median and 60% in those with calcium below the median.) Discuss how this differential participation would be likely to have affected the hypothetical results, which show that women with calcium intake below the median have a 24% 10-year incidence of hip fractures whereas those with calcium intake above the median have a 16% 10-year incidence of hip fracture.

5

Retrospective Cohort, Nested Case-Control, and Case-Cohort Studies: Planning and Execution

Chapter 4 pointed out that one of the major advantages of prospective cohort studies is that the exposure is measured before the disease is diagnosed, while one of the main limitations is the high cost of most studies. Chapter 5 presents three types of study designs that may be considered modifications of the traditional prospective cohort study: the retrospective cohort study, the nested case-control study, and the case-cohort study. When the appropriate circumstances occur such that one of these designs can be implemented, the cost is generally considerably decreased, yet exposure is still measured before the disease is diagnosed.

RETROSPECTIVE COHORT STUDIES

In a retrospective cohort study, also called an historical cohort study or noncurrent prospective study, the investigator identifies a cohort of individuals based on their characteristics in the past and then reconstructs their subsequent disease experience up to some defined point in the more recent past or up to the present time (or occasionally into the future). A study of this type thus differs from a prospective cohort study, in which the cohort is identified on the basis of *current* characteristics and is then followed forward in time.

One frequent use of retrospective cohort studies is to assess the effects of exposures at the workplace, such as among cohorts of workers exposed to asbestos or benzene (Infante et al., 1977; Newhouse and Berry, 1973), or farmers exposed to herbicides and other agents (Morrison et al., 1993). Other cohorts have included college students followed retrospectively for evidence of subsequent risk of coronary heart disease according to participation in college sports (Paffenbarger et al., 1978), and for possible relationships between curvature of the spine identified in college and the subsequent development of back pain (Dieck et al., 1985). In Denmark, cohorts of schoolchildren have been followed retrospectively in order to study the relationship between measles virus infection in childhood and the occurrence of a variety of diseases during adulthood (Ronne, 1985). Cohorts undergoing medical procedures such as tubal sterilization have been followed to determine their subsequent risk for other procedures such as hysterectomy (Goldhaber et al., 1993). Pregnant women exposed to diethylstilbestrol (DES) have been followed to assess their subsequent risk of cancer (Hadjimichael et al., 1984). Results from this study of DES exposure are shown in Table 5–1. In this instance, none of the rate ratios was statistically significantly different from 1.0 when the cohort of exposed women was compared to women who were patients of the same group of physicians but who did not receive DES during pregnancy. However, as in many cohort studies, the number of disease events is rather small, so that there is considerable uncertainty about the numerical value of the rate ratio in the underlying population. This uncertainty is reflected in the relatively wide confidence intervals for the rate ratios. Confidence intervals, which give a range of plausible values for the population value of a measure, will be described in Chapter 6.

Retrospective cohort studies have some distinct advantages over prospective cohort studies; in particular, they can be completed in a much more timely fashion and are therefore considerably less expensive. For example, the effects of many carcinogens can be observed only after a 15- or 20-year latent period. If a cohort exposed some 30 years ago can be identified, then the appropriate latent period will already have passed and the epidemiologic questions of interest can be addressed solely on the basis

Table 5–1. Cancer Incidence and Rate Ratios for Women Exposed to DES during Pregnancy

Type of Cancer	Number of Cancers among Exposed Women (31,279 Woman-Years[a])	Number of Cancers among Nonexposed Women (29,570 Woman-Years[a])	Rate ratio	95% Confidence Interval
Breast	38	24	1.50	0.88–2.49
Cervix	9	6	1.40	0.51–3.84
Uterus	9	11	0.77	0.32–1.86
Ovary	6	2	2.83	0.57–14.00
Colon-rectum	11	7	1.48	0.57–3.82
Brain	4	1	3.77	0.42–33.70
Lymphatic-hematopoietic	5	1	4.71	0.55–40.30

[a]The number of woman-years varies slightly, depending on the cancer under consideration.

Source: Hadjimichael et al. (1984).

of historical information. One need not wait for decades to observe the eventual effects of the suspected carcinogen, as would be necessary in a prospective cohort study.

Because of the magnitude of time and money needed for prospective cohort studies, investigators often find themselves trying to decide not so much between prospective and retrospective cohort studies as between a retrospective cohort study and a case-control study. Case-control studies share with retrospective cohort studies the advantage that the investigator usually need not wait many years for a sufficient number of cases of the disease of interest to develop. The key difference between these two study designs is that in a retrospective cohort study, the investigator selects participants on the basis of their exposure status. Therefore, for exposures of extremely low prevalence, this type of sampling may be the only practical way of ensuring that the number of exposed individuals is adequate for a meaningful statistical evaluation of possible effects of the exposure on disease incidence. In contrast, in a case-control study the investigator selects participants according to whether or not they have the disease, so that for rare diseases the case-control approach may be the only way to identify enough cases for meaningful analysis. Sometimes a case-control study is the only option, for in order to undertake a retrospective cohort study, information on past exposure must be available. Lack of such information greatly limits the number of instances in which retrospective cohort studies can be carried out.

Selection of Groups for Study

As in prospective cohort studies, selection of the most appropriate groups to study in retrospective cohort studies requires careful attention to both practical and theoretical issues. The factors to be considered in selecting a group depend both on the specific exposure and disease under investigation and on the nature of the population groups potentially available to the investigator for study.

The group selected must be one in which a large number of people has been exposed to the agent of interest. A sufficient number of these people must have been exposed at high enough levels that important excess incidence for the diseases under investigation is likely to be detected. Also, reasonably accurate data on the levels of exposure of individual cohort members should be available. Finally, an exposed cohort must be selected in such a manner that an appropriate unexposed comparison group can be identified. Studies of the relationship between exposure to ionizing radiation and the incidence of cancer of various body sites will be used to illustrate the application of these principles.

Several occupational groups have been exposed in the past to relatively large amounts of radiation on the job. These include uranium miners, radium dial painters, and radiologists who practiced in the early part of this century (Boice and Land, 1982). For each of these occupational groups, thousands of exposed individuals have been available for study through retrospective cohort methods. Although precise quantification of dose is not possible, each group is known to have had certain organs exposed to hundreds of rads, the units in which absorbed dose of radiation is expressed. This degree of exposure is many times larger than the variation in exposure stemming from individual differences in routine diagnostic x-rays and terrestrial radiation sources. Consequently, if radiation did have an effect on the incidence of a particular disease, these occupational groups would be reasonable cohorts in which to search initially for epidemiologic evidence of such a relationship.

Specification of appropriate groups for comparison with each of these occupational cohorts is complicated by the healthy worker effect (Chapters 3 and 4) and possibly by other behavioral differences between these workers and other segments of the population. These potential biases are of particular concern when studying an occupational group such as radiologists, who are a highly selected group in terms of sociodemographic factors, awareness of health issues, and likely access to a thorough diagnostic work-up when ill. Consequently, radiologists in the United States have been compared with internists and other medical specialists (Matanoski et al., 1975). As discussed earlier in this chapter, in an industrial setting one might attempt to identify a comparison industry in which the workers are generally similar to the exposed cohort except in terms of exposure. The major drawback of such an approach is that the comparison groups may in fact be exposed to other risk factors for the disease, thereby reducing or reversing an association between the exposure of interest and the disease. Use of unexposed workers within the same industry as the comparison group is another approach, such as clerical workers in the nuclear industry. In retrospective cohort studies, however, such comparisons may often be suspect because of strong selection factors determining assignment to jobs that involve direct exposure. Historically, for instance, in many industries, persons holding the clerical positions are nearly all women, whereas other jobs have been filled entirely by men. In light of these problems and of the added expense of including an unexposed cohort, a majority of retrospective cohort studies of occupationally exposed groups use disease incidence or mortality rates among the general population as the basis for comparison (Archer et al., 1976; Mancuso et al., 1977).

Occupational exposure to radiation is only one of many exposures that have been studied by means of a retrospective cohort design in groups of workers. For example, a large collaborative retrospective cohort was initiated in 1962 to examine mortality among 59,072 men employed in the steel plants of Pennsylvania (Lloyd and Ciocco, 1969). All but 97 of the men were successfully followed from 1953 to 1962 for determination of vital status. The study provided important new information on the relationship between exposure to coke oven fumes and mortality from respiratory cancer (Lloyd et al., 1970).

Because of the wide variety of medical uses for radiation, medically irradiated cohorts provide a valuable source of information on the risks of radiation. Until the carcinogenic effects of radiation were suspected, radiation was used widely for the treatment of a number of nonmalignant conditions, including ankylosing spondylitis, postpartum mastitis, thymus hypertrophy, tinea capitis, and metropathia hemorrhagica (Boice, 1981). Such medical exposures are usually well documented, and other persons with the same disorder treated by means other than radiation can be used as a comparison group, provided that factors related to cancer incidence do not influence the choice of treatment for individual patients. Persons treated for cancer with radiotherapy provide another source of information on radiation-induced disease. However, particular caution is needed in this type of retrospective cohort study because those composing the exposed group already have a demonstrated tendency to develop cancer. Medically exposed cohorts are also obviously important when the exposure of interest is a constituent of a particular prescription drug. For the majority of exposures one might hope to study, however, medically exposed groups are simply not available.

General population groups, some of whose members have had exposures of interest, are useful in retrospective cohort studies only when there is wide variability in the level of exposure, when exposure levels are high for a sufficient number of cohort members, and when the exposure levels have been documented. The populations of Hiroshima and Nagasaki have provided a great deal of information about effects of radiation, for instance. The average radiation dose was substantial, and the magnitude of the dose to which residents were exposed varied considerably because of their differing distances from the point of impact of the bomb. Other general population groups without such an exceptional exposure would provide little information on radiation risks. As Land (1980) has illustrated, the numbers of cohort members required from most general population groups would have to be extremely large for detecting the modest increases in risk associated with slight exposure differences, such as those for persons living close to nuclear power plants as compared to persons living elsewhere.

As was described for prospective cohort studies, prepaid health care plans can facilitate linkage of exposures such as surgical procedures and pharmacologic agents to a variety of subsequent outcomes (Goldhaber et al., 1993). Not only is follow-up facilitated in such a setting, but exposures and outcomes are likely to be documented on the records of cohort members.

Measurement of Exposure

When the exposure took place many years before the initiation of the study, measurement may be exceedingly difficult and only a crude classification may be possible. For example, in studying an occupational exposure, one might regard all workers in a particular industry as exposed and all workers outside that industry as unexposed. Such crude measures of exposure are obviously far short of optimal. Errors of measurement are likely to attenuate the observed magnitude of the association (Chapter 13). Also, without a more refined classification, it is impossible to assess whether a dose-response relationship between the exposure and disease exists. Such a relationship is an important criterion for inferring causality.

Frequently, it is possible to achieve only modestly more refined measurement of exposure than a crude dichotomy of exposed versus not exposed. In an occupational study, length of employment in the industry of interest may be used as an indirect measure of cumulative exposure to the particular agent. Such a measure at least permits some assessment of dose-response relationships, although length of employment is likely to be a poor proxy for the actual level of exposure for individual cohort members. Another major drawback of indicators such as length of employment is that exposure is measured in units other than the actual physical units in which the exposure itself would more properly be measured, such as rads or parts per million. Therefore, the study results may have limited value for setting standards and for other policy issues.

Direct measures of exposure levels in individual cohort members can sometimes be approximated by synthesis of data available from various sources. One example is a study by Boice and Monson of radiogenic breast cancer among women receiving multiple fluoroscopic examinations of the chest in the course of air-collapse therapy for tuberculosis (Boice and Monson, 1977). The primary measure of radiation exposure for this study was the number of times that a particular tuberculosis patient had received an air refill to maintain the desired degree of collapse of the lung. Surviving physicians, technicians, and patients were interviewed in order to obtain more specific information about the nature of the exposure that might permit refinement of the measure. Data were collected regarding the usual duration of fluoroscopic examinations, the use of filtration, and the orientation of the patient during examination (Boice et al., 1978). This latter factor is particularly important to consider for breast cancer because the absorbed dose to the breast is reduced greatly when radiation enters the body from the back rather than the front. In combination with physical measurements taken from fluoroscopic machines of the type that had been used when the patients were treated, an equation was developed that permitted estimates of the number of rads of radiation received by each exposed woman in the cohort.

It is apparent that the need to obtain exposure data from historical materials places important limitations on the quality of the data in many retrospective cohort studies. Often adequate data are simply not available, and a retrospective cohort study cannot be done. However, in those instances where extensive information on exposure happens to have been collected, the quality of the data may rival that which would be collected in a prospective cohort study.

Measurement of Disease

The historical nature of retrospective cohort studies often places constraints on the measurement of disease occurrence as well as of exposure. Because the investigator usually must rely on information collected for other purposes, death certificates may be the only available source of data on disease occurrence. The limitations of death certificates have been discussed in Chapter 3. Death certificates are dependable as documentation of the fact that a person has died, but their accuracy for cause-specific mortality is highly variable.

Complete information on disease incidence, as opposed to mortality, is available for only a minority of retrospective cohort studies. In Connecticut, the existence of a population-based cancer registry dating from 1935 makes it possible to ascertain virtually all diagnoses of cancer since that time, as long as cohort members remain residents of the state. This registry has been used, for example, to investigate the incidence of cancer among workers at a nuclear materials fabrication plant (Hadjimichael et al., 1983). In the absence of a registry, incidence data can only be approximated. In their study of breast cancer among women treated with lung-collapse therapy, Boice and Monson (1977) mailed questionnaires to surviving members of their cohort and asked about history of cancer and other chronic diseases. The information obtained concerning cancer among living patients was then combined with the information from death certificates. Some cancers were probably missed, however, because 22% of living cohort members did not respond and because some women who survive several years following a diagnosis of breast cancer may die of other causes without the cancer being noted on their death certificates.

This underascertainment of disease occurrence invariably diminishes the precision of estimation of exposure-disease associations in retrospective (or prospective) cohort studies. As discussed in Chapter 13, when the extent of misclassification on disease status differs according to exposure status, serious bias in the apparent magnitude and even the direction of the association may result. Consequently, it is especially important that the same procedures to identify disease occurrence be followed for exposed and unexposed cohort members. If accurate general population rates are used for comparison with incomplete incidence data collected for the exposed cohort, substantial underestimation of the magnitude of association or even an apparent protective effect for an exposure that is in fact deleterious can result.

Measurement of Confounding Variables

Given the many problems in obtaining adequate information on exposure and disease in retrospective cohort studies, it is not surprising that information on important confounding variables is often lacking. Consequently, the results of many retrospective cohort studies are far from definitive regarding causal relationships. However, because a confounding variable must be related to *both* the exposure and the disease, it is not essential that information on all risk factors for the disease be measured and included in the analysis. If it is known from a previous study that a particular risk factor for the disease under investigation is unrelated to the exposure of interest, then the risk factor can be ignored without biasing the results. To take an extreme example, it is possible to obtain valid estimates of the association between an exposure and lung cancer in the absence of information on smoking, if it is known that exposed and unexposed cohort members have similar smoking histories. For a retrospective cohort study of the possible association between radiotherapy for primary breast cancer and subsequent primary cancer of other sites, Schwartz (1984) used ancillary data from a recent case-control study to assess whether the probability of receiving radiotherapy was related to a woman's smoking status. Because no such relationship was found, Schwartz was able to compare irradiated and nonirradiated breast cancer patients in terms of subsequent incidence of lung cancer with a certain degree of confidence that the results were unlikely to be confounded by smoking. However, because the clinical use of radiotherapy for the treatment of breast cancer has changed considerably over time, information from a recent case-control study may not be generalizable to the long time interval spanned by the retrospective cohort study. Direct measurement of confounding variables in the study itself is of course always preferable.

Another means for dealing with confounding variables in retrospective cohort studies involves obtaining information on the potentially confounding variables through direct interview or mail questionnaires from the members of the cohort who are still alive and who can be located at the time the study is conducted. Boice and Monson (1977) used this approach to obtain information on known risk factors for breast cancer from the surviving members of their cohort of tuberculosis patients. Because such information is obtained for survivors only, it cannot be used directly in the analysis as a potential confounding variable. Instead, one considers the likelihood of confounding by comparing the distribution of the potential confounding variable among exposed and unexposed survivors. A finding of similar distributions of the potential confounding variables among exposed and unexposed survivors constitutes fairly strong evidence that the variables are unrelated to exposure and therefore do not confound the exposure-disease association.

Methods for Tracing Cohort Members

Tracing of cohort members constitutes a major portion of the field work for retrospective cohort studies. For recent years, many of the follow-up methods described in Chapter 4 for prospective cohort studies can be applied. From 1979 on, deaths can be identified through the National Death Index. Computer files from credit bureaus and state departments of motor vehicles can also serve as productive and cost-effective means for tracing cohort members. Follow-up has become much more efficient in recent years because of the advent of computers and the computerization of large files. For years prior to 1970, tracing efforts are more difficult and labor-intensive. Searching early vital records for possible deaths of cohort members may require manual review of each of several annual listings of deaths, each of which may be arranged only approximately in alphabetical order.

Resources of particular value for tracing subjects in retrospective cohort studies are city directories. These are produced annually for most municipalities, and for many areas they are available for a period of several decades. Individuals are listed alphabetically by surname and also by street address. City directories make it possible to identify relatives living with the cohort members. When further efforts to trace the cohort member fail, these relatives may be traced and the cohort member located through them. Notations are often made in the city directory if an individual has died; the new place of residence is sometimes noted when a person has moved. For cohort members who are especially difficult to trace, city directories are useful for identifying neighbors who might be contacted about the current whereabouts of cohort members.

The complexity of the process of tracing cohort members is illustrated in Figure 5-1. The figure shows schematically the procedures used in the Massachusetts study of tuberculosis patients (Boice, 1978). To a much greater extent than in prospective cohort studies, the follow-up of cohort members in retrospective cohort studies requires individualized tracing efforts. As discussed in Chapter 4, however, the only way to ensure that differential losses to follow-up have not biased study results is to hold all losses to an absolute minimum. Thus, the effort spent in locating cohort members has important implications for the validity of the study. Also, because more complete follow-up leads to the identification of additional disease events, it enhances precision of estimation.

Addition of a Prospective Component to a Retrospective Cohort Study

Once a cohort has been assembled for a retrospective cohort study, valuable additional information can often be obtained inexpensively by adding a prospective component. For example, the cohort of tuberculosis patients in Massachusetts has been followed prospectively in order to identify additional incident cases of cancer and additional deaths. Because of the long latent period for cancer and the increasing incidence and mortality rates with age, considerably more precise estimates of radiation effects will be possible with this relatively modest additional effort.

Analysis of Retrospective Cohort Studies

The same methods of analysis that are used for prospective cohort studies can be used for retrospective cohort studies. When an internal comparison group is available, Poisson regression (described in Chapter 6) or the Cox proportional hazard model (described in Chapter 7) can be used. If the cohort contains only exposed individuals and is compared to published incidence or mortality rates as the reference population, then standardized mortality (or incidence) ratios can be computed as the measure of association. If person-years at risk are unavailable or inappropriate, then proportional mortality (or incidence) ratios can be calculated. Standardized mortality ratios and proportional mortality ratios are described in Chapter 7.

NESTED CASE-CONTROL STUDIES

It is sometimes expedient to design a case-control study within either a retrospective or prospective cohort study. Consider a traditional cohort study in which an investigator wishes to find out whether a positive result

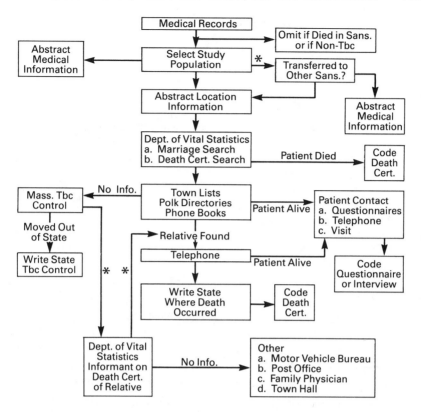

* Contingency Procedure That Depends on Outcome of Previous Source

Figure 5-1. Procedure for locating cohort members in a retrospective cohort study of women treated for tuberculosis in Massachusetts (from Boice, 1978).

from a certain expensive serologic test is associated with an increased risk of rheumatoid arthritis. In such a traditional cohort study, either prospective or retrospective, the investigator might start with blood samples drawn from 10,000 people free of rheumatoid arthritis. The cohort might then be followed for 10 years, either prospectively or retrospectively, to determine the incidence rate of rheumatoid arthritis in those positive and in those negative on the serologic test.

A modification of this traditional cohort design, called a nested case-control study, is illustrated in Figure 5-2. The blood samples from the 10,000 people could be frozen and stored. Suppose that after 10 years has elapsed, 200 people had developed rheumatoid arthritis and 9800 had not. The stored serum samples from the 200 cases and a sample of, say, 400 of the 9800 without the disease could then be tested. This sampling of non-diseased individuals would greatly reduce the cost from what it would be if

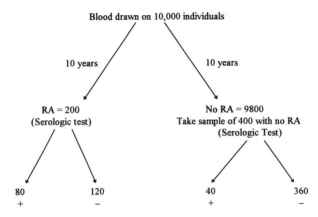

Figure 5–2. Hypothetical example of a nested case-control study. RA denotes rheumatoid arthritis (from Kelsey, 1983).

the sera from all 10,000 cohort members had to be tested, yet the serologic status before disease occurrence would be measured. The proportion testing positive among the cases could then be compared to the proportion testing positive among the controls, as in a usual case-control study.

Nested case-control studies are being used increasingly in studies relating risk factors measured in blood to incidence of disease. When a sufficient number of cases of a disease of interest accrue, controls are selected from unaffected cohort members who are still alive and under surveillance at the time the cases developed the disease; typically the controls are matched by age, gender, and time of entry into the cohort. A person who is selected as a control may later become a case, although this will occur infrequently unless the disease of interest is common. An example of a nested case-control study is one undertaken to identify possible relationships between Epstein-Barr virus (EBV) and Hodgkin's disease. Cases of Hodgkin's disease were identified through cancer registries and hospital records in a cohort of over 240,000 persons from whom blood had been drawn and stored in one of five serum banks several years earlier. Tests were carried out on the sera of cases for antibody patterns to EBV and cytomegalovirus and results of the tests compared with tests on coded sera from matched controls who did not develop Hodgkin's disease (Mueller et al., 1989). Controls were matched to cases on serum bank, gender, race, date of collection of index serum sample ± 6 months, and date of birth ± 1 year. The results confirmed an association between the presence of EBV antibodies and Hodgkin's disease and also indicated that the altered patterns of EBV antibody preceded the diagnosis of Hodgkin's disease by some 3 to 5 years.

Nested case-control studies may be used to reduce cost regardless of whether testing of blood samples is needed. For instance, in a nested case-control study to assess whether exposure to electromagnetic fields among Norwegian railway workers is related to an increased risk of brain tumors or leukemia, 39 railway workers with brain tumors and 52 workers with leukemia were each matched on age to four or five controls from the same cohort of railway workers (Tynes et al., 1994). Since determination of exposure to electromagnetic fields and to certain potential confounding variables was time-consuming and expensive, obtaining exposure data on a sample of cohort members who did not develop these cancers was considerably less expensive than ascertaining exposure status on the entire cohort of 13,030 railway workers.

The availability of a variety of banks of stored sera around the world and the current interest in serologic predictors of disease make nested case-control studies an attractive and economical approach, as long as the serologic marker of interest has not undergone degradation over time. In many instances it may also be necessary to obtain information on important confounding variables from the cases and controls. Analysis of nested case-control studies generally involves techniques similar to those used in other case-control studies, as described in Chapters 7 and 9.

CASE-COHORT STUDIES

A case-cohort study (also occasionally called a case-base study) is another method of increasing efficiency compared to a traditional retrospective or prospective cohort study. In a case-cohort study (Kupper et al., 1975; Prentice, 1986), cases are cohort members who develop the disease(s) of interest, and controls are a random sample of members of the same cohort. Thus, the same person can be included in the study as both a case and control, although this will occur infrequently for uncommon diseases. Similar to the nested case-control design, information on exposure and covariates is needed for all of the cases and for only a sample of cohort members selected for the control group. However, unlike a nested case-control study in which a control is matched to a case on membership in the cohort at the time the case developed the disease (and frequently on other variables as well), in a case-cohort study, time and other relevant variables are not matched in the design but are taken into account in the analysis. Also, in a case-cohort study, the same controls may be used for more than one case group.

Suppose an investigator were interested not only in whether the serologic test in Figure 5–2 is predictive of rheumatoid arthritis, but also whether it is predictive of systemic lupus erythematosus and ankylosing spondylitis as well. Suppose that in the cohort, 200 cases of rheumatoid arthritis, 100 cases of systemic lupus erythematosus, and 150 cases of ankylosing spondylitis developed over a 10-year period (Fig. 5–3), and suppose that 400 people from the original cohort were randomly chosen to serve as a control group. The serologic test then need be performed only on the cohort members who were actually selected for the study as cases or controls. In this hypothetical example, when the cases are compared to the control group (10% of whom were positive on the serologic test), the serologic marker is strongly associated with rheumatoid arthritis (40% of cases positive), moderately associated with systemic lupus erythematosus (20% of cases positive), but not associated with ankylosing spondylitis (10% of cases positive).

The case-cohort design can be used to obtain rate ratio, risk ratio, and odds ratio estimates within a cohort (Kupper et al., 1975; Prentice, 1986). It can also be used to compare rate and risk estimates in exposed groups within the cohort to rate and risk estimates in an external population (Wacholder and Boivin, 1987). For instance, in a recent case-cohort study to address the question of whether certain fertility drugs increase the risk for ovarian and certain other cancers (Rossing et al., 1994), the incidence of

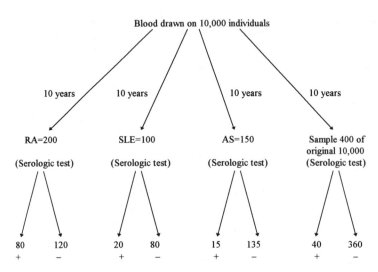

Figure 5–3. Hypothetical example of a case-cohort study. RA denotes rheumatoid arthritis, SLE denotes systemic lupus erythematosus, and AS denotes ankylosing spondylitis.

these cancers in women who had used ovulation-inducing drugs was assessed in relation to the incidence of the cancers in infertile women in the same cohort who had not used these drugs and in relation to the incidence in the general population of the geographic area.

Methods of analyzing case-cohort studies have been described by Greenland (1986), Flanders et al. (1990), Sato (1992a,b), Wacholder and Boivin (1987), and Prentice (1986).

The relative advantages and disadvantages of case-cohort and nested case-control designs are discussed by Wacholder (1991). He points out that the major advantages of the case-cohort design are consequences of the random sampling of controls, whereas those of the nested case-control study are a consequence of matching on time. Advantages of the case-cohort design are the ability to use the same control group for comparison with several disease groups, flexibility in the analysis in choice of time scale (since such time-related variables as age or time since entry into the cohort are frequently matched in nested case-control studies), use of the same control group for purposes other than those initially planned, use of the same control group for future studies, and more rapid control selection. On the other hand, the nested case-control approach will be somewhat more efficient statistically (meaning that it will have the ability to detect differences as being statistically significant with a smaller sample size than a case-cohort study), unless most cohort members enter the study at about the same time and are followed for about the same length of time, uses methods of analysis familiar to most epidemiologists, allows easier calculation of needed sample size, and does not require ascertainment of data on a control beyond the time data are collected for the matched case.

STUDYING A RARE EXPOSURE AND A RARE DISEASE

Finally, White (1982) has proposed a two-stage design to reduce costs when an investigator wants to study the relationship between a rare exposure and a rare disease. In the first stage, exposure and disease status are ascertained in a large sample of individuals, and in the second stage, covariates are measured in smaller samples of individuals who have been subdivided according to exposure and disease status. To increase efficiency, large proportions are sampled from the exposure-disease groups with smaller numbers of people, and relatively small proportions are sampled from the exposure-disease groups with larger numbers of people. Methods of analyzing data from such a two-stage design have been described by White (1982) and also Cain and Breslow (1988).

REFERENCES

Archer VE, Gillam JD, Wagoner JK. 1976. Respiratory disease and mortality among uranium miners. *Ann NY Acad Sci* 271:280–293.

Boice JD Jr. 1978. Follow-up methods to trace women treated for pulmonary tuberculosis, 1930–1954. *Am J Epidemiol* 107:127–139.

Boice JD Jr. 1981. Cancer following medical irradiation. *Cancer* 47:1081–1090.

Boice JD Jr, Land CE. 1982. Ionizing radiation. In: D Schottenfeld, JF Fraumeni Jr, Eds. Cancer Epidemiology and Prevention. Philadelphia, WB Saunders Co.

Boice JD Jr, Monson RR. 1977. Breast cancer in women after repeated fluoroscopic examinations of the chest. *J Natl Cancer Inst* 59:823–832.

Boice JD Jr, Rosenstein M, Trout ED. 1978. Estimation of breast doses and breast cancer risk associated with repeated fluoroscopic chest examinations of women with tuberculosis. *Radiat Res* 73:373–390.

Cain KC, Breslow NE. 1988. Logistic regression analysis and efficient design for two-stage studies. *Am J Epidemiol* 128:1198–1206.

Dieck GS, Kelsey JL, Goel VK, Panjabi MM, Walter SD, Laprade MH. 1985. An epidemiologic study of the relationship between postural asymmetry in the teen years and subsequent back and neck pain. *Spine* 10:872–877.

Flanders WD, Dersimonian R, Rhodes P. 1990. Estimation of risk ratios in case-base studies with competing risks. *Stat Med* 9:423–435.

Goldhaber MK, Armstrong MA, Golditch IM, Sheehe PR, Petitti DB, Friedman GD. 1993. Long-term risk of hysterectomy among 80,007 sterilized and comparison women at Kaiser Permanente, 1971–1987. *Am J Epidemiol* 138:508–521.

Greenland S. 1986. Adjustment of risk-ratios in case-base studies (hybrid epidemiologic designs). *Stat Med* 5:579–584.

Hadjimichael OC, Meigs JW, Falcier FW, Thompson WD, Flannery JT. 1984. Cancer risk among women exposed to exogenous estrogens during pregnancy. *J Natl Cancer Inst* 73:831–834.

Hadjimichael OC, Ostfeld AM, D'Atri DA, Brubaker RE. 1983. Mortality and cancer incidence experience of employees in a nuclear fuels fabrication plant. *J Occup Med* 25:48–61.

Infante PF, Rinsky RA, Wagoner JK, Young RJ. 1977. Leukemia in benzene workers. *Lancet* 2:76–79.

Kelsey JL. 1983. Cohort studies. *J Rheumatol* 10:96–99.

Kupper LL, McMichael AJ, Spirtas R. 1975. A hybrid epidemiologic study design useful in estimating relative risk. *J Am Stat Assoc* 70:524–528.

Land CE. 1980. Cancer risks from low doses of ionizing radiation. *Science* 209:1197–1203.

Lloyd JW, Ciocco A. 1969. Long-term mortality study of steelworkers. I. Methodology. *J Occup Med* 11:299–310.

Lloyd JW, Lundin FE Jr, Redmond CK, Geiser PB. 1970. Long-term mortality study of steelworkers. IV. Mortality by work area. *J Occup Med* 12:151–157.

Mancuso TF, Stewart A, Kneale G. 1977. Radiation exposures of Hanford workers dying from cancer and other causes. *Health Phys* 33:369–384.

Matanoski GM, Seltzer R, Sartwell PE, Diamond EL, Elliott EA. 1975. The current mortality rates of radiologists and other physician specialists: specific causes of death. *Am J Epidemiol* 101:199–210.

Morrison H, Savitz D, Semenciw R, Hulka B, Mao Y, Morison D, Wigle D. 1993. Farming and prostate cancer mortality. *Am J Epidemiol* 137:270–280.

Mueller N, Evans A, Harris NL, Comstock GW, Jellum E, Magnus K, Orentreich N, Polk F, Vogelman J. 1989. Hodgkin's disease and Epstein-Barr virus. Altered antibody pattern before diagnosis. *N Engl J Med* 320:689–695.

Newhouse ML, Berry G. 1973. Asbestos and laryngeal carcinoma. *Lancet* 2:615.

Paffenbarger RS Jr, Wing AL, Hyde RT. 1978. Physical activity as an index of heart attack risk in college alumni. *Am J Epidemiol* 108:161–175.

Prentice RL. 1986. A case-cohort design for epidemiologic cohort studies and disease prevention trials. *Biometrika* 73:1–11.

Ronne T. 1985. Measles virus infection without rash in childhood is related to disease in adult life. *Lancet* 1:1–4.

Rossing MA, Daling JR, Weiss NS, Moore DE, Self SG. 1994. Ovarian tumors in a cohort of infertile women. *N Engl J Med* 331:771–776.

Sato T. 1992a. Estimation of a common risk ratio in stratified case-cohort studies. *Stat Med* 11:1599–1605.

Sato T. 1992b. Maximum likelihood estimation of the risk ratio for case-cohort studies. *Biometrics* 48:1215–1221.

Schwartz SM. 1984. An Evaluation of the Risk of Second Primary Malignant Neoplasms Following Breast Cancer Radiotherapy. M.P.H. Essay, Yale University.

Tynes T, Jynge H, Vistnes AI. 1994. Leukemia and brain tumors in Norwegian railway workers, a nested case-control study. *Am J Epidemiol* 139:645–653.

Wacholder S. 1991. Practical considerations in choosing between the case-cohort and nested case-control designs. *Epidemiology* 2:155–158.

Wacholder S, Boivin J-F. 1987. External comparisons with the case-cohort design. *Am J Epidemiol* 126:1198–1209.

White JE. 1982. A two-stage design for the study of the relationship between a rare exposure and a rare disease. *Am J Epidemiol* 115:119–128.

Exercises

1. Design a retrospective cohort study to test one of the following hypotheses. Discuss the strengths and weaknesses of your proposed study.

a. High serum uric acid levels (which are associated with gout) protect against cancer.

b. Hormone replacement therapy protects against death from all causes combined in women.

c. Hormone replacement therapy alters the risk for certain common cancers in women.

2. Give an example (other than any mentioned previously in this chapter) of a hypothesis that you could test by means of

a. a retrospective cohort study

b. a nested case-control study

c. a case-cohort study

In each instance, give reasons for your choice and discuss any potential limitations of the study design as a means of testing the hypothesis.

6

Cohort Studies:
Statistical Analysis I

Because all cohort studies, whether prospective or retrospective, monitor the disease status of cohort members over time, it is essential to account for the time at risk for disease by each member while he or she is monitored. A cohort member is said to be at risk for the disease of interest during a given time period if he or she is both under observation and susceptible to the disease during that period; therefore, if he or she does develop the disease, its occurrence will be documented.

Some cohort members will be at risk during only part of the study period, for several reasons. First, not all participants are enrolled in the study at its start. If the total duration of a study is 10 years and if the first 3 years are needed to identify participants and to obtain information on the risk factors of interest, then the period of observation for individual cohort members would vary from 7 to 10 years. Second, some cohort members may be removed from the population at risk because they died of causes unrelated to the disease of interest. Finally, some participants may be lost to follow-up because the investigator cannot trace them over the entire study period. These individuals may differ systematically from the rest of the cohort, and their numbers should be minimized to the extent possible.

Analysis of cohort data must account for the unequal lengths of time that participants are observed for the occurrence of the outcome of interest. A natural way to do so is to use the incidence rate of the disease, defined in Chapter 2 as the number of occurrences of the disease per unit time, per person. If an estimate of the probability of disease during the study period is desired, it can be obtained from the incidence rate using equation (2.1) given in Chapter 2. However, the incidence rate itself and its variation with exposure are often of direct interest.

The terms used in the statistical analysis of cohort data reflect its origins in reliability theory, which is the study of times to failure of equipment parts and components. Thus, individuals who develop the disease of interest are said to "fail," individuals who are withdrawn from observation because of death or loss to follow-up are said to be "censored," incidence rates are called "hazard rates," and risks (probabilities) are called "cumulative hazard."

We begin by describing how to estimate the probability of failure during the study period in the cohort as a whole.

ESTIMATING RISK FOR A COHORT

A simple way to estimate the probability of failure in the study period using data from a cohort is the product-limit or Kaplan-Meier method (1958). We illustrate this method with the hypothetical data in Figure 6–1. In this example a cohort of 20 individuals is observed from a starting time, which we call time $t = 0$, to some later time, called $t = T$. The occurrence of a particular disease is the outcome of interest. For each individual, a horizontal line indicates the time period when he or she is at risk for the disease. Each cohort member is assumed to be free of disease initially. An X indicates the onset of the disease of interest (a failure), and a vertical line indicates withdrawal due to death or loss to follow-up (a censored observation). A total of five members of the cohort fail (i.e., develop the disease of interest) at times t_1, t_2,..., t_5 marked on the horizontal axis. Ten members

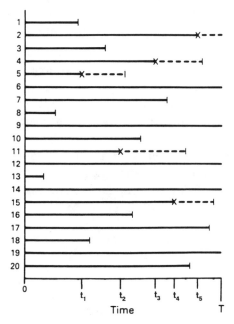

Figure 6–1. Hypothetical cohort of twenty individuals, followed from time 0 to time T. X marks an onset of the disease of interest. A vertical bar marks a censored observation.

are withdrawn from observation before disease onset or study termination, and the remaining five members are alive at the end of the study. (The withdrawal of four members after they failed is irrelevant to the analysis, because the withdrawals occurred when the individuals were no longer at risk for failure and thus were no longer contributing time at risk or failure events to the study.)

Because of withdrawals, only 25.0% of the cohort has actually been observed to develop the disease. This value underestimates the probability of failure in the period, because it incorrectly assumes that everyone was at risk for the whole period. The product-limit estimate of the probability of failure during the study period allows for the possibility that some of the failure times may be censored. It is obtained by calculating a product of terms, one term for each disease occurrence. Suppose there are m_1 individuals at risk for failure just before the first failure at time t_1. Because one of these individuals failed and the remaining $m_1 - 1$ of them avoided failure at t_1, an estimate of the probability of avoiding failure in a small time interval around t_1 is $(m_1 - 1)/m_1$. In the figure there are 17 individuals at risk for failure just before the first failure; therefore the probability of avoiding failure in a small time interval around time t_1 is 16/17. Similarly, the probability of avoiding failure in a small time interval about t_2 is 13/14 because 14 individuals were at risk just before the failure occurred. The probability of avoiding failure in the entire time period is estimated as the product of these terms: (16/17) (13/14) (10/11) (8/9) (6/7) = 0.605. The product-limit estimate of the probability of failure in the time period is one minus the probability of avoiding failure, or 0.395. Thus, if disease risk in individuals who are censored by death or loss to follow-up does not differ systematically from that in the rest of the cohort, one would expect an estimated 39.5% of the entire cohort to develop the disease in the period. This value is considerably higher than the 25% estimate obtained by ignoring the censoring.

In general, if there are D failures in the period from time 0 to time T, and there are m_1 cohort members at risk just before the first failure, m_2 members at risk just before the second failure, and so on, the product limit estimate of the probability of failure is

$$P(T) = 1 - \left[\frac{m_1 - 1}{m_1} \cdot \frac{m_2 - 1}{m_2} \cdots \frac{m_D - 1}{m_D} \right]. \qquad (6.1)$$

The set of cohort members at risk just before a given failure is sometimes called the *risk set* for that failure. Risk sets will be discussed further in Chapter 7.

The Kaplan-Meier method can be used to estimate the probability $P(t)$

of failure at any time t during the study, simply by restricting the formula to the failures occurring before time t. Figure 6–2A shows a plot of the failure probability as a function of time for the hypothetical data of Figure 6–1. Notice that the plot is a step function, with jumps at the failure times. Figure 6–2B shows a plot of the complementary probability of avoiding failure during the study period; this plot is called the *Kaplan-Meier survival curve*. The height of the curve at any time on the horizontal axis gives the probability of surviving beyond that time. Methods for calculating the standard error of the product-limit estimate are given in standard texts on survival analysis (Kalbfleisch and Prentice, 1980; Lee, 1980).

The product limit estimate is particularly simple for cohorts with no withdrawals; such cohorts are most likely to occur when death from any cause is the outcome. In this case it is simply the number of failures divided by the number of cohort members. Data of Zuckerman et al. (1984) from a cohort study of psychosocial influences on mortality in a low-income population over the age of 61 years illustrate this calculation. The outcome of interest is all-cause mortality over a 2-year period. The cohort consists of 398 members, 47 of whom died (i.e., failed) during this period; the remaining 351 members were alive at the end of the period. Because there are no withdrawals, in formula (6.1) the numerator of each ratio (i.e., the number

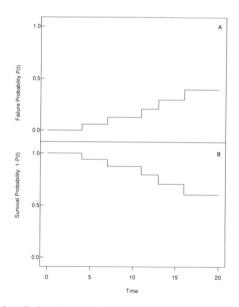

Figure 6–2. (A) Product-limit estimate P(t) as a function of time t from start of study and (B) estimated survival function 1-P(t), also called a Kaplan-Meier survival curve, for the hypothetical data of Figure 6–1.

of individuals at risk after a failure) equals the denominator of the next ratio (i.e., the number at risk just before the next failure). Thus, after cancellation, the product limit estimate of the probability of death in the 2-year period reduces to $1 - (351/398) = 47/398 = 0.118$.

An alternative estimate of the probability of failure during the study period is obtained by first computing the hazard rate for failure (or, in this instance, mortality rate) and then converting it to an estimate of the probability of failure (or, in this instance, death), using the relation (2.1) from Chapter 2. As an example, we estimate the average annual mortality rate in the population studied by Zuckerman et al. In doing so, we need the total number of person-years at risk contributed by the 398 individuals. Lacking the exact death dates of the 47 cohort members who died, we shall assume that during the 2-year follow-up period, each of them contributed 1 year at risk of death. (In fact, some contributed more than 1 year and some contributed less, but the assumption that, on average, each contributed half the length of the study period is usually a good approximation for studies of short duration.) Then during the 2-year period, the 47 deceased individuals contributed 1 year each and the $398 - 47 = 351$ surviving individuals contributed 2 years each. Thus, the entire cohort contributed $1 \times 47 + 2 \times 351 = 749$ person-years at risk. An estimate of the average annual mortality rate is 47 deaths/749 person-years $= 0.0627$ deaths per year per person. We use this estimate in relation (2.1) from Chapter 2 to estimate the probability of death in the $T = 2$-year follow-up period as:

$$P(2) = 1 - \exp(-0.0627 \text{ deaths/year} \times 2 \text{ years}) = 0.118.$$

This value agrees with the product limit estimate. In many cases of practical importance, the product limit estimate and the one obtained via the hazard rate will be in good agreement, even if some of the failure times are censored.

COMPARISONS BETWEEN TWO EXPOSURE GROUPS

Until now we have focused on estimating the probability of failure in a single population. Usually, however, we want to compare failure probabilities in two or more subgroups having different exposures, while adjusting for potential confounding variables. We can do this conveniently by estimating the hazard rate for each subgroup, and then, if we wish, converting it to an estimate of the probability of failure during the study period. In addition, the hazard rate itself and its variation with exposure are often of interest. For example, if the cohort was sampled from a population containing occupationally exposed individuals, it is useful to compare the death rate in exposed versus unexposed persons. We now describe analysis of data for two exposure groups in a cohort. We assume that time at risk and measures of exposure and confounding variables are available for all cohort members. Chapter 7 covers methods appropriate when time at risk is unavailable.

Comparison without Control for Possible Confounding

To illustrate the hazard rate comparison for two exposure groups, we return to the data of Zuckerman et al. (1984). For one of the analyses reported by the authors, the cohort members were divided into those who during an initial interview scored high on an index of religiousness and those who scored low. The index was constructed from a number of questionnaire items concerning participation in religious services and the importance of religion in one's daily life. The outcome of interest was all-cause mortality over the next 2 years. Table 6–1 shows the data.

The question at this point is whether there is an association between religiousness and mortality. We will consider this question statistically in two ways: by hypothesis testing and by estimation. For hypothesis testing, a *null hypothesis* must be specified. For this example, the null hypothesis is that religiousness (the exposure of interest) is unrelated to mortality over the next 2 years. In the sample, the mortality rates are clearly not equal (8.8 vs. 4.3 deaths per 100 person-years at risk), but the null hypothesis relates to the population, not the sample. Therefore, the statistical question to be addressed is whether the sample might plausibly have come from a population in which the null hypothesis is true.

The statistical basis for deciding whether to reject the null hypothesis is the probability that a test statistic as large or larger than that observed in the sample would occur if the null hypothesis were true. This probability depends on the sampling distribution of the data when the null hypothesis is true. An accurate approximation to the sampling distribution of the data in Table 6–1 is to assume that the numbers of deaths in the two groups are independent Poisson variables[1] with means $331 \times I_1$ and $418 \times I_2$. Here I_1 and I_2 represent the unknown death rates in the population for nonreligious

Table 6–1. Deaths and Person-Years According to Religiousness[a]

	Deaths	Person-Years	Average Annual Death Rate
Not religious	29	331	0.088
Religious	18	418	0.043
Total	47	749	0.063

[a]Adapted from Zuckerman et al. (1984).

and religious individuals, respectively. The null hypothesis is H_O: $I_1 = I_2$. Under the null hypothesis, one would expect the 47 deaths to be distributed over the two groups in proportion to the numbers of person-years at risk in the two groups. Thus, the expected number of deaths in the religious group would be $47 \times 418/749 = 26.23$, and the expected number of deaths in the nonreligious groups would be $47 \times 331/749 = 20.77$. These numbers are combined with the observed numbers of deaths to yield a test statistic for assessing whether the death rates I_1 and I_2 are equal. The test statistic is

$$\chi^2 = \frac{(O - E)^2}{D p_1 p_2} = 5.84. \tag{6.2}$$

Here $O = 18$ is the observed number of deaths among the religious, $E = 26.23$ is the expected number of deaths among the religious, $D = 47$ is the total number of deaths in the cohort, and $p_1 = 331/749$ and $p_2 = 418/749$ are the proportions of the total person-years at risk that are contributed by the nonreligious and religious groups, respectively. When the null hypothesis is true, the sampling distribution of χ^2 is approximately that of a chi-squared variable with one degree of freedom. The mean of a chi-squared variable equals its number of degrees of freedom. Therefore, in this example, a value substantially larger than one would give evidence against the null hypothesis. Referring the value $\chi^2 = 5.84$ to a table of values of the chi-squared distribution (found in the back of many statistics textbooks), we find that the probability of obtaining a value this large or larger is less than 2% under the null hypothesis. Thus, the data provide evidence against the null hypothesis of no association between religiousness and mortality.

In most epidemiologic settings it is important to carry the analysis beyond hypothesis testing. The investigator usually is interested not only in whether there is an association, but also in the magnitude of the association. Two commonly used measures of association for data such as those in Table 6–1 are (1) the *ratio* of death rates for religious and nonreligious groups and (2) the *difference* in death rates for religious and nonreligious groups. These are estimated by the corresponding quantities in the sample. For example, an estimate of the ratio of death rates in religious versus nonreligious groups in the population is the rate ratio in the sample: $\hat{r} = 0.043/0.088 = 0.489$. (A hat over a quantity denotes a sample estimate of the quantity.) Thus, the data suggest that the death rate of those scored religious is about half that of those scored not religious.

By itself, a point estimate of the rate ratio is difficult to interpret because it does not indicate the extent to which chance may have played a role. This additional information is provided by calculating a *confidence interval*. A confidence interval is a range of plausible values for the population value of the measure of association. An approximate confidence interval for the rate ratio is obtained by first estimating its variance and then using the square root of the variance (the standard error) to construct the confidence interval. Because the estimated rate ratio must be positive and its distribution is skewed, we can get a more accurate confidence interval by working with the natural logarithm[2] of the rate ratio, hereafter called the *log rate ratio*. We assume a normal distribution for our estimate. The approximate 95% confidence interval for the log rate ratio is obtained by multiplying the standard error (SE) by the standard normal deviate (1.96 for a 95% confidence interval), and (a) subtracting this quantity from and (b) adding this quantity to the log rate ratio to obtain the lower and upper confidence limits, respectively:

$$\text{Lower limit} = \ln \hat{r} - 1.96 \times \text{SE}\{\ln \hat{r}\}$$
$$\text{Upper limit} = \ln \hat{r} + 1.96 \times \text{SE}\{\ln \hat{r}\}, \qquad (6.3)$$

We shall use this method for constructing confidence intervals several times in this volume.

The approximate variance of the log rate ratio is estimated by the sum of the reciprocals of the numbers of deaths. For the data in Table 6–1, this calculation yields a variance of $(1/18) + (1/29) = 0.0900$. The estimated standard error of the log rate ratio is $\sqrt{0.0900} = 0.300$. For our example, we have:

$$\text{Lower limit} = \ln (0.489) - (1.96 \times 0.300) = -1.3041$$
$$\text{Upper limit} = \ln (0.489) + (1.96 \times 0.300) = -0.1281$$

Exponentiation of these two values yields 95% confidence limits for the rate ratio itself of $e^{-1.3041} = 0.27$ and $e^{-0.1281} = 0.88$.

A confidence interval provides more information about the association than does a test of the null hypothesis. The latter, if statistically significant at the 5% level, indicates only that the null value of 1.0 can be ruled out with a 5% chance of error. By contrast, the upper confidence limit in the example indicates not only that a value of 1.0 for the rate ratio is unlikely, but also that any value larger than 0.88 is unlikely. Additionally, the lower confidence limit indicates that any value less than 0.27 is unlikely. A confidence interval of 0.27 to 0.88, in which the upper limit is less than one, provides evidence there is a statistically significant negative association of exposure (religiousness) with the outcome (death).

Stratified Comparison to Account for Possible Confounding

Now that statistical techniques for a simple exposed-unexposed comparison have been introduced, an analysis that takes account of possible con-

founding variables will be illustrated. A common technique for controlling
the effects of potential confounding variables (also called covariates) is to define strata based on their levels. For instance, Zuckerman et al. (1984) considered gender and initial health status as two factors that might confound
the association between religiousness and mortality. Table 6–2 shows the
notation for a general two-way classification of deaths and person-years. The
rows represent exposure groups and the columns represent strata of potential confounding variables. Table 6–3 illustrates how such strata could be
formed from more detailed data from the study of Zuckerman et al. (1984).

Consider now the counts of deaths among exposed and unexposed
persons in each stratum formed by the covariates in Tables 6–2 and 6–3.
We assume that the sampling distributions of these counts are independent
Poisson[1] distributions. For this reason the methods of this chapter are
sometimes called Poisson regression methods. The population mean for the
death count among the unexposed in stratum k is assumed to be $I_{1k}n_{1k}$,
where I_{1k} is the unknown death rate in stratum k among the unexposed,
and n_{1k} is the number of person-years at risk. Similarly, the mean for the
count among the exposed in stratum k is taken as $I_{2k}n_{2k}$, where I_{2k} and n_{2k}
are defined analogously.

We wish to evaluate the stratum-specific rate ratios $r_k = I_{2k}/I_{1k}$ for
exposed versus unexposed. Three hypotheses of interest are shown in Table
6–4. Our objectives are to (a) test the null hypothesis H_0 that rates for
exposed and unexposed in the population are equal in each stratum of the
covariates; (b) estimate the ratio of exposed to unexposed rates assuming
provisionally that this ratio is common to all strata (hypothesis H_1); and (c)
evaluate the hypothesis H_1 of a common rate ratio relative to the alternative
H_2 that the rate ratios vary across strata.

Testing the null hypothesis. The hypothesis H_0 can be tested by considering the statistic

$$\chi^2 = \frac{(O - E)^2}{\Sigma_k D_k \pi_{1k} \pi_{2k}}. \tag{6.4}$$

Table 6–2. Notation for a General Two-Way Classification of Deaths and Person-Years
(P-Y) according to Two Exposure Levels, Stratified by K Levels of One or More Potential
Confounding Variables

	\multicolumn{8}{c}{Stratum of Potential Confounding Variables}
	1		2		k		K	
Exposure	Deaths	P-Y	Deaths	P-Y	Deaths	P-Y	Deaths	P-Y
Unexposed	d_{11}	n_{11}	d_{12}	n_{12} $\cdots$	d_{1k}	n_{1k} $\cdots$	d_{1K}	n_{1K}
Exposed	d_{21}	n_{21}	d_{22}	n_{22} $\cdots$	d_{2k}	n_{2k} $\cdots$	d_{2K}	n_{2K}
Total	D_1	N_1	D_2	N_2 $\cdots$	D_k	N_k $\cdots$	D_K	N_K

Table 6-3. Deaths and Person-Years (P-Y) according to Religiousness, Stratified by Gender and Initial Health Status[a]

| | Stratum Determined by Gender and Health Status | | | | | | | | |
| | 1. Male Well | | 2. Male Ill | | 3. Female Well | | 4. Female Ill | | Total | |
	Deaths	P-Y	Deaths	P-Y	Deaths	P-Y	Deaths	P-Y	Deaths	P-Y
Not religious	5	79	13	49	2	122	9	81	29	331
Religious	4	66	4	38	2	176	8	138	18	418
Total	9	145	17	87	4	298	17	219	47	749

[a]Adapted from Zuckerman et al. (1984).

Table 6–4. Hypotheses for a Stratified Analysis: Two Exposure Groups

H_0: $r_k = 1$ (null hypothesis), rates for exposed and unexposed are equal in each stratum of confounding variables

H_1: $r_k = r$, exposed-unexposed rate ratios are common to all strata

H_2: the general alternative that exposed-unexposed rate ratios may vary across strata.

Here $O = d_{21} + ... + d_{2k}$ is the observed number of deaths among the exposed, π_{1k} and π_{2k} are the proportions of the total person-years at risk in stratum k that are contributed by the unexposed and exposed, respectively, $E = D_1 n_{21}/N_1 + ... + D_k n_{2k}/N_k$ is the expected number of deaths among the exposed, and Σ_k denotes summation over the strata $k = 1,2,...,K$. When the null hypothesis is true, the sampling distribution of χ^2 is approximately that of a chi-squared variable on one degree of freedom. For the data in Table 6–3, the observed and expected numbers of deaths in the religious are, respectively, $O = 18$ and $E = (9 \times 66/145) + (17 \times 38/87) + (4 \times 176/298) + (17 \times 138/219) = 24.60$. Similar substitution gives the denominator in (6.4) as 11.4. Thus, $\chi^2 = (18 - 24.6)^2/11.4 = 3.8$. Using a table of chi-squared values, we find that the probability of obtaining a value this large or larger under the null hypothesis is $p = 0.05$.

The test statistic for the unstratified data of the previous section was obtained by substituting the totals over strata into formula (6.4), with $K = 1$. That is, substituting $O = 18$, $E = 47 \times 418/749 = 26.23$, $D_1 = 47$, $\pi_{11} = 331/749$, and $\pi_{12} = 418/749$ into the formula gives the previously noted value

$$\chi^2 = \frac{(O - E)^2}{D_1 \pi_{11} \pi_{12}} = 5.84.$$

Estimating the Common Rate Ratio.[3] We wish to estimate the ratio of death rates among exposed versus unexposed, assuming provisionally that it does not vary with gender or initial health status. (In the next section we will test this assumption.) The Mantel-Haenszel estimate,

$$r_{MH} = \frac{(d_{21}n_{11}/N_1) + \cdots + (d_{2K}n_{1K}/N_K)}{(d_{11}n_{21}/N_1) + \cdots + (d_{1K}n_{2K}/N_K)}, \tag{6.5}$$

has good statistical properties, and it can be calculated without a computer. For the data in Table 6–3, we find that

$$r_{MH} = \frac{(4 \times 79/145) + (4 \times 49/87) + (2 \times 122/298) + (8 \times 81/219)}{(5 \times 66/145) + (13 \times 38/87) + (2 \times 176/298) + (9 \times 138/219)}$$

$$= 0.554.$$

Because this value for the rate ratio is rather close to the unstratified value of 0.489 calculated from the data of Table 6–1, gender and initial health status seem not to be strong confounders of the association between religiousness and mortality.

As in the unstratified analysis, it is desirable to calculate confidence limits for the common rate ratio r via its natural logarithm. The standard error of the logarithm of the Mantel-Haenszel estimate can be estimated as

$$\text{SE}(\ln r_{\text{MH}}) = \frac{(A_1 + A_2 + \cdots + A_k)^{1/2}}{r_{\text{MH}}^{1/2}(B_1 + \cdots + B_k)} \qquad (6.6)$$

(Breslow and Day, 1987). Here $A_k = D_k n_{1k} n_{2k}/N_k^2$ and $B_k = A_k N_k/(n_{1k} + r_{\text{MH}} n_{2k})$, $k = 1,...,K$. For the data in Table 6–3, $K = 4$ and $A_1 = 9 \times 79 \times 66/(145)^2 = 2.232$, $A_2 = 17 \times 49 \times 38/(87)^2 = 4.182$, $A_3 = 4 \times 122 \times 176/(298)^2 = 0.967$, and $A_4 = 17 \times 81 \times 138/(219)^2 = 3.962$. Thus, $(A_1 +...+ A_4)^{1/2} = (2.232 + 4.182 + 0.967 + 3.962)^{1/2} = (11.343)^{1/2} = 3.368$. Moreover, $B_1 = 2.23 \times 145/(79 + 0.554 \times 66) = 2.232 \times 145/115.56 = 2.800$, and similarly, $B_2 = 5.194$, $B_3 = 1.313$, and $B_4 = 5.511$. Substituting these values in formula (6.6) gives

$$\text{SE}(\ln r_{\text{MH}}) = \frac{(2.232 + 4.182 + 0.967 + 3.962)^{1/2}}{(0.554)^{1/2}(2.800 + 5.194 + 1.313 + 5.571)} = 0.305$$

The estimate for $\ln r_{\text{MH}}$ is $\ln (0.554) = -0.590$. The upper and lower limits of the 95% confidence interval for log rate ratio are calculated by adding and subtracting 1.96 times the standard error from the estimate as follows:

$$\text{Lower limit} = -0.590 - (1.96 \times 0.305) = -1.188$$
$$\text{Upper limit} = -0.590 - (1.96 \times 0.305) = 0.008.$$

Exponentiating leads to confidence limits of $e^{-1.188} = 0.305$ and $e^{0.008} = 1.008$ for the rate ratio itself. Because the upper confidence limit is slightly greater than one, the null hypothesis of no association between religiousness and mortality cannot be rejected at the 5% level of statistical significance. Obviously, however, the result falls only slightly short of achieving this level of statistical significance.

The preferred estimate of the common rate ratio is one obtained by the method of maximum likelihood, because in large samples it tends to have the smallest standard error. However, an iterative computer algorithm is needed to calculate the maximum likelihood estimate. The maximum likelihood estimate r_{ML} is the solution of an equation obtained by setting the observed number of deaths among the exposed (i.e., religious) equal to the expected number under the hypothesis H_1. This expected number is the sum over the covariate strata of terms $D_k p_k$, $k = 1,...,K$. Here D_k is the total number of individuals who died in covariate stratum k, and p_k is the fraction of all deaths in stratum k predicted to occur among exposed individuals:

$$p_k = \frac{rn_{2k}}{n_{1k} + rn_{2k}} = \frac{I_{2k}n_{2k}}{I_{1k}n_{1k} + I_{2k}n_{2k}}. \tag{6.7}$$

Solving the resulting equation for r_{ML} requires a computer program. For the data in Table 6–3, the maximum likelihood estimate obtained using the computer software EGRET (Mauritsen, 1994) is $r_{ML} = 0.555$; thus, $\ln r_{ML} = -0.589$.

An estimate for the standard error of $\ln r_{ML}$ is $1/(\Sigma_k D_k \hat{p}_k \hat{q}_k)^{1/2}$. Here $\hat{p}_k = 1 - \hat{q}_k$ is the fitted proportion of exposed among the dead in stratum k, given by formula (6.7) with the estimate r_{ML} in place of the unknown rate ratio r. Application of this formula to the data in Table 6–3 gives $p_1 = 0.555 \times 66/(79 + 0.555 \times 66) = 0.317$, $p_2 = 0.555 \times 38/(49 + 0.555 \times 38) = 0.301$, and similarly $p_3 = 0.444$ and $p_4 = 0.486$. Thus, SE($\ln r_{ML}$) = $1/[9 \times 0.317 \times (1 - 0.317) + 17 \times 0.301 \times (1 - 0.301) + 4 \times 0.444 \times (1 - 0.444) + 17 \times 0.486 \times (1 - 0.486)]^{1/2} = 1/(10.906)^{1/2} = 0.305$. The resulting 95% confidence limits for r, obtained by using formula (6.3) and then exponentiating, are $\exp[-0.589 - 1.96 \times 0.305] = 0.305$ and $\exp[-0.589 + 1.96 \times 0.305] = 1.009$.

For the data in Table 6–3, the Mantel-Haenszel and maximum likelihood estimates of the common rate ratio agree well ($r_{MH} = 0.554$; $r_{ML} = 0.555$). In general, the Mantel-Haenszel estimate is a good approximation to the maximum likelihood estimate when the unknown rate ratio r is close to one; in practice, the two estimates usually agree even when r departs from one.

Testing homogeneity of the rate ratios across covariate strata. Until now, we have assumed that the rate ratio relating the religious to the nonreligious does not vary with gender and initial health status (hypothesis H_1). The last row of Table 6–5 shows the observed death rate ratios for religious versus nonreligious persons in the four gender/health status strata. There is some variation in these ratios, and one might question whether it is due to chance or whether the rate ratios in the population differ by stratum.

Table 6–5 also shows the expected numbers E of deaths under the assumption of a common rate ratio. Using the notation of Table 6–2, we label the expected numbers of deaths among nonreligious and religious in stratum k as $\hat{d}_{1k}$ and $\hat{d}_{2k}$, respectively. These were calculated as $\hat{d}_{1k} = D_k - \hat{d}_{2k}$, and $\hat{d}_{2k} = D_k \hat{p}_k$ where D_k is the total number of deaths in covariate stratum k, and where $\hat{p}_k$ is given by formula (6.7) with either the Mantel-

Table 6–5. Observed (O) and Expected[a] (E) Numbers of Deaths, Person-Years (P-Y) at Risk, Residuals[b] and Death Rates according to Religiousness, Stratified by Gender and Initial Health Status, for the Data of Table 6–3

| | Stratum Determined by Gender and Health Status | | | | | | | | | | | |
| | 1. Male Well | | | 2. Male Ill | | | 3. Female Well | | | 4. Female Ill | | |
	$\frac{O}{E}$	P-Y Residual[b]	Death Rate · 10²	$\frac{O}{E}$	P-Y Residual	Death Rate · 10²	$\frac{O}{E}$	P-Y Residual	Death Rate · 10²	$\frac{O}{E}$	P-Y Residual	Death Rate · 10²
Not religious	5 / 6.15	79 / −0.464	6.329	13 / 11.89	49 / 0.322	26.531	2 / 2.22	122 / −0.148	1.639	9 / 8.74	81 / 0.088	11.111
Religious	4 / 2.85	66 / 0.681	6.061	4 / 5.11	38 / −0.492	10.526	2 / 1.78	176 / 0.165	1.136	8 / 8.26	138 / −0.090	5.797
Rate ratio			0.958			0.397			0.693			0.522

[a] Estimated by maximum likelihood assuming a common rate ratio for the four strata determined by gender and initial health status.
[b] (Observed deaths−Expected deaths)/(Expected deaths)$^{1/2}$.

Haenszel or maximum likelihood estimate in place of the unknown rate ratio r. For example, referring back to Table 6–3 and using r_{ML} in place of r in formula (6.7), we find that the expected number of deaths among religious males whose health status was well is $\hat{d}_{21} = D_1\hat{p}_1 = 9 \times 0.317 = 2.85$, while the expected number of deaths among nonreligious males whose health status was well is $9 - 2.85 = 6.15$. Similarly, the expected number of deaths among religious and nonreligious males classified as ill are, respectively, $17 \times 0.30 = 5.11$ and $17 - 5.11 = 11.89$.

To test for heterogeneity in the rate ratios, we substitute these observed and expected numbers of deaths into the formula

$$\chi^2_{\text{HET}} = \sum_k \sum_j \frac{(d_{jk} - \hat{d}_{jk})^2}{\hat{d}_{jk}}, \tag{6.8}$$

where $\sum_j$ denotes summation over the two indices $j = 1$ and $j = 2$, and, as usual, $\sum_k$ denotes summation over the covariate strata $k = 1,...,K$. If the hypothesis H_1 of a common rate ratio is valid, the statistic χ^2_{HET} has approximately a chi-squared distribution on $K - 1$ degrees of freedom. For the data in Table 6–5 we find $\chi^2_{\text{HET}} = (5-6.15)^2/6.15 + (4-2.85)^2/2.85 + (13-11.89)^2/11.89 + (4-5.11)^2/5.11 + (2-2.22)^2/2.22 + (2-1.78)^2/1.78 + (9-8.74)^2/8.74 + (8-8.26)^2/8.26 = 1.09$ on $K - 1 = 3$ degrees of freedom. The probability of obtaining a chi-squared value this large or larger is 0.78. This small value of χ^2_{HET} suggests that the observed variation in the rate ratios across gender or health status is most likely due to chance.

However, agreement between the test statistic and its number of degrees of freedom does not guarantee that the rate ratio is constant across strata of the covariates, particularly when the number of degrees of freedom is large and the numbers of deaths in some of the cells are small. More thorough scrutiny can be based on the set of *residuals* for the JK cells. The residual for the $(j,k)^{th}$ cell is the difference $d_{jk} - \hat{d}_{jk}$ between the observed and predicted numbers of deaths for that cell. Because of small numbers of deaths, the test statistic χ^2_{HET} may not achieve statistical significance despite systematic trends in the residuals with increasing levels of a covariate, or large residuals in a single cell. It is useful to examine the standardized residuals, which are the square roots $(d_{jk} - \hat{d}_{jk})/(\hat{d}_{jk})^{1/2}$ of the terms in expression (6.8). (Actually, these are studentized standardized residuals, as defined by McCullagh and Nelder [1989]). In the absence of heterogeneity, their sampling distribution is approximately that of a standard normal variable, and thus 95% of the time they should fall within the range ±1.96. Table 6–5 shows the standardized residuals for the data in Table 6–3; because none are greater in absolute value than 1.96, they are within the acceptable range.

If the data show marked heterogeneity in the rate ratios that cannot be attributed to chance, then attempts to summarize them with a single rate ratio can obscure important features of the underlying rates and should be avoided. For example, if in Table 6–5 the ratio of death rates for those scored religious relative to those scored not religious were greater than one for males and less than one for females, then estimates of a common rate ratio would be close to unity. This overall rate ratio would incorrectly suggest no association between religiousness and mortality, when in fact a positive association is seen in males and a negative one in females.

If the effect of exposure were to add a constant amount to the rates I_{1k} among unexposed individuals in stratum k, then the rate differences $I_{2k} - I_{1k}$, and not the rate ratios, would be constant across strata. The assumption of a constant rate difference is called an *additive* or *absolute risk model*, while the assumption of a constant rate ratio is called a *multiplicative* or *relative risk model*. The multiplicative model also is called a *proportional hazards model*, because it assumes that exposure (religiousness) multiplies the unexposed hazard rate by the same fixed proportion in each stratum. Figure 6–3 shows hypothetical age-specific death rates under each of these models, when age is represented continuously, rather than stratified.

Unless the data are extensive or the effects of exposure strong, it is

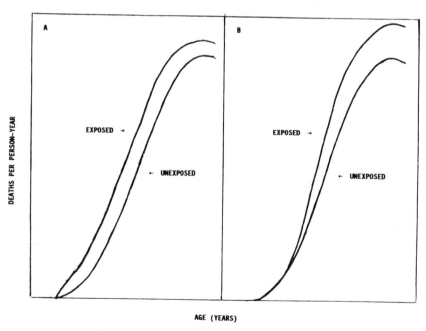

Figure 6–3. Plots of death rates versus age for two hypothetical groups of individuals: those exposed to an agent that increases the risk of death, and those unexposed to the agent. The effect of exposure is (A) to add a fixed amount to the unexposed death rate (additive model); (B) to multiply the unexposed death rate by a fixed amount (multiplicative model).

difficult to discriminate between additive and multiplicative models on the basis of the data alone. Instead, the choice of model must be motivated either by biological plausibility (although we seldom have biological mechanisms to guide us), or by analytical convenience. We restrict attention to multiplicative models because analytic methods are simpler for them.

COMPARISONS AMONG MORE THAN TWO EXPOSURE GROUPS

In the previous section when dealing with two exposure groups, we estimated the rate ratio relating the exposed group to the unexposed group, assuming it did not vary across strata of the other variables. Then we tested the hypothesis that the rate ratio does not vary across strata of the covariates. We now generalize these notions to cohort studies such as the study of smoking and mortality among U.S. veterans conducted by Kahn et al. (1966), where interest centers on the relation between an outcome (say, death from respiratory cancer) and several exposure groups (where exposure is cigarette smoking). Table 6–6 shows data for cohort members who at enrollment were either lifelong nonsmokers or current cigarette smokers. The data are stratified into smoking and age groups, where the former are determined by cigarette smoking status at the time of study enrollment. Again we wish to adjust for covariates such as age, and again we do so by stratifying the data jointly by exposure and covariates, as in Table 6–6.

In the general case, we shall think for concreteness of j as indexing J exposure (smoking) groups and k as indexing K confounder (age) groups. Table 6–7 shows notation for a typical two-dimensional layout. Within the cell formed by the jth row and k^{th} column one records the number d_{jk} of deaths and the number n_{jk} of person-years at risk. Referring again to Table 6–6 we see that the respiratory cancer data of Kahn et al. have been stratified into $J = 6$ exposure groups and $K = 5$ age groups.

Table 6–6 differs from Table 6–3 in the allocation of person-years at risk to the cells. For the data of Zuckerman et al. (1984), each cohort member contributed all of his or her person-years to a single cell. For the respiratory cancer data, by contrast, the person-years contributed by a veteran may be distributed across several cells. A cohort member contributes time to a cell only when his values of the variables fall within the boundaries defining the cell. For instance, an occasional smoker who entered the study on his 48th birthday and died three months after his 63rd birthday contributed 7 years (from age 48 years to age 54 years) to the cell (2,2) corresponding to the second age row and second smoking column, and 8.25 years (from age 55 years until death) to cell (3,2). The two studies differ in this way because the variables of interest differ with respect to their

Table 6-6. Observed (*O*) and Expected[a] (*E*) Respiratory Cancer Deaths, Person-Years (P-Y) at Risk and Death Rates among U.S. Veterans[b] according to Cigarette Consumption, by Age

Age (Years)

Smoking Group	(Index)	35–44 O/E	35–44 P-Y / Rate·10^5	45–54 O/E	45–54 P-Y / Rate·10^5	55–64 O/E	55–64 P-Y / Rate·10^5	65–74 O/E	65–74 P-Y / Rate·10^5	75–84 O/E	75–84 P-Y / Rate·10^5	Total O/E	Total P-Y / Rate·10^5
Nonsmokers	(0)	0 / 1.4	35,164 / 0	0 / 4.2	15,134 / 0	25 / 215.8	213,858 / 11.69	49 / 264.7	171,211 / 28.62	4 / 18.2	8,480 / 47.12	78 / 504.24	443,847 / 17.57
Smokers Occasional	(.5)	0 / 0.1	3,657 / 0	0 / 0.4	1,283 / 0	6 / 14.8	14,624 / 41.03	10 / 15.5	10,053 / 99.47	1 / 1.1	512 / 195.31	17 / 31.90	30,129 / 56.42
Cigarettes/day 1–9	(5)	0 / 0.3	8,063 / 0	0 / 0.9	3,129 / 0	31 / 45.6	45,217 / 68.56	44 / 57.4	37,130 / 118.50	5 / 4.1	1,923 / 260.01	80 / 108.34	95,462 / 83.80
10–20	(15)	2 / 2.4	59,965 / 3.34	2 / 4.5	16,392 / 12.20	183 / 153.0	151,664 / 120.66	239 / 157.2	101,731 / 234.93	15 / 8.3	3,867 / 387.90	441 / 325.50	333,619 / 132.19
21–39	(30)	4 / 1.6	40,643 / 9.84	10 / 3.5	12,839 / 77.89	245 / 104.0	103,020 / 237.82	194 / 77.4	50,045 / 387.65	7 / 2.7	1,273 / 549.88	460 / 189.20	207,820 / 221.35
40+	(50)	0 / 0.2	3,992 / 0	2 / 0.5	1,928 / 103.73	63 / 19.8	19,649 / 320.63	50 / 13.8	8,937 / 559.47	3 / 0.5	232 / 1,293.10	118 / 34.83	34,738 / 339.69
Total		6 / 6.0	151,484 / 3.96	14 / 14.0	50,705 / 27.61	553 / 553.0	548,032 / 100.91	586 / 586.0	379,107 / 154.57	35 / 35.0	16,287 / 214.90	1,194 / 1,194.0	1,145,615 / 104.22

[a]Based on the assumption that the death rate is independent of smoking, and calculated as the total number D_k of deaths in age group k multiplied by the fraction n_{jk}/N_k of all person-years in age group k that belong to smoking category j.

[b]Adapted from Kahn (1966).

Table 6–7. Notation for a General Two-Way Classification of Observed (O) and Expected (E) Deaths and Person-Years (P-Y) according to J Exposure Levels, Stratified by K Levels of One or More Potential Confounding Variables

| | Stratum of Potential Confounding Variable (e.g., Age) | | | | | | | | Total | |
| | 1 | | 2 | | $\cdots$ k $\cdots$ | | K | | | |
Exposure Group	$\dfrac{O}{E}$	P-Y Rate	$\dfrac{O}{E}$	P-Y Rate	$\dfrac{O}{E}$	P-Y Rate	$\dfrac{O}{E}$	P-Y Rate	$\dfrac{O}{E}$	P-Y Rate
1	d_{11} / $D_1 n_{11}/N_1$	n_{11} / d_{11}/n_{11}	d_{12} / $D_2 n_{12}/N_2$	n_{12} / d_{12}/n_{12}	d_{1k} / $D_k n_{1k}/N_k$	n_{1k} / d_{1k}/n_{1k}	d_{1K} / $D_K n_{1K}/N_K$	n_{1K} / d_{1K}/n_{1K}	d_{1+}[a] / $D_+ n_{1+}/N_+$	n_{1+} / d_{1+}/n_{1+}
2	d_{21} / $D_1 n_{21}/N_1$	n_{21} / d_{21}/n_{21}	d_{22} / $D_2 n_{22}/N_2$	n_{22} / d_{22}/n_{22}	d_{2k} / $D_k n_{2k}/N_k$	n_{2k} / d_{2k}/n_{2k}	d_{2K} / $D_K n_{2K}/N_K$	n_{2K} / d_{2K}/n_{2K}	d_{2+} / $D_+ n_{2+}/N_+$	n_{2+} / d_{2+}/n_{2+}
j	d_{j1} / $D_1 n_{j1}/N_1$	n_{j1} / d_{j1}/n_{j1}	d_{j2} / $D_2 n_{j2}/N_2$	n_{j2} / d_{j2}/n_{j2}	d_{jk} / $D_k n_{jk}/N_k$	n_{jk} / d_{jk}/n_{jk}	d_{jK} / $D_K n_{jK}/N_K$	n_{jK} / d_{jK}/n_{jK}	d_{j+} / $D_+ n_{j+}/N_+$	n_{j+} / d_{j+}/n_{j+}
J	d_{J1} / $D_1 n_{J1}/N_1$	n_{J1} / d_{J1}/n_{J1}	d_{J2} / $D_2 n_{J2}/N_2$	n_{J2} / d_{J2}/n_{J2}	d_{Jk} / $D_k n_{Jk}/N_k$	n_{Jk} / d_{Jk}/n_{Jk}	d_{JK} / $D_K n_{JK}/N_K$	n_{JK} / d_{JK}/n_{JK}	d_{J+} / $D_+ n_{J+}/N_+$	n_{J+} / d_{J+}/n_{J+}
Total	D_1 / D_1	N_1 / D_1/N_1	D_2 / D_2	N_2 / D_2/N_2	D_k / D_k	N_k / D_k/N_k	D_K / D_K	N_K / D_K/N_K	D_+ / D_+	N_+ / D_+/N_+

[a] $d_{1+} = d_{11} + d_{12} + \cdots + d_{1K}$, with similar notation for d_{2+}, n_{2+}, etc.

dependence on follow-up time. The variables considered in Table 6–3 (gender, initial health status and index of religiousness) do not assume different values during the study period. However, one of the variables considered in Table 6–6 (age) changes value with time since start of follow-up. If the exposure variable had been total packs of cigarettes smoked during one's lifetime, then the exposure variable also would change value during follow-up, as cohort members accrue additional exposure. Construction of tables such as Table 6–6 requires, for each cohort member, age at start and end of follow-up, and, if the exposure variable(s) change with time, an exposure measurement during each year of follow-up.

Analysis of data such as those in Table 6–6 typically begins with inspection of the observed death rates d_{jk}/n_{jk}, and their variation with exposure in each age group. Interest also may focus on the variation of death rates with age in each exposure group. We see in Table 6–6 that the observed respiratory cancer death rates tend to increase with both age and smoking level. Although this display of observed rates helps us understand their underlying structure, we usually will need summary measures of association relating death rates to exposure and possibly also to age.

Summary measures of association are useful because the detailed results are often too lengthy to be communicated and interpreted easily. Summary measures are especially desirable when the numbers of deaths are sparse, because the $J \times K$ cell-specific rates are based on small numbers and are therefore imprecise, making inference difficult. When $J \times K$ is large, summary measures also help us interpret the many observed rates, by highlighting trends and other features that might otherwise be missed.

To illustrate, we might assume a multiplicative model for the joint effects of age and smoking in Table 6–6, and summarize the $J \times K = 6 \times 5 = 30$ death rates as follows. First, we specify the five age-specific death rates $I_{11}, \ldots, I_{15}$ for the nonsmokers, which we call age parameters. Parameters are unknown constants whose values determine the death rates. Having done so, we need only specify the rate ratio r_j for the jth smoking group to obtain all the age-specific rates $I_{j1} = r_j I_{11}, \ldots, I_{j5} = r_j I_{15}$ for that group. Therefore, the five age parameters $I_{11}, \ldots, I_{15}$ and the five rate ratios $r_2, \ldots, r_6$ (parameters that determine the effects of smoking) specify all 30 death rates in Table 6–6.

As noted previously, summary measures such as those available from the multiplicative model are useful only if the effects of exposure are consistent across the age groups. If, for example, death rates increased with increasing exposure among the young and decreased with increasing exposure among the old, no single set of summary measures of exposure effects could adequately describe the death rates for all age groups.

The most commonly used summary parameters are those of the multiplicative model. In its most general form, this model states that the death rate I_{jk} in exposure group j and age group k is the product of an exposure parameter r_j and an age parameter s_k:

$$I_{jk} = r_j s_k, j = 1,...,J; k = 1,...,K. \tag{6.9}$$

This model, although nominally dependent on J exposure parameters $r_1,...,r_J$ plus K age parameters $s_1,...,s_K$, actually requires only $J + K - 1$ nonredundant parameters. Therefore we must fix one of the $J + K$ parameters in equation (6.9); it is convenient to do so by designating one exposure group as the *referent* group, giving it the index $j = 1$, and then setting the exposure parameter $r_1 = 1$. Then we see from equation (6.9) that $I_{11} = s_1,...,I_{1K} = s_K$ are the age-specific rates in the referent group. The non-smokers form a natural, unexposed referent group for the data in Table 6-6. However, if no natural referent group is available one can be selected arbitrarily, as its choice will not affect tests of the null hypothesis or estimates of parameters in the models described below.

For individuals in the jth exposure group and the kth age group, we let $r_{jk} = I_{jk} = I_{jk}/I_{1k}$ denote the rate ratio relative to the referent group. Referring to the respiratory cancer data of Table 6-6, there are five rate ratios for each of the $K = 5$ age groups, which are the population death rates in each of the five categories of smokers divided by the population death rate in non-smokers. The hypotheses of interest, framed in terms of these unknown ratios, are shown in Table 6-8. Hypothesis H_1 is just another formulation of the multiplicative model given by equation (6.9); it specifies that the rate ratios for the different exposure groups do not vary with age. Hypothesis H_2 also is a multiplicative model; in addition, it specifies that the (common) rate ratio relating exposure group j to the referent is a function of some exposure index x_j. The functional form f usually is specified but may depend on unknown parameters. For example, we might assign a smoking index to each smoking group in Table 6-6, such as the mean or median smoking rate for individuals in the group, or the midpoint of the range of smoking rates for the group. Then to test the hypothesis that the death rates depend linearly on the smoking indices, we would take the $f(x_j)$ to be a linear function of x_j, whose intercept and slope parameters are estimated from the data. Hypotheses H_1 and H_2 are examples of *proportional hazards models*, because they specify that exposure multiplies the age-specific baseline rate in the referent group by a fixed amount, independent of age.

Formal analysis of data with several exposure levels is similar to that described for two exposures in the previous section. The death counts d_{jk} are assumed to be independent Poisson[1] variables with means $I_{jk}n_{jk}$. Here I_{jk} is the unknown death rate for cohort members in exposure group j and age group k. A basic assumption is that the death rate does not vary with age or exposure within the boundaries of each cell. For instance, the death

Table 6-8. Hypotheses for a Stratified Analysis: K Exposure Groups

H_0: $r_{jk} = 1$ (null hypothesis), age-specific rates are the same in all J exposure groups
H_1: $r_{jk} = r_j$, exposure rate ratios do not vary across K age strata
H_2: $r_{jk} = f(x_j)$, exposure rate ratios are independent of age and are a specified function of exposure levels x_j
H_3: the general alternative of unrestricted rate ratios.

---

rate in cell (1,3) of Table 6-6 (smokers of 1-9 cigarettes per day, aged 35-44 years) is assumed to be the same for all men in this 10-year age range and for all average smoking rates between one and nine cigarettes per day. The goals now are (a) to test the null hypothesis H_0 that death rates differ for none of the J exposure groups; (b) if the null hypothesis is rejected, to estimate parameters that indicate how the rates vary with exposure (the latter task usually involves fitting a model, such as those assumed by the hypotheses H_1 and H_2, describing how the rates vary with both age and exposure); and (c) to evaluate how well the model fits the data. To accomplish these goals, we first describe some methods of analysis that do not require computer programming. Then we conclude with a discussion of the more optimal but computationally intensive maximum likelihood methods.

Analysis by Hand or Calculator

To test the null hypothesis that the death rates do not depend on exposure we could use an extension of the chi-squared statistic given in formula (6.4) for data with just two exposure groups (see Breslow and Day, [1987]). However, calculating this statistic requires multiplying matrices and computing their inverses, which, for more than three exposure groups, is not feasible without a computer. For rough work it can be approximated by the easily calculated statistic χ^2 of Table 6-9. When the null hypothesis of no exposure effect is true, χ^2 has a chi-squared sampling distribution with $J - 1$ degrees of freedom. When it is false, χ^2 tends to be smaller than the extension described by Breslow and Day (1987) (particularly when the exposure distributions vary appreciably with age), making it somewhat less likely that the null hypothesis will be rejected. For the respiratory cancer data in Table 6-6, with $J = 6$ smoking groups, we find from the extreme right columns that $O_1 = 78$ and $E_1 = 504.30$, $O_2 = 17$ and $E_2 = 31.89$, $O_3 = 80$ and $E_3 = 108.34$, $O_4 = 441$ and $E_4 = 325.50$, $O_5 = 460$ and $E_5 = 189.20$, and finally, $O_6 = 118$ and $E_6 = 34.83$. Substituting these numbers into the formula for χ^2 in Table 6-9 gives

$$\chi^2 = \frac{(78 - 504.3)^2}{504.3} + \frac{(17 - 31.89)^2}{31.89} + \cdots + \frac{(118 - 34.83)^2}{34.83}$$

$$= 360.3 + 7.0 + 7.4 + 41.0 + 387.6 + 198.6 = 1001.9.$$

Table 6–9. Chi-Squared Statistics for Hypothesis Testing

NOTATION:

d_{jk} = number of deaths in exposure group j and confounder (e.g., age) stratum k

n_{jk} = number of person-years in exposure group j and age stratum k

$O_j = d_{j1} + d_{j2} + \cdots + d_{jK}$ = total number of deaths in exposure group j

$D_k = d_{1k} + d_{2k} + \cdots + d_{Jk}$ = total number of deaths in age stratum k

N_k = total number of person-years in age stratum k

$\hat{d}_{jk}$ = expected number of deaths in exposure group j and age stratum k under null hypothesis. For null hypothesis of no exposure effect, $\hat{d}_{jk} = D_k n_{jk}/N_k$

$E_j = \hat{d}_{j1} + \hat{d}_{j2} + \cdots + \hat{d}_{jK}$ = expected number of deaths in exposure group j under null hypothesis

x_j = index of exposure level in exposure group j

TEST OF H_o: NO ASSOCIATION WITH EXPOSURE

$$\chi^2 = \frac{(O_1 - E_1)^2}{E_1} + \cdots + \frac{(O_J - E_J)^2}{E_J}.$$

Under H_o, χ^2 is distributed as a chi-square variable with $J - 1$ degrees of freedom.

TEST OF H_o: NO TREND IN DEATH RATES WITH EXPOSURE

$$\chi^2_{\text{TREND}} = \frac{[\Sigma_{j=1}^{J} x_j(O_j - E_j)]^2}{\Sigma_{j=1}^{J} x_j^2 E_j - \Sigma_k [(\Sigma_{j=1}^{J} x_j \hat{d}_{jk})^2/D_k]}.$$

Under H_o, χ^2_{TREND} is distributed as a chi-square variable with one degree of freedom.

TEST OF H_o: SMALL MODEL FITS DATA (DEVIANCE)

$$\chi^2_{DEV} = 2 \sum_k \sum_j \hat{d}_{jk}^{(b)} \log(\hat{d}_{jk}^{(b)}/\hat{d}_{jk}^{(s)}) + \hat{d}_{jk}^{(s)} - \hat{d}_{jk}^{(b)},$$

where $\hat{d}_{jk}^{(b)}$ and $\hat{d}_{jk}^{(s)}$ are the expected numbers of deaths in cell (j,k) for big and small models, respectively. For either model, $\hat{d}_{jk} = n_{jk}\hat{l}_{jk}$, where $\hat{l}_{jk}$ is given by the model with maximum likelihood estimates in place of the unknown parameters. Under H_o, the deviance χ^2_{DEV} is distributed as a chi square variable with degrees of freedom equal to the number of parameters in the big model minus the number of parameters in the small model.

This value, as expected, is slightly smaller than the value of 1014.0 of the more complicated statistic calculated by the matrix method (Breslow and Day, 1987). Both values are highly unlikely for a chi-squared variable with $J - 1 = 5$ degrees of freedom ($p < 0.001$). Thus, we reject the null hypothesis of no difference in respiratory cancer death rates among the smoking groups.

There is a natural ordering for the exposure groups in Table 6–6, which can be captured by assigning an index x_j of exposure to each group. For example, we have assigned to the jth smoking group a smoking index x_j, shown in column 2 of the table. Here x_j is the median smoking rate in cigarettes per day of veterans in smoking group j. If there is a trend in the death rates with increasing levels of exposure, then a more powerful test of the null hypothesis than the one based on χ^2 is obtained by referring the statistic χ^2_{TREND} of Table 6–9 to a chi-squared distribution on one degree of freedom. Calculations for the data in Table 6–6 are shown in Table 6–10. We find that $\chi^2_{\text{TREND}} = 999.8$, extremely unlikely for a chi-squared variable on one degree of freedom ($p < 0.001$).

This test for trend in death rates with increasing exposure levels serves two purposes. First, it increases the likelihood of correctly rejecting the null hypothesis when it is false and when the rates change monotonically with exposure. Second, it summarizes the evidence either supporting or refuting a causal association between exposure and risk of death (see Chapter 2). If, for example, the death rates in Table 6–6 were larger for smokers than for nonsmokers but did not vary among the smokers, then one might question the causal nature of the association between smoking and mortality from respiratory cancer. That is, with no trend found, the higher death rates among smokers could have occurred because they differed systematically from the nonsmokers with respect to some other attribute that itself increased their risk. This scenario of an abrupt jump followed by a plateau in death rates can itself produce a significant value of the trend test statistic χ^2_{TREND}. This problem can be avoided by excluding the referent group when calculating χ^2_{TREND} (i.e., by applying the formula in Table 6–9 to the subcohort consisting only of individuals in the exposed groups $j = 2,...,J$). Excluding the nonsmokers from the test for trend gives a value of 869.4 for χ^2_{TREND}, still highly unlikely ($p < 0.001$) for a chi-squared variable on one degree of freedom, and lending support to a causal role for cigarette smoking in respiratory cancer.

We now turn to the problem of *estimating the magnitudes of association* between risk of death and the various levels and types of exposure. Estimates of the common rate ratios $r_2,...,r_J$ and 95% confidence intervals under hypothesis H_1 can be obtained by applying the Mantel-Haenszel formulas (6.5) and (6.6) separately to each of the $J - 1$ exposed groups, treating the referent group as unexposed. That is, the Mantel-Haenszel estimate of rate-ratio r_j in the jth group is obtained from formula (6.5) by replacing the number d_{2k} of deaths and the number n_{2k} of person-years by the corresponding numbers d_{jk} and n_{jk} in exposure group j. Table 6–11 shows the Mantel-Haenszel estimates and confidence intervals for the rate ratios associated with cigarette smoking for the respiratory cancer data of Table 6–6. For example, the numerator of the Mantel-Haenszel estimate of the death rate ratio r_2 for occasional smokers relative to nonsmokers is, from formula (6.5), $N = [0 \times 35,164/(35,164 + 3,657)] + [0 \times 15,134/(15,134 + 1,283)] + [6 \times 213,858/(213,858 + 14,624)] + [10$

Table 6-10. Calculations for Trend Test Statistic χ^2_{TREND} from Veterans' Data of Table 6-6

$$\chi^2_{TREND} = \frac{[\sum_{j=1}^{6} x_j(O_j - E_j)]^2}{\sum_{j=1}^{6} x_j^2 E_j - \sum_{k=1}^{5} [(\sum_{j=1}^{6} x_j \hat{d}_{jk})^2 / D_k]}$$

Smoking Group j	O_j	E_j	x_j	$x_j(O_j - E_j)$	$x_j^2 E_j$
1	78	504.3	0	0	0
2	17	31.9	0.5	-7.4	7.8
3	80	108.3	5	-141.5	2707.5
4	441	325.5	15	1732.5	73,237.5
5	460	189.2	30	8127.0	170,190.0
6	118	34.8	50	4160.0	87,000
Total	1194	1194.0	—	13,870.6	333,142.8

Age Group k	\multicolumn{6}{c}{$x_j\hat{d}$ for smoking group j}			
	1	2	3	4	5	6	Total	Deaths D_k	$(\sum_{j=1}^{6} x_j \hat{d}_{jk})^2 / D_k$
1	0	0.05	1.5	36.0	48.0	10.0	95.6	6	1521.6
2	0	0.2	4.5	67.5	105.0	25.0	202.2	14	2920.3
3	0	7.4	228.0	2295.0	3117.0	990.0	6651.4	553	79,665.6
4	0	7.8	287.0	2359.5	2322.0	690.0	5666.3	586	54,789.1
5	0	0.6	20.5	124.5	81.0	25.0	251.6	35	1807.9
Total									140,704.6

$$\chi^2_{TREND} = \frac{(13,870.6)^2}{333,142.8 - 140,704.6} = 999.8$$

Table 6–11. Estimates and Confidence Intervals (CIs) for Common Rate Ratios for Data of Table 6–6

	Mantel-Haenszel[a] Rate Ratio	95% CI	Maximum Likelihood[b] Rate Ratio	95% CI
Nonsmokers	1.0	—	1.0	—
Smokers				
Occasional	3.52	2.08–5.95	3.47	2.05–5.87
Regular (cigarettes per day)				
1–9	4.76	3.48–6.50	4.77	3.49–6.51
10–20	9.00	7.07–11.46	8.87	6.97–11.29
21–39	16.66	12.99–21.37	16.62	12.74–20.64
40+	23.68	17.63–31.80	22.62	16.99–30.12

[a]Obtained from formula (6.5) with separate comparison of each smoking group to nonsmokers.
[b]Obtained by using EGRET software (Mauritsen, 1994).

$\times$ 171,211/(171,211 + 10,053)] + [1 $\times$ 8,480/(8,480 + 512)] = 5.6160 + 9.4453 + 0.9431 = 16.0044. The denominator is [0 $\times$ 3,657/(35,164 + 3,657)] + [0 $\times$ 1,283/(15,134 + 1,283)] + [25 $\times$ 14,624/(213,858 + 14,624)] + [49 $\times$ 10,053/(171,211 + 10,053)] + [4 $\times$ 512/(8,480 + 512)] = 1.6001 + 2.7176 + 0.2278 = 4.5454. Thus, the Mantel-Haenszel estimate for r_2 is N/D = 16.0044/4.5454 = 3.52.

Having estimated the rate ratios $r_2,...,r_J$, the next step is *testing the hypothesis H_1* of common rate ratios across age strata. This can be done by evaluating the sum of squared standardized residuals given by χ^2_{HET} in formula (6.8), where the inner summation is now taken over the range $j = 1$ to $j = J$. Also in (6.8), $\hat{d}_{jk} = D_k n_{jk} r_j/(n_{1k}r_1 + n_{2k}r_2 + ... + n_{jK}r_J)$ is the fitted number of deaths in a cell, with $r_1 = 1$ and with Mantel-Haenszel estimates for $r_2,...,r_J$. For the respiratory cancer data of Table 6–6 we find for nonsmokers aged 35–44 years, for example, that $d_{11} = 0$ and $\hat{d}_{11} = 6 \times 35,164 \times 1.0/(35,164 \times 1.0 + 3.657 \times 3.52 + 8,063 \times 4.76 + 59,965 \times 9.00 + 40,643 \times 16.66 + 3,992 \times 23.68) = 210,984/1,397,744.5 = 0.15$, where the Mantel-Haenszel estimates $r_1 = 1.0$, $r_2 = 3.52$, $r_3 = 4.76$, $r_4 = 9.00$, $r_5 = 16.66$, $r_6 = 23.68$ are obtained from Table 6–11. Thus, in formula (6.8) the first summand is $(d_{11} - \hat{d}_{11})^2/\hat{d}_{11} = (0 - 0.15)^2/0.15 = 0.15$. Continuing in this way, we compute the $J \times K = 6 \times 5 = 30$ summands in formula (6.8), finally obtaining $\chi^2_{\text{HET}} = 10.67$. The number of degrees of freedom associated with χ^2_{HET} is the number of cells with nonzero person-years of observation, minus the number $J + K - 1$ of fitted parameters in the multiplicative model. For the respiratory cancer data with $K = 5$ and $J = 6$, the number of degrees of freedom is $J \times K - (J + K - 1) = 30 - 10 = 20$. The probability that a chi-squared variable with 20 degrees of freedom achieves the value 10.67 or higher is $p = 0.95$; thus the data agree well with the hypothesis that rate ratios associated with the smoking categories do not vary with age.

As discussed in an earlier section (Testing homogeneity of rate ratios across confounder strata) in the context of two exposure groups, agreement between model predictions and the data can be checked by examining the (studentized) standardized residuals for the cells of the table. If the hypothesis of common rate ratios adequately summarizes the data, these residuals should be distributed approximately as independent normal variables, each with mean zero and variance one. Table 6–12 shows the residuals for the respiratory cancer data. None falls outside the range $\pm$ 1.96 (the range of plausible values for a standard normal variable), and collectively they show no systematic trends with age or smoking status. Thus, the standardized residuals provide further evidence that rate ratios associated with the smoking categories do not vary with age.

Model Fitting by the Method of Maximum Likelihood

We have seen that relatively simple methods that do not require a computer program can be used to test the null hypothesis, to obtain estimates of the exposure effects under the multiplicative model given by hypothesis H_1, and to examine the fit of this model. However, an analysis usually will have several additional objectives. For example, the investigator may wish to describe how the rates vary with levels of both exposure and age (or other covariates). In particular, the investigator may wish to introduce and compare several specific functions describing how the death rates vary with exposure (sometimes called fitting a "dose-response curve") in order to select one that adequately fits the data. Finally, because there are many possible ways of summarizing the joint effects of exposure and age, the investigator will want to choose among them and evaluate the adequacy of

Table 6–12. Studentized Standardized Residuals[a] for the Multiplicative Model Fit to the Data of Table 6–6

Age (years)	35–44	45–54	55–64	65–74	75–84
Nonsmokers	−0.389	−0.692	−0.805	0.948	0.174
Smokers					
Occasional	−0.235	0.378	−0.402	0.387	0.250
Regular					
(cigarettes per day)					
1–9	−0.406	−0.687	0.269	−0.023	0.525
10–20	−0.208	−1.237	−0.323	0.671	−0.126
21–39	0.641	1.236	0.605	−1.000	−0.717
40+	−0.637	0.459	−0.112	−0.399	0.405

[a](Observed deaths − expected deaths)/(Expected deaths)$^{1/2}$, where the expected deaths are fitted under the assumption that smoking rate-ratios do not vary with age.

fit of the preferred model. All of these objectives can be accomplished by fitting to the data a series of models by the method of maximum likelihood, and comparing the goodness-of-fit of the various models by evaluating statistics called deviances. These procedures require a computer and software such as GLIM (Baker and Nelder, 1978), EGRET (Mauritsen, 1994), or SAS (1990).

As noted earlier in this chapter, maximum likelihood estimates are optimal in the sense of tending to have less variability than other estimates. The method of maximum likelihood (and other methods based on estimating equations that are beyond the scope of this book) offer an additional advantage: they provide sets of tools for a systematic approach to all goals of the analysis. Specifically, by fitting and evaluating a series of models, the investigator can accomplish simultaneously all three objectives of testing the null hypothesis of no exposure effect, of estimating measures of association relating death rates to exposures and covariates, and of evaluating goodness of model fit.

To describe these methods, we need the notion of nested models. One model is said to be *nested* in another larger one if it arises by restricting some of the parameters in the larger model, either by specifying values for them or by requiring that they satisfy certain constraints. For the data in Table 6–1, for example, we consider two models. The larger one allows two unknown parameters, the death rate I_1 for the nonreligious, and the death rate I_2 for the religious. The smaller model, which is specified by the null hypothesis that death rates are unrelated to religiousness, involves only one unknown parameter: the common death rate for both religious and nonreligious. The second model is nested in the first larger one, because it arises from the first one by specifying $I_1 = I_2$.

For such a pair of nested models, a test of the small model relative to the larger one can be based on the *deviance* between them. The deviance is a statistic that reflects the probability of observing the data when their sampling distribution is determined by the small model, relative to the corresponding probability under the large model. Specifically, the deviance is twice the logarithm of the ratio of the likelihood of the data under the large model divided by the likelihood of the data under the small model. For this reason deviances are also called likelihood ratio statistics.[4]

In calculating the deviance, the unknown parameters in large and small models are replaced by their maximum likelihood estimates. If the death rates underlying the data follow the small model, the sampling distribution of the deviance is approximately that of a chi-squared variable. The number of degrees of freedom of its distribution is the difference between the number of fitted parameters in the large model and that of the small model. The deviance has a convenient additive property when applied to three nested models (large, medium, and small): the deviance between large and small models is the sum of the deviance between large and medium models and the deviance between medium and small models.

Table 6–13 shows a series of nested models for analyzing data such as those of Zuckerman in Tables 6–1 and 6–3, and the respiratory cancer data of Table 6–6. Table 6–13 is similar to the layout for an analysis of variance in linear regression. Model 5 stipulates that all $J \times K$ death rates are unrestricted; this largest model involves $J \times K$ parameters (a death rate for each cell) and it contains all the other models. The multiplicative Model 4 is nested in Model 5 because it restricts the JK death rates: it requires that the rate ratios relating exposure group j to the referent ($j = 1$) be independent of age (indexed by k): $I_{j1}/I_{11} = I_{j2}/I_{12} = \ldots = I_{jK}/I_{1K}$. In Table 6–13 this common rate ratio is denoted simply by r_j. Models 2 and 3 are both nested in Model 4. Model 2 specifies that the $J - 1$ rate ratios relating the exposed to the referent are all one: $r_2 = \ldots = r_J = 1$. Thus, Model 2 specifies that there is no effect of exposure. Model 3 specifies that the K age-specific rates in the referent group are equal: $s_1 = s_2 = \ldots = s_K$. Neither one of Models 2 and 3 is nested in the other. Model 1 stipulates that all $J \times K$ death rates are equal; this smallest model involves only one parameter (the single death rate). Model 1 arises from Model 2 by stipulating that the age-specific rates are all equal, and from Model 3 by stipulating that the exposure-specific rates are all equal. Because Models 2 and 3 are themselves nested in Model 4, which is in turn nested in Model 5, we see that

Table 6–13. Models for General Data of Table 6–7

Model for Rates in Sampled Population	Rate for Cell (j,k)[a]	Number of Parameters	Degrees of Freedom of Deviance[b]
1. No effects of confounder (e.g., age) or exposure	Constant, independent of age and exposure	1	$JK - 1$
2. No exposure effect	Equals age-specific rate s_k in referent group	K	$JK - K$
3. No age effect	Equals rate in youngest age group at exposure level j	J	$JK - J$
4. Multiplicative effects of age and exposure	Product of referent rate s_k times common rate ratio r_j	$J + K - 1$	$JK - J - K + 1$
5. Unrestricted rates	Arbitrary variation with age and exposure	JK	0

[a]Corresponding to exposure level j and age category k.

[b]Relative to the unrestricted Model 5.

Model 1 is nested in all the other models. Also shown in Table 6–13 for each model is the number of fitted parameters in the model, and the number of degrees of freedom relative to that of the largest Model 5.

Application to data of Zuckerman et al. We illustrate the strengths of the maximum likelihood method by reexamining the mortality data of Zuckerman et al. (1984), presented previously in Tables 6–1 and 6–3. Table 6–14 shows a series of nested models and, for each, the deviance between the model and Model 5.

To compute the deviance between two models we use the formula for χ^2_{DEV} in Table 6–9. This formula requires the expected number of deaths $\hat{d}_{jk}$ in each of the JK cells, where $\hat{d}_{jk} = n_{jk}\hat{I}_{jk}$ is the product of the n_{jk} of person-years in cell (j,k) times the maximum likelihood estimate (MLE) $\hat{I}_{jk}$ of the rate for the cell. The MLEs $\hat{I}_{jk}$ vary from one model to another. Under Model 1, the MLE for $I_{jk} \equiv I$ is the total number of deaths divided by the total number of person-years. From Table 6–1, $\hat{I} = 47/749 = .063$, and the $\hat{d}_{jk}$ are obtained by multiplying the person-years n_{jk} by .063. Under Model 2, the MLE for $I_{jk} \equiv I_k$ for the kth stratum defined by gender and health status is the number $d_{1k} + d_{2k}$ of deaths in the stratum divided by the number $n_{1k} + n_{2k}$ of person-years in the stratum. Thus, from Table 6–3, $\hat{I}_1 = 9/145 = .062$, $\hat{I}_2 = 17/87 = .195$, $\hat{I}_3 = 4/298 = .013$, and $\hat{I}_4 = 17/219 = .078$. Similarly, the MLEs for $I_{1k} = I^{(1)}$ and $I_{2k} = I^{(2)}$ under Model 3 are $\hat{I}^{(1)} = 29/331 = .088$ and $\hat{I}^{(2)} = 18/418 = .043$. The maximum likelihood estimate of the common rate ratio for the religious relative to the non-religious is simply the maximum likelihood estimate of $r = r_2$ in the multiplicative Model 4, which we had computed earlier using EGRET software (Mauritsen, 1994) as 0.555. Finally, the maximum likelihood estimates of the $J \times K$ death rates in the unrestricted Model 5 are just the observed rates $\hat{I}_{jk} = d_{jk}/n_{jk}$. Therefore, the fitted numbers of deaths $\hat{d}_{jk} = \hat{I}_{jk}n_{jk}$ for this model are just the observed numbers d_{jk}.

Once we have estimated the expected numbers $\hat{d}_{jk}$ under each of the models, we use the formula of Table 6–9 to compute deviances between pairs of models, with the large model taken as Model 5 and the small model taken as the one under test. For example, referring to the data in Table 6–3, the deviance between Models 1 and 5 is $\chi^2_{\text{DEV}} = 2 (Y + Z)$, where

$$Y = 5 \ln \left(\frac{5}{79 \times .063} \right) + 4 \ln \left(\frac{4}{66 \times .063} \right) + 13 \ln \left(\frac{13}{49 \times .063} \right)$$

$$+ 4 \ln \left(\frac{4}{38 \times .063} \right) + 2 \ln \left(\frac{2}{122 \times .063} \right) + 2 \ln \left(\frac{2}{176 \times .063} \right)$$

$$+ 9 \ln \left(\frac{9}{81 \times .063} \right) + 8 \ln \left(\frac{8}{138 \times .063} \right) = 18.93,$$

Table 6–14. Models for Data of Tables 6–1 and 6–3; $J = 2$ Exposure Groups; $K = 4$ Covariate Strata

Model for Rates in Sampled Population	Rate for Cell (j,k) [a]	Number of Parameters	Degrees of Freedom	Deviance [b]
1. No effect of gender, health status, or religiousness	Constant, independent of gender, health status and religiousness	1	$JK - 1 = 7$	38.2
2. No effect of religiousness	Specific for gender and health status, independent of religiousness	$K = 4$	$JK - K = 4$	4.9
3. No effect of gender or health status	Specific for religiousness, independent of gender and health status	$J = 2$	$JK - J = 6$	32.4
4. Multiplicative effect of religiousness with gender and health status	Specific for gender and health status, times a common rate-ratio r_2 for religiousness	$J + K - 1 = 5$	$JK - J - K + 1 = 3$	1.1
5. Unrestricted death rates	Arbitrary variation with gender, health status and religiousness	$JK = 8$	0	0

[a] Corresponding to religiousness ($j = 1$: nonreligious, $j = 2$: religious) and gender/health status ($k = 1$: male well, $k = 2$: male ill; $k = 3$: female well, $k = 4$: female ill).
[b] Relative to the unrestricted Model 5.

and

$$Z = (79 \times .063) - 5 + (66 \times .063) - 4 + \cdots + (138 \times .063) - 8 = 0.19.$$

So $\chi^2_{\mathrm{DEV}} = 2(18.93 + .19) = 38.24$.

Figure 6–4 shows how these deviances can be used to construct a hierarchy of tests for model criticism. First, an unstratified test of the null

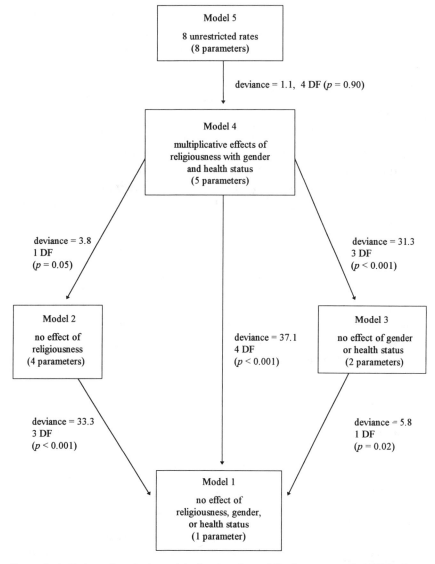

Figure 6–4. Series of nested models for the data of Zuckerman et al. (1984) shown in Table 6–3. The models are described further in Table 6–14.

hypothesis that rates do not vary with exposure (religiousness) is based on the deviance between Model 3 (no effect of gender, health status but possibly an exposure effect) and Model 1 (no effect of gender, health status or religiousness). The deviance for Model 1 (small model) versus Model 3 (large model) is $5.8 = 38.2 - 32.4$, the difference in deviances for Models 1 and 3 in Table 6–14. The number of degrees of freedom associated with this deviance is $J - 1 = 1$. The value 5.8 agrees with the value $\chi^2 = 5.843$ obtained earlier from the chi-squared test statistic given by formula (6.2).

Next, a stratified test of the null hypothesis that rates do not vary with religiousness is based on the deviance between Model 4 (possible effects of both confounders and religiousness) and Model 2 (possible confounder effects but no religiousness effect). Subtracting the deviances for Models 2 and 4 in Table 6–14, we find a deviance of 3.8 on $J + K - 1 - K = J - 1$ $= 1$ degree of freedom. This value agrees with the value 3.8 previously obtained for the stratified test statistic χ^2 of formula (6.4).

Finally, a test for heterogeneity in the rate ratios of Table 6–4 is based on the deviance between Model 5 and Model 4. For the data of Table 6–3, we find in Table 6–14 and Figure 6–4 a deviance of 1.1 on $JK - K - J + 1$ $= K - 1 = 3$ degrees of freedom. This value agrees with the value 1.09 for the sum of squared standardized residuals given by χ^2_{HET} of equation (6.8).

In summary, the deviances for the nested series of models in Figure 6–4 suggest that a multiplicative model for the joint effects of religiousness and gender/health status (Model 4) is adequate, but that no smaller model is adequate. That is, death rates vary both with religiousness and with gender/health status.

This example shows that the succinct set of nested models and deviances shown in Table 6–14 and Figure 6–4 provides all of the results of the various tools described in the previous sections.

REFERENCES

Baker RJ, Nelder JA. 1978. The GLIM System: Release 3. Oxford, Numerical Algorithms Group.

Breslow NE, Day NE. 1987. Statistical Models in Cancer Research. Vol. 2. The analysis of cohort studies. Lyon, IARC Press.

Chang H-GH, Morse DL, Noonan C, Coles B, Mikl J, Rosen A, Putnam P, Smith PF. 1993. Survival and mortality patterns of an acquired immunodeficiency syndrome (AIDS) cohort in New York State. *Am J Epidemiol* 138: 341–349.

Jacobsen SJ, Sargent DJ, Atkinson EJ, O'Fallon WM, Melton LJ III. 1995. Population-based study of the contribution of weather to hip fracture seasonality. *Am J Epidemiol* 141:79–83.

Kahn H. 1966. The Dorn study of smoking and mortality among U.S. veterans: report on eight and one-half years of observation. *NCI Monogr* 19:1–125.

Kalbfleisch J, Prentice RL. 1980. The Statistical Analysis of Failure Time Data. New York, Wiley.

Kaplan EL, Meier P. 1958. Nonparametric estimation from incomplete observations. *J Am Stat Assoc* 53:457–481.

Lee ET. 1980. Statistical Methods for Survival Analysis. Belmont, CA, Lifetime Learning Publications.

Mauritsen R. 1994. EGRET. Seattle, WA., Statistics and Epidemiology Research Corporation.

McCullagh P, Nelder JA. 1989. Genealogical Linear Models. 2nd Ed. London, New York, Chapman Hall.

SAS Language. 1990. Version 6.x. First Edition. Cary, NC., SAS Institute Inc.

Zuckerman DM, Kasl SV, Ostfeld AM. 1984. Psychosocial predictors of mortality among the elderly poor: the role of religion, well-being, and social contacts. *Am J Epidemiol* 119:419–423.

Exercises

1. A small group of individuals was followed prospectively from January 1, 1995, to February 1, 1995, to monitor the incidence of adverse reactions to a drug. The results were as follows:

Patient	Date of Outcome	Outcome
1	2/1	No reaction
2	2/1	No reaction
3	1/9	Adverse reaction
4	2/1	No reaction
5	1/13	Dropped out of study
6	1/15	Adverse reaction
7	1/18	Adverse reaction
8	2/1	No reaction
9	1/25	Dropped out of study
10	2/1	No reaction

Assuming that the two patients who dropped out of the study had not had a reaction as of the time they dropped out, calculate the product-limit estimate of the risk of developing an adverse reaction during the month of January.

2. In a study of survival of people diagnosed with AIDS in New York State, Chang et al. (1993) used the Kaplan-Meier method to estimate the cumulative proportions surviving 1, 2, and 3 years after diagnosis. They obtained the following results:

Variable	Cumulative Proportion Surviving		
	1 Year Proportion (SE)[a]	2 Years Proportion (SE)	3 Years Proportion (SE)
Age (years) at diagnosis			
<30	0.538 (0.018)	0.321 (0.018)	0.211 (0.018)
30–34	0.509 (0.017)	0.311 (0.016)	0.189 (0.016)
35–39	0.485 (0.017)	0.291 (0.017)	0.177 (0.016)
≥40	0.441 (0.014)	0.253 (0.013)	0.164 (0.013)
AIDS risk factor			
Men who had sex with men (MSWM) only	0.517 (0.012)	0.292 (0.012)	0.164 (0.011)
Injecting drug user (IDU) only	0.466 (0.014)	0.295 (0.013)	0.205 (0.014)
Both MSWM and IDU	0.432 (0.036)	0.228 (0.033)	0.145 (0.030)
Other	0.472 (0.021)	0.293 (0.021)	0.203 (0.021)
Total	0.488 (0.008)	0.290 (0.008)	0.183 (0.008)

[a] Standard error.

    a. What proportion of the total cohort survived until 1 year? 2 years? 3 years?
    b. How did survival vary by age?
    c. How did survival vary by AIDS risk factors?
    d. Note the standard errors for the estimates of (i) the proportion of the entire cohort surviving for 3 years and (ii) the proportion of those in the "both MSWM and IDU" category surviving for 3 years. Why do you think one standard error is larger than the other?
    e. Why was the Kaplan-Meier method used in this table?

3. Use the data in Table 6–3 to consider the following:
    a. Calculate an estimate of the summary (common) rate ratio for the association between religiousness and morality when stratification is on the basis of gender but not initial health status.
    b. Calculate a 95% confidence interval for this rate ratio.
    c. Calculate the corresponding rate ratio and 95% confidence interval when stratification is on the basis of initial health status but not gender.
    d. What do these results indicate about the nature of any confounding of the association between religiousness and mortality?

4. Is there any evidence that health status modifies the association between religiousness and mortality? Examine this question by (a) testing for heterogeneity in the rate ratios and (b) examining residuals.

5. In a retrospective cohort study of the effects of season and weather on hip fracture incidence in Rochester, Minnesota, Jacobsen et al. (1995) used Poisson regression analysis to examine the association between weather and season and hip fracture incidence. Incidence rates were calculated as the number of fractures divided by person-days at risk. Incidence rates were calculated for each calendar day of year, aggregating the number of fractures and person-time at risk over the 38-year follow-up period. When the investigators examined the effect of season alone on hip fracture incidence, they obtained the following results for women in the age group 45–74 years.

Season	Crude Rate Ratio	95% Confidence Interval
Summer	1.00[a]	
Fall	1.05	0.76–1.46
Winter	1.44	1.06–1.96
Spring	1.10	0.80–1.52

[a]Reference category.

a. What do the rate ratio and 95% confidence interval of 1.44 (1.06–1.96) for winter mean?

The investigators then used Poisson regression to construct a multivariate model in which several variables representing season and weather type were all adjusted for simultaneously:

Season or Weather Type	Adjusted Rate Ratio[a]	95% Confidence Interval
Summer, clear	1.00[b]	
Season		
Fall	0.95	0.67–1.33
Winter	1.16	0.81–1.65
Spring	1.08	0.78–1.50
Weather type		
Snow or blowing snow	1.22	0.91–1.63
Freezing rain, freezing drizzle, or glaze	1.60	1.06–2.41
Rain	0.87	0.67–1.13
High wind	0.79	0.32–1.92

[a]Each rate ratio is adjusted for the effects of all other variables in the table.

[b]Referent category.

b. What do the rate ratio and 95% confidence interval of 1.16 (0.81–1.65) for winter mean?

Among women age 75 years and older, the following results were reported regarding season:

Season	Crude Rate Ratio	95% Confidence Interval
Summer	1.00[a]	
Fall	1.03	0.85–1.25
Winter	1.16	0.96–1.40
Spring	0.81	0.66–0.99

[a]Referent category.

c. What do the rate ratio and 95% confidence interval of 1.16 (0.96–1.40) for winter mean?

When a multivariate model was constructed in which several variables representing season and weather type were adjusted for simultaneously, the following results were obtained:

Season or Weather Type	Adjusted Rate Ratio[a]	95% Confidence Interval
Summer, clear	1.00[b]	
Season		
Fall	1.03	0.84–1.25
Winter	1.15	0.93–1.43
Spring	0.80	0.65–0.98
Weather type		
Snow or blowing snow	1.01	0.84–1.22
Freezing rain, freezing drizzle, or glaze	0.89	0.65–1.21
Rain	0.96	0.82–1.13
High wind	1.35	0.88–2.08

[a]Each rate ratio is adjusted for the effects of all other variables in the table.

[b]Referent category.

d. What do the rate ratio and 95% confidence interval of 1.15 (0.93–1.43) for winter mean?

e. What are possible explanations of these findings regarding the effect of season and weather on hip fracture incidence?

NOTES

1. A Poisson sampling distribution for a count of events gives the probability of observing n events by the formula $M^n e^{-M}/n!$. Here M is the mean number of events in the population. If a count of events has a Poisson distribution, its variance equals its mean.

2. The natural logarithm of a quantity, often denoted in formulas by ln or $\log_e$, is the logarithm to the base e. In formulas, we shall use the notation "ln" for the natural logarithm, which should not be confused with the logarithm to the base 10, denoted $\log_{10}$. Exponentiating ln x gives x: $e^{\ln x} = x$.

3. Depending on the context, the common rate ratio (or risk ratio or odds ratio) is also called the *summary* or *adjusted* rate ratio (or risk ratio or odds ratio).

4. The term *deviance* is used because this statistic is the logarithm of a ratio and therefore represents the difference between two quantities.

7

Cohort Studies:
Statistical Analysis II

Chapter 6 described Poisson regression methods for analysing cohort data, implemented by stratifying counts of death and person-years of observation into a two-dimensional table of exposure levels (rows) and covariates (columns), and examining death rates in the cells of the table. In this chapter we consider an alternative to Poisson regression, called Cox regression (Cox, 1972), and other methods useful in special situations when the methods of Chapter 6 are inappropriate or impractical. The first of these special situations occurs when information on the exposures and/or potential confounding variables of interest are readily available only at great expense, relative to the disease or death data. For example, in a retrospective cohort study of the relation between prostate-specific antigen (PSA) and subsequent incidence of prostate cancer, the "exposures" were PSA levels in sera drawn and stored at the time of repeated medical examinations (Whittemore et al., 1995). Because of the expense of retrieving and analyzing the large number of serum samples, PSA levels were assayed for only two small subsets of cohort members: men who subsequently developed prostate cancer and a sample of men who did not. The analytic methods appropriate here are based on *nested case-control* and *case-cohort* designs. These designs were described in Chapter 5.

The second situation requiring special methods occurs when interest centers on the effects of one or more exposures but the cohort contains no unexposed subcohort for comparison. Instead, death rates in the cohort must be compared to national or regional rates, or rates in some other comparison population. In a study of radiogenic cancers in patients with tuberculosis who received multiple fluoroscopic chest examinations (Boice and Monson, 1977), cancer death rates in patients were compared to Massachusetts mortality rates. The methods appropriate for this situation are based on *standardized mortality ratios* (SMRs) or *standardized incidence ratios* (SIRs).

The third situation requiring special methods occurs when person-years at risk are unavailable or inappropriate for the cohort. Milham (1982) used death certificates to code the occupations of all white male residents of Washington State aged 20 years or older who died between 1950 and 1979. The occupations of interest were those involving exposures to electrical and magnetic fields. Thus, the exposed group consisted of men whose occupations (as recorded on their death certificates) could have involved these exposures. The outcome of interest was death from leukemia. Person-years at risk were unavailable, so the author compared the proportion of all deaths from leukemia in the exposed group to the corresponding proportion among all other deceased white male Washington State residents. A similar situation arises when person-years at risk, though available from some source, cannot be applied to the population contributing the deaths. For instance, when working with registry-based cancer counts, person-years at risk based on census data for Hispanics in the region covered by the registry may not pertain to the same population as the one designated Hispanic by the registry. This discrepancy can occur because the census uses self-reported ethnicity, whereas the registry uses ethnicity as indicated by hospital staff. Because cause-specific death rates may vary with age, gender, race/ethnicity and time of death, it is important that the analysis accommodate possible differences in these characteristics between the exposed and comparison groups. The methods appropriate for this situation are based on *proportional mortality ratios* (PMRs) or *proportional incidence ratios* (PIRs).

COX REGRESSION FOR ANALYSIS OF AN ENTIRE COHORT

As noted in Chapter 6, an essential feature of the analysis of cohort data is accounting for the time at risk for disease that is contributed by individuals while they are under observation. A key assumption underlying the methods of Chapter 6 is that the death or disease rate does not vary within the boundaries of each cell of the two-dimensional table defined by stratifying exposures and confounding variables. In principle, this approximation could be improved by finer stratification of the variables, giving smaller cells. In practice, however, a large proportion of cells containing few or no deaths compromises the statistical approximations underlying the inferences. Other methods, based on modeling the death rates as varying functions of time considered as a continuous variable, do not assume that the rates are constant within discrete categories. These are called "continuous time methods," or "Cox regression methods" (Cox, 1972), and they are useful for the analysis of nested case-control and case-cohort designs, as well as for cohort studies. However, they can be computationally intensive when used to analyze large cohort studies, yet are unlikely to yield inferences that differ appreciably from those based on the methods of Chapter 6 (Breslow et al., 1983).

The Cox regression method assumes that the death or disease rate for the population from which the cohort is sampled depends on a continuous time variable, denoted as t. It also depends on risk factors through some unknown constants that represent measures of association between the outcome of interest and the risk factors. Typically, the investigator has several choices for the time variable, such as age, time since start of observation, or time since first employment in an occupation. Detailed guidelines for choosing among the time variables is beyond the scope of this book. In general, however, a good time variable is one for which the death or disease rate increases or decreases strongly. In a study of lung cancer among uranium miners, for example, the time variable might be age (which is highly correlated with lung cancer death rates) rather than time since first underground mining; in a study of predictors for breast cancer survival, the most appropriate time variable might be time since diagnosis.

For a given time variable, the investigator records the times at which cohort members fail (i.e., die of the cause of interest, or develop the disease or other outcome of interest). We call these cohort members *cases*. The investigator also records the risk factors and potential confounding variables for each cohort member. We use the term *predictor variables* to denote the risk factors of interest, the potential confounding variables, and any variables that may modify the effects of the risk factors. Let $x_1, \ldots, x_p$ denote a particular person's values of the p predictor variables to be examined in a Cox regressional model. Also, let $I(t,x)$ denote that person's death or disease rate at time t. The Cox regression model specifies that

$$\ln[I(t,x)/I(t, x^*)] = b_1(x_1 - x_1^*) + \ldots + b_p(x_p - x_p^*). \quad (7.1)$$

Here $x^* = x_1^*, \ldots, x_p^*$ represents arbitrary values for the predictor variables, chosen as baseline values of comparison. $I(t, x^*)$ is called the *baseline rate*. Also $b_1, \ldots, b_p$ are unknown constants estimated from the data, and are called *regression coefficients*.

Notice that the left side of equation (7.1) is the logarithm of the death rate ratio for a person with variables x relative to someone with baseline values x^*. By exponentiating both sides of equation (7.1) we see that the death rate at time t for a person with predictor variables x is

$$I(t, x) = I(t, x^*)\exp[b_1(x_1 - x_1^*) + \ldots + b_p(x_p - x_p^*)]. \quad (7.2)$$

If the regression coefficient b_j for the jth predictor variable is close to zero ($j = 1, \ldots, p$), then variation of that variable will not contribute much to the variation in the death rate $I(t, x)$ as calculated from equation (7.2). On the other hand, if the coefficient for that variable is a large number (positive

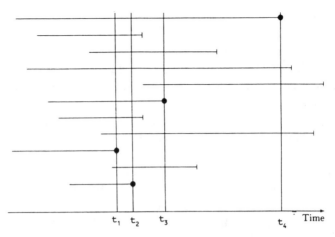

Figure 7-1. Illustration of risk sets in a hypothetical cohort study of 11 persons (horizontal lines). Four individuals (cases, represented by solid circles) developed the disease of interest (i.e., failed), at times t_1, t_2, t_3, t_4. The risk set of a case consists of those individuals whose lines intersect the vertical line at his or her failure time. Notice that cohort members may enter and exit from follow-up at varying times, and that cases belong to the risk sets of other cases who fail before they do.

or negative), then that variable will contribute strongly to the magnitude of the death rate.

The regression coefficients $b_1, \ldots, b_p$, which are of primary interest, are estimated by maximizing a "partial likelihood," so called because it does not involve any unknown constants in the baseline rate $I(t, x^*)$, which usually are not of interest to the investigator. The maximization is accomplished by comparing the risk factors of each case to those of all cohort members who are at risk just before he or she fails. The collection of these individuals includes the case himself or herself, and is called the *risk set* for the case. Figure 7-1 shows the composition of the risk sets for four cases (solid dots) at time t_1, t_2, t_3, t_4. Notice that the risk sets include future cases, i.e., cohort members who subsequently develop the disease.

The partial likelihood is a product of terms, one from each cohort member who fails (i.e., each case). To describe the contribution from a typical case who fails at time t, let R_{it} be the death rate ratio for the ith person in this case's risk set. That is, if person i has predictor variable $x = x_{i1}, \ldots, x_{ip}$ at time t, then

$$R_{it} = \frac{I(t,x)}{I(t,x^*)} = \exp[b_1(x_{i1} - x_1^*) + \cdots + b_p(x_{ip} - x_p^*)]. \quad (7.3)$$

The case's contribution to the partial likelihood is his or her rate ratio divided by the sum of the rate ratios of all subjects in his or her risk set:

$$\frac{R_{0t}}{R_{0t} + R_{1t} + \cdots + R_{Nt}}. \tag{7.4}$$

Here the subscript $i = 0$ denotes the case, and there are N other members in the risk set. Finding regression coefficients to maximize the likelihood requires a computer and software such as SAS (1990), EGRET (Mauritsen, 1994), or GLIM (Baker and Nelder, 1978).

Once the regression coefficients have been estimated, standard errors can be obtained by standard methods whose description is beyond the scope of this book. Confidence limits for the regression coefficients can then be computed in the usual way, and exponentiated to give a confidence interval for the corresponding rate ratios.

Table 7–1 illustrates the results of a Cox regression analysis of the relation between 5-year mortality and several measures of physical and mental health and cognitive functioning among 1118 elderly male participants of the Western Collaborative Group Study (Swan et al., 1995). The estimated regression coefficients for the $p = 8$ predictor variables are shown in column 2. The primary predictor variable of interest was cognitive functioning, as measured by a man's score on a standardized test called the Digit Symbol Substitution test. The investigators chose for their time variable the time from test administration to death or study completion. Information on the other predictor variables in Table 7–1 was obtained at the time of testing.

The first four variables $x_1, \ldots, x_4$ were coded as continuous variables. The baseline values $x_1^*, \ldots, x_4^*$ are typically taken to be their means among all cohort members, but the choice is arbitrary, as it does not affect the estimated regression coefficients. Thus, according to equation (7.2), $b_1, \ldots, b_4$ estimate the change in the logarithm of the death rate per unit change in the associated variable. For example, the death rate ratio of 0.96 associated with the digit symbol score was obtained by exponentiating -0.041; it suggests a 4% decrease in death rate with each unit increase in the raw test score, adjusting for the effects of all the other variables in the table. Confidence limits were obtained from the regression coefficient, standard error, and standard normal deviate (1.96) in a manner similar to that described in Chapter 6. Education (x_5) was coded as an ordinal variable assuming seven levels, with level 1 as the baseline level. Thus b_5 estimates the change in logarithm of the death rate per increase of one point on the education scale. The remaining variables, x_6, x_7, x_8 were coded as dichotomies, assuming the value 1 if the attribute was present and zero if it was absent. Thus, b_6, b_7, b_8 estimate the logarithm of the death rate ratio among those with the attribute relative to those without it. For example, the death rate ratio of 2.78 associated with a cancer history indicates that men

Table 7–1. Results of Cox Regression Analysis Relating Physical and Mental Status to All-Cause Mortality among Elderly Men in the Western Collaborative Group Study

	Variable	Regression Coefficient	(Standard Error)	Death Rate Ratio	95% Confidence Interval	p Value
x_1	Age (years)	0.058	(.024)	1.06	1.01–1.11	0.016
x_2	Digit symbol score[a]	−0.041	(.011)	0.96	0.94–0.98	0.004
x_3	Serum cholesterol (mg/dl)	−0.223	(.249)	0.80	0.49–1.30	>0.05
x_4	Systolic blood pressure (mm Hg)	0.157	(.228)	1.17	0.75–1.83	>0.05
x_5	Education[b]	0.049	(.220)	1.05	0.68–1.61	>0.05
x_6	Cancer history (yes/no)	1.022	(.248)	2.78	1.71–4.52	<0.001
x_7	Cardiovascular disease (yes/no)	0.652	(.226)	1.92	1.23–2.99	0.004
x_8	Cigarette smoking (ever/never)	0.068	(.187)	1.07	0.74–1.54	>0.05

[a]See Swan et al. (1995) for description of units of the score.

[b]Ordinal variable assuming seven values, ranging from 1 = less than 8th grade to 7 = doctoral level.

Source: Swan et al., 1995.

with such a history were almost three times more likely to die than were men without a history of cancer, adjusting for the effects of all the other variables in the table.

The analysis shown in Table 7–1 is sometimes called Cox multivariate regression, since all eight predictor variables were included in the same model. In this way each variable is adjusted for all the others. The p-value for each coefficient in Table 7–1 represents the probability of obtaining an estimate with an absolute value as large or larger than the one actually observed, if the true coefficient for the population were zero.

NESTED CASE-CONTROL AND CASE-COHORT ANALYSES

Mantel (1973) suggested that for large cohort studies, considerable savings in cost with very little loss of efficiency can be gained from analyzing data for only certain subsets of individuals in the cohort. The subsets consist of all cases and a sample of other cohort members.

Two examples of this strategy are nested case-control and case-cohort designs, as described in Chapter 5. Cox's regression method can be used to analyze data from these two designs. To do so, one evaluates exposures for only a sample of individuals in the cases' risk sets. For both designs, the sum in the denominator of expression (7.4) includes the case and only a subset of the other members of the risk set. The members of the subset serve as controls for the case. In the nested case-control design, the investigator samples the risk sets in such a way that members of the different risk sets (i.e., cases and noncases) do not overlap. For the case-cohort design, by contrast, the investigator selects all cases and a random sample of the entire cohort (cases and noncases) for the comparison subset. The investigator then uses the Cox regression method on the data for this "subcohort" to estimate the regression coefficients. The variances of these estimates must be modified to account for the sampling.

We illustrate the application of the method for analyzing a nested case-control study by considering a retrospective cohort study of lung cancer deaths among some 3300 white, male U.S. uranium miners who were employed in mines in Arizona, Colorado, New Mexico, and Utah. The exposure of interest is inhalation of radon and its radioactive decay products. A nested case-control analysis using age as the time variable was conducted (Whittemore and McMillan, 1983; Halpern and Whittemore, 1987). Four control miners were chosen from the risk set of each case (miner who died with lung cancer). The risk set for a case consisted of all miners who were alive and under follow-up at the same age the case was when he died. For the case and each of his four matched controls, esti-

Table 7-2. Results of a Nested Case-Control Analysis of Lung Cancer Mortality among U.S. Uranium Miners in Relation to Radon Exposure and Cigarette Smoking

Variable	Regression Coefficient	(Standard Error)	Death Rate Ratio	95% Confidence Interval
RADON EXPOSURE (WORKING-LEVEL-MONTHS)				
x_1 0–21	0	—	1.00	—
x_2 22–119	0.513	(.299)	1.67	0.93–3.00
x_3 120–359	0.867	(.261)	2.38	1.43–3.97
x_4 360–839	1.235	(.218)	3.44	2.24–5.27
x_5 840–1799	1.444	(.226)	4.24	2.72–6.60
x_6 1800+	2.637	(.222)	13.98	9.04–21.59
CIGARETTE SMOKING (PACK-YEARS)				
z_1 0–9	0	—	1.00	—
z_2 10–19	1.435	(.221)	4.20	2.72–6.48
z_3 20–29	1.153	(.246)	3.17	1.96–5.13
z_4 30+	2.019	(.211)	7.53	4.98–11.39

mated exposures to radon daughters and to cigarette smoke (an important potential confounding variable and a possible modifier of the effect of radon), were cumulated up to the year of the case's lung cancer death. Radon exposures, measured in working-level-months, were stratified into $J = 6$ increasing levels. Tobacco exposures, measured in pack-years of cigarette smoking, were stratified into $K = 4$ increasing levels. These are shown in Table 7-2.

The objective was to estimate the death rate ratio for men in each of the $J - 1 = 5$ highest radon categories relative to the rate in the lowest category of 0–21 working-level-months, while adjusting for the effects of cigarette smoking. To achieve this aim, the authors used five dichotomous predictor variables $x_2, \ldots, x_6$ to code the five highest categories. For example, they coded $x_2 = 1$ if a man's radon exposure was between 22 and 119 working-level-months, and $x_2 = 0$ otherwise. Similarly, three dichotomous predictor variables z_2, z_3, z_4 were used to code the three highest smoking categories. This coding scheme gives a representation of the death rate ratio (equation 7.3) for the ith miner in the risk set of a case who fails at time t in terms of the $5 + 3 = 8$ predictor variables as

$$R_{it} = \exp[b_2 x_{i2} + \ldots + b_6 x_{i6} + c_2 z_{i2} + c_3 z_{i3} + c_4 z_{i4}].$$

[Here the subscript i denotes the ith miner's values of the predictor variables.] Notice that miners with baseline levels of radon and smoking exposure are coded

$$x_{i2} = \cdots = x_{i6} = z_{i2} = z_{i3} = z_{i4} = 0,$$

so that for them, the ratio $R_{it} = \exp(0) = 1$. Notice also that $\exp(b_j)$ represents the death rate ratio in radon category j relative to that in category

1, for $j = 2, \ldots, 6$, while $\exp(c_k)$ is the corresponding ratio for the kth smoking category, $k = 2, 3, 4$. The estimated regression coefficients and the corresponding death rate ratios are shown in Table 7–2. One can see that the rate ratio for lung cancer increases markedly with greater radon exposure independent of the effect of cigarette smoking on risk of death from lung cancer.

For a case-cohort analysis of the uranium miner data, one would select a random sample of the 3300 miners and if necessary, add to this sample any men who died with lung cancer who were excluded from the sample. The analysis would proceed as if this subcohort were the entire cohort; however, the variances of the estimated rate ratio parameters must be adjusted to accommodate the sampling design (Prentice, 1986). Both the nested case-control analysis and the case-cohort analysis require computer software such as that used for Cox regression analysis.

We conclude this section with the observation that the risk factors of interest in the uranium mining example (cumulative exposures to radon and to cigarette smoke) differ from those in the previous example of mortality among men in the Western Collaborative Group Study. In the uranium mining example, the measured levels of both risk factors changed as the time variable increased. In the first example, by contrast, the risk factor levels were measured only at the start of follow-up. Variables of the latter type, whose values do not change with time, are called *time-independent,* or *fixed,* whereas the former are called *time-dependent.* As we have seen, Cox regression analysis and Poisson regression analysis can handle both types of variables.

STANDARDIZED MORTALITY RATIOS (SMRs) AND STANDARDIZED INCIDENCE RATIOS (SIRs)

The Cox regression method and the Poisson regression method of Chapter 6 are appropriate for comparing death or disease rates among exposed and unexposed cohort members. In contrast, methods based on the SMR and SIR are used when the cohort contains only exposed persons, and comparisons are based on published incidence or mortality rates for a reference population. For concreteness we shall call this reference population the general population. For these analyses, expected numbers of deaths or disease occurrences frequently are calculated on the basis of gender-specific, age-specific, and occasionally race-specific rates for the general population. If these rates have changed over time, it is important that the rates be time-specific as well.

To clarify ideas, we refer to the general two-way table of disease counts and person-years shown in Table 6–7. All exposure groups (rows) of the

Table 7–3. Calculation of Standardized Mortality Ratio (SMR) for Respiratory Cancers among White U.S. Uranium Miners

Age (Years)	Observed Deaths	Person-Years	National[a] Death Rate	Expected Deaths
30–44	16	34936.9	11.5	4.0
45–49	31	9485.2	46.8	4.4
50–54	28	8003.8	90.2	7.2
55–59	46	6308.8	162.9	10.3
60–64	33	4443.0	242.3	10.8
65–69	16	2580.4	325.2	8.4
70–74	18	1174.3	371.0	4.4
75+	6	726.7	336.0	2.4
Total	194	67659.1	132.7[b]	
SMR = O/E = 194/51.9 = 3.74				51.9

[a]U.S. respiratory cancer death rate (deaths per 100,000 persons) in white males in 1970. Source: Vital Statistics of the United States, 1970 (1974).

[b]Crude death rate in U.S. white males aged 30+ years.

Source: Halpern and Whittemore (1987).

table now represent exposed subsets of the cohort. The columns of the table represent strata of covariates such as gender, race, age and year of death. For example, Table 7–3 shows lung cancer deaths and person-years at risk among the cohort of white, male U.S. uranium miners studied by Halpern and Whittemore (1987). In this example uranium mining is treated as a dichotomous variable. Amount of exposure is not considered. There are eight age groups (here represented as rows) and one exposure group (the entire group). Under the null hypothesis that the lung cancer death rates among uranium miners equal those among the general population of U.S. white males, we can compute the expected number of deaths for each age group by multiplying the number of person-years at risk in that age group by the age-specific death rate among U.S. white males. For example, the expected number of deaths among miners aged 30–44 years in Table 7–3 is $34936.9 \times 11.5/100,000 = 4.0$. The death rate $11.5/100,000$ is that of U.S. white males of that age in 1970, a typical year when deaths among the miners occurred. The total expected number of deaths is the sum of expected numbers over all age groups. Accordingly, in Table 7–3 we find that the expected number of respiratory cancer deaths for miners is $E = 51.9$.

If we were to ignore possible age differences between the miners and the general population of U.S. white males in 1970, we would simply multiply the total person-years at risk ($N = 67,659.1$ in Table 7–3) by the crude U.S. death rate $132.7/100,000$ to obtain the value 89.8 for the expected number of deaths. This value is considerably larger than the age-adjusted value 51.9, because the miners tended to be younger than the general population.

A test of the null hypothesis that the miners had the same respiratory cancer death rates as those of U.S. white males is obtained by referring the statistic $\chi^2 = (O-E)^2/E$ to a chi-squared distribution on one degree of freedom. Here O and E represent, respectively, the observed and expected number of deaths in the entire cohort. For the data in Table 7–3, $\chi^2 = (194-51.9)^2/51.9 = 389.1$. A value this large or larger is highly unlikely ($p < 0.0001$) to have occurred by chance.

An estimate of the SMR for uranium miners is the ratio of observed to expected deaths $O/E = 194/51.9 = 3.74$. Approximate 95% confidence limits for the SMR are given by

$$\text{Lower limit} = \frac{O}{E}\left(1 - \frac{1}{90} - \frac{1.96}{3\sqrt{O}}\right)^3;$$

$$\text{Upper limit} = \frac{(O+1)}{E}\left(1 - \frac{1}{9(O+1)} + \frac{1.96}{3\sqrt{O+1}}\right)^3$$

(Rothman and Boice, 1979). For the uranium miner data, these formulas give a confidence interval of (3.23, 4.30). Thus, death rates from respiratory cancer among the miners are three to four times higher than those of the general population.

The strengths and weaknesses of the SMR as a summary measure of association between exposure and risk of death can be seen by considering the model fitting of Chapter 6. Table 7–4 shows three nested models for the age-specific death rates underlying the uranium miner data in Table 7–3. The smallest Model 1 completely specifies these rates as equal to those of the general population of U.S. white males. Model 1 involves no unknown parameters. Model 1 is nested in Model 2, which specifies that the rates among the uranium miners are proportional to those of the general population, with proportionality factor c. Model 2 involves the single unknown parameter c; the smaller Model 1 arises by specifying $c = 1$. Models 1 and 2 both are nested in Model 3, which puts no restriction on the $J \times K$ rates

Table 7–4. Models for Data of Table 7–3

Model for Rates in Sampled Population	Rate for Cell (j,k)	Number of Parameters	Degrees of Freedom of Deviance[a]
1. Equal to external rates	I_{jk}^*	0	JK
2. Proportional to external rates	cI_{jk}^*	1	$JK - 1$
3. Unrestricted rates	I_{jk}	JK	0

[a] Relative to Model 3.

(where J is the number of exposure groups and K is the number of covariate strata). Thus Model 3 involves $J \times K = 1 \times 8 = 8$ fitted parameters.

Tests of hypotheses are based on the deviance between pairs of models, defined in Table 6–9. The deviance between Model 2 and Model 1 provides a test of the null hypothesis that the miners have the same respiratory cancer death rates as the U.S. population. To calculate this deviance, we need the expected numbers of deaths $\hat{d}_1^{(1)}, \ldots, \hat{d}_8^{(1)}$ for each of the eight age groups under Model 1, which are given in the last column of Table 7–3. We also need the expected numbers of deaths under the bigger Model 2, which are $\hat{d}_1^{(2)} = c\hat{d}_1^{(1)}, \ldots, \hat{d}_8^{(2)} = c\hat{d}_8^{(1)}$. The estimated SMR $= O/E$ is the maximum likelihood estimate of the unknown parameter c in Model 2. We have seen that for the miner data this value is $c =$ SMR $= 3.74$. Substituting these numbers into the formula for χ^2_{DEV} in Table 6–9, we obtain, after cancellation and simplification, $\chi^2_{DEV} = 2 \times 51.9 \times [3.74 \times \ln 3.74 + 1 - 3.74] = 228.1$. This value is very large ($p < 0.0001$) when compared to a chi-squared statistic on one degree of freedom, providing strong evidence that the miners' rates do not equal those of the general population.

The deviance between Model 3 and Model 2 provides a test of Model 2; that is, the assumption that miners' respiratory cancer death rates are proportional to rates in the general population. Several authors (e.g., Gaffey, 1976; Breslow and Day, 1984; Whittemore, 1985) have noted pitfalls in the use of the SMR when Model 2 fails to hold. In particular, ratios of SMRs for two exposure groups can be misleading, and may even lie completely outside the range of age-specific rate ratios (Breslow and Day, 1984). It is thus important to test the assumption of proportionality between age-specific rates of the cohort and those of the general population when using the SMR or SIR as a summary measure of risk. For the data in Table 7–3, the deviance between Model 2 and Model 3 is calculated by taking $\hat{d}_1^{(2)}, \ldots, \hat{d}_8^{(2)}$ to be the expected numbers of deaths under Model 2, which are obtained by multiplying the last column of Table 7–3 by 3.74. The expected numbers of death $\hat{d}_1^{(3)}, \ldots, \hat{d}_8^{(3)}$ under the bigger Model 3 are just the observed numbers of deaths, shown in column 2 of Table 7–3. Substituting these values into the formula for χ^2_{DEV} in Table 6–9, we find that $\chi^2_{DEV} = 22.2$. When compared to a chi-squared statistic on $8 - 1 = 7$ degrees of freedom, this value is statistically significant ($p < 0.01$), suggesting poor fit of Model 2 to the miner data. The largest contributions to this deviance come from the age group 45–49 years, for which the observed 31 deaths exceed the expected number 4.6 by a factor of 6.7, and from the age group 65–69 years, for which the observed 16 deaths exceed the expected number 8.4 by a factor of only 1.9. Thus, the summary SMR of 3.73 provides an inadequate overall summary of the rate ratios in each age group (which vary from 1.9 to 6.7), and it should be used with caution. A more informative report would specify all eight age-specific SMRs.

PROPORTIONAL MORTALITY (INCIDENCE) ANALYSES

Analyses similar to those of Chapter 6 for stratified cohort data can be carried out using only disease or death counts. Such analyses are useful for data such as the leukemia mortality data among workers exposed to electrical and magnetic fields analyzed by Milham (1982), for which the person-years at risk are unavailable.

To illustrate the use of proportional mortality analyses, we apply them to the veterans data discussed in Chapter 6, ignoring the person-years information at hand. At issue is the relationship between cigarette smoking and death from respiratory cancer. A group of deaths from other cancers (colorectal cancer, prostate cancer, lymphoma and leukemia, hereafter called selected cancers) has been chosen for comparison. All other deaths are ignored. Table 7–5 shows the numbers of deaths by cause, age, and smoking status (nonsmokers versus the combined group of all smokers).

Proportional mortality analysis of these data rests on the following argument: if mortality from both respiratory cancer and the selected cancers is unrelated to cigarette smoking, then in Table 7–5 respiratory cancer deaths should account for the same fraction of all deaths among smokers as among nonsmokers. If, on the other hand, cigarette smoking increases the risk of respiratory cancer death but is unrelated to mortality from the selected cancers, then respiratory cancer deaths should make up a higher fraction of all deaths among smokers than among nonsmokers. The validity of this argument requires that risk of death from the selected cancers be unrelated to cigarette smoking, the exposure of interest.

To formalize this argument, we begin by ignoring the potential confounding effects of age, and consider only the 2×2 table formed by the numbers of respiratory cancer deaths and deaths from selected cancers among nonsmokers and smokers, given by the totals in the extreme right columns of Table 7–5. Let I_N and I_S denote the respiratory cancer death rate among nonsmokers and smokers, respectively, and let I_N^* and I_S^* be the corresponding death rates for the selected cancers. The expected proportion of deaths due to respiratory cancer in a given smoking category is $p = I/(I + I^*)$. Within each smoking group, the odds that a death was due to respiratory cancer, given that it was due to one of the two types of malignancies, is $p/(1 - p) = I/I^*$. The proportional mortality ratio (PMR) is defined as the ratio of odds in smokers to odds in nonsmokers:

$$\text{PMR} = \frac{p_S}{1 - p_S} \div \frac{p_N}{1 - p_N} = \frac{I_S}{I_S^*} \cdot \frac{I_N^*}{I_N}. \tag{7.5}$$

If smoking is unrelated to risk of the other causes of death, i.e., if $I_N^* = I_S^*$, then the PMR in equation (7.5) is just the respiratory cancer death rate ratio $r = I_S/I_N$ for smokers relative to nonsmokers. If, on the other hand,

Table 7-5. Numbers of Deaths from Specific Causes among U.S. Veterans according to Cause of Death, Age and Cigarette Consumption

Age (Years)	35-44		45-54		55-64		65-74		75+		Total	
	RSP[a] CA	SLCT[b] CA	RSP CA	SLCT CA	RSP CA	SLCT CA	RSP CA	SLCT CA	RSP CA	SLCT CA	RSP CA	SLCT CA
Smoking												
Smoker	6	16	14	12	528	446	537	505	31	42	1116	1021
Nonsmoker	0	2	0	1	25	254	49	308	4	45	78	610
Total	24		27		1253		1399		122		2825	

Cause of Death

[a] Respiratory cancer.

[b] Selected cancers: colorectal cancers, prostate cancer, lymphomas and leukemias.

smoking increases risk of the other causes of death, that is, if $I_S^* > I_N^*$, then the PMR is less than the rate ratio, and is biased downward.

For the pooled data in the last columns of Table 7–5, estimates of p_N and p_S are $\hat{p}_N = 78/(78 + 610) = 0.113$ and $\hat{p}_S = 1116/(1116 + 1021) = 0.522$. That is, 11.3% of the nonsmokers' deaths and 52.2% of the smokers' deaths are due to respiratory cancer. Notice that $\hat{p}_N/(1 - \hat{p}_N) = 78/610$, and $\hat{p}_S/(1 - \hat{p}_S) = 1116/1021$. Substituting these ratios in the left side of equation (7.5) gives an estimated PMR of $(1116/1021)/(78/610) = 8.548$. This value is rather close to the estimated crude death rate ratio $\hat{r} = (1116/701,768)/(78/443,856) = 9.049$ calculated using the actual person-years in Table 6–6. The similarity suggests that the selected cancers are not strongly related to cigarette smoking.

To illustrate the downward bias in the PMR associated with a comparison group of outcomes that are themselves associated with the exposure of interest, we consider the group of deaths from all causes other than respiratory cancer, many of which are smoking-related. There was a total of 6854 such deaths among nonsmoking veterans and 14,528 such deaths among smoking veterans. Therefore, the proportion of deaths due to respiratory cancer among nonsmokers is $\hat{p}_N = 78/(78 + 6854)$, giving $\hat{p}_N/(1 - \hat{p}_N) = 78/6854$. The corresponding proportion among smokers is $\hat{p}_S = 1116/(1116 + 14,528)$, with $\hat{p}_S/(1 - \hat{p}_S) = 1116/14,528$. Substituting these values into formula (7.5) gives the associated PMR estimate as $(1116/14,528) / (78/6854) = 6.750$. As expected, this value is considerably smaller than both the value 9.049 obtained from Table 6–6 using person-years at risk and the value 8.548 obtained when causes of death known to be related to smoking are excluded.

The preceding discussion highlights an analogy between proportional mortality analysis of cohort data and odds ratio analysis of case-control data (to be discussed in Chapter 9). The analogy can be seen by regarding individuals who die from the disease of interest as "cases" and those who die from the other diseases as "controls." The PMR is then the odds of being a "case" among the exposed (e.g., the smokers) divided by the corresponding odds among the unexposed (the nonsmokers). In Chapter 8 we shall see that the controls in a case-control study should be representative of the population from which the cases were drawn with respect to the exposure of interest. Similarly, the "controls" (i.e., those who die from other causes in this PMR analysis) should be representative of the population from which the cases came with respect to smoking (which would not be true if smoking were related to their deaths).

We can construct a confidence interval for the PMR (and for other types of odds ratio) in the same way that we did in Chapter 6 for the rate ratio. It is again advantageous to work with logarithms, so we consider the natural logarithm of the PMR. To estimate the variance of our estimate of ln $(8.548) = 2.1457$, we take the sum of the reciprocals of the numbers of deaths of each type among the exposed (smokers) and unexposed (non-smokers). For our data this is $(1/78) + (1/610) + (1/116) + (1/1021) = 0.02406$. The standard error of the logarithm PMR is thus $\sqrt{.02406} = 0.15511$. A 95% confidence interval for the logarithm of the PMR is:

$$\text{Lower limit} = 2.1457 - (1.96 \times 0.15511) = 1.8417$$

$$\text{Upper limit} = 2.1457 + (1.96 \times 0.15511) = 2.4497$$

Exponentiating these values gives the confidence interval for the PMR itself as $e^{1.8417} = 6.31$ and $e^{2.4497} = 11.59$.

The preceding analyses do not account for the possible confounding effects of age. Age may confound the analysis because the death rates for the two causes may differ in their relations to age (e.g., respiratory cancer deaths may occur at older ages than do deaths from the selected cancers), and smoking habits also may differ by age. To control confounding, we stratify the cause-specific and exposure-specific data into K age strata. Table 7–5 gives the setup for the veterans' data with $K = 5$ age strata. Among smokers, we let I_{Sk} and I^*_{Sk} denote, respectively, the death rate in age group k for respiratory cancer and selected cancers. Among non-smokers, I_{Nk} and I^*_{Nk} are defined similarly. Interest centers on the rate ratio I_{Sk}/I_{Nk} relating respiratory cancer death rates in smokers to rates in non-smokers in age stratum k. We let $p_{Nk} = I_{Nk}/(I_{Nk} + I^*_{Nk})$ denote the proportion of deaths among nonsmokers in age stratum k that were due to respiratory cancer. Also, we let $p_{Sk} = I_{Sk}/(I_{Sk} + I^*_{Sk})$ denote the same proportion for smokers. The PMR in stratum k, defined as the odds ratio relating respiratory cancer deaths in smokers relative to nonsmokers in that stratum, is

$$\text{PMR} = \frac{p_{Sk}}{1 - p_{Sk}} \div \frac{p_{Nk}}{1 - p_{Nk}} = \frac{I_{Sk}}{I^*_{Sk}} \cdot \frac{I^*_{Nk}}{I_{Nk}}. \tag{7.6}$$

If the PMR does not vary across age strata, then its common value (equation 7.6) gives a summary measure of association between smoking and respiratory cancer death. Again we see that if smoking is unrelated to the other causes of death (i.e., if $I^*_{Sk} = I^*_{Nk}$), then the PMR equals the desired ratio of respiratory cancer death rates in smokers relative to nonsmokers.

Having defined a summary PMR for stratified data, it remains to describe estimates and confidence intervals for it and tests of the null hypothesis that its value is one. A reliable and easily calculated estimate is the Mantel-Haenszel estimate (Mantel-Haenszel, 1959) of a summary odds ratio in a series of K 2 × 2 tables. This estimate is defined in Chapter 9, where it is introduced as a tool for the analysis of case-control data. For the data in Table 7–5, the Mantel-Haenszel estimate is 8.451. This value is close to the unstratified value of 8.548, suggesting that age is not a strong confounder of this analysis. Chapter 9 also describes how to calculate a confidence interval for the summary odds ratio based on the Mantel-Haenszel estimate.

If there are more than two exposure groups, the PMR relating each exposed group to the unexposed referent group can be estimated separately using the Mantel-Haenszel method. For a more complex analysis, the method of maximum likelihood is preferable. The use of model fitting by the method of maximum likelihood for odds ratio estimation and hypothesis testing is discussed in Chapter 9.

If a cohort lacks both an unexposed subcohort and appropriate person-years at risk, then cause-specific deaths (or incidence) in the cohort can be contrasted with those in an external population to estimate the rate ratio associated with exposure. The underlying assumptions are now twofold: (a) the death rates of the population from which the cohort was sampled and those of the external population are proportional, for both the cause of death of interest and the comparison group of other causes of death, and (b) the exposure of interest is unrelated to risk of death from the other causes. The analysis is similar to the one described above that uses an internal unexposed group; the reader is referred to Breslow and Day (1984) for details.

REFERENCES

Baker RJ, Nelder JA. 1978. The GLIM System: Release 3. Oxford, Numerical Algorithms Group.

Bobstick RM, Potter JD, Sellers TA, McKenzie DR, Kushi LH, Folsom AR. 1993. Relation of calcium, vitamin D, and dairy food intake to incidence of colon cancer among older women: The Iowa Women's Health Study. *Am J Epidemiol* 137:1302–1317.

Boice JD Jr, Monson RR. 1977. Breast cancer in women after repeated fluoroscopic examinations of the chest. *J Natl Cancer Inst* 59:823–832.

Breslow NE, Day NE. 1984. Statistical Methods in Cancer Research. Vol. 2. The analysis of case-control studies. Lyon, IARC Press.

Breslow NE, Lubin JH, Marek P, Langholz B. 1983. Multiplicative models and cohort analysis. *J Am Stat Assoc* 78:1–12.

Collins JA, Garner JB, Wilson EH, Wrixon W, Casper RF. 1984. A proportional hazards analysis of the clinical characteristics of infertile couples. *Am J Obstet Gynecol* 148:527–532.

Cox DR. 1972. Regression models and life table (with discussion). *J Roy Stat Soc B* 34:187–220.

Gaffey WR. 1976. A critique of the standardized mortality ratio. *J Occup Med* 18:157–160.

Halpern J, Whittemore AS. 1987. Methods for analyzing occupational cohort data with application to lung cancer mortality in uranium miners. *J Chron Dis* 40:79S–88S.

Knekt P, Reunanen A, Järvinen R, Seppänen R, Heliövaara M, Aromaa A. 1994. Antioxidant vitamin intake and coronary mortality in a longitudinal population study. *Am J Epidemiol* 139:1180–1189.

Mantel N. 1973. Synthetic retrospective studies and related topics. *Biometrics* 29:479–486.

Mantel N, Haenszel W. 1959. Statistical aspects of the analysis of data from retrospective studies of disease. *J Natl Cancer Inst* 22:719–748.

Mauritsen R. 1994. EGRET. Seattle WA. Statistics and Epidemiology Research Corporation.

Milham S. 1982. Mortality from leukemia in workers exposed to electrical and magnetic fields. (Letter to the Editor) *N Engl J Med* 307:249.

Prentice RL. 1986. A case-cohort design for epidemiologic cohort studies and disease prevention trials. *Biometrika* 73:1–11.

Rothman KJ, Boice JD Jr. 1979. Epidemiologic Analysis with a Programmable Calculator. (NIH Publ 79–1649). Washington, DC, U.S. Government Printing Office.

SAS Language. 1990. Version 6.x. First Ed. Cary, NC, SAS Institute Inc.

Swan GE, Carmelli D, LaRue A. 1995. Performance on the digit symbol substitution test and 5-year mortality in the Western Collaborative Group Study. *Am J Epidemiol* 141:32–40.

Vital Statistics of the United States, 1970. 1974. Vol. II. Mortality, Part A. Rockville, MD: U.S. Department of Health, Education and Welfare, Public Health Service, Health Resources Administration, National Center for Health Statistics. (HRA) 74–1102.

Whittemore AS. 1985. Methods old and new for analyzing occupational cohort data. *Am J Ind Med* 12:233–248.

Whittemore AS, Lele C, Friedman GD, Stamey T, Vogelman JH, Orentreich N. 1995. Prostate-specific antigen as predictor of prostate cancer in black men and white men. *J Natl Cancer Inst* 87:354–360.

Whittemore AS, McMillan A. 1983. Lung cancer mortality among U.S. uranium miners. *J Natl Cancer Inst* 71:489–499.

Exercises

1. Knedt et al. (1994) reported the following results from a cohort study of the relation between dietary intakes of antioxidant vitamins and subsequent mortality from coronary heart disease. They used Cox regression analysis to adjust for age, smoking (current vs. not current smoker), serum cholesterol, hypertension (four categories), body mass index, and energy intake at baseline.

Tertile[a] of Consumption Antioxidant Vitamin	Adjusted Rate Ratio (95% Confidence Interval)					
	Carotenoids		Vitamin C		Vitamin E	
MALES						
Lowest[b]	1.00		1.00		1.00	
Middle	1.06	(0.74–1.50)	0.87	(0.61–1.25)	0.97	(0.67–1.40)
Highest	1.02	(0.70–1.48)	1.00	(0.68–1.45)	0.68	(0.42–1.11)
p value for test for linear trend	0.36		0.94		0.01	
FEMALES						
Lowest[b]	1.00		1.00		1.00	
Middle	1.46	(0.82–2.61)	0.51	(0.26–0.99)	0.73	(0.38–1.39)
Highest	0.62	(0.30–1.29)	0.49	(0.24–0.98)	0.35	(0.14–0.88)
p value for test for linear trend	0.60		0.06		<0.01	

[a]Tertile means that the study population has been divided into three groups of approximately equal size.
[b]Referent category.

a. What antioxidant vitamins show an inverse association with coronary heart disease mortality?

b. Is there any evidence of effect modification by gender?

c. Why did the investigators adjust for age, smoking, serum cholesterol, hypertension, body mass index, and energy intake?

d. Do you think they should adjust for any other variables? If so, which ones?

e. What does the p value of 0.06 under Vitamin C intake for females mean?

2. Bobstick et al. (1993) reported the following results from a cohort study that examined the relation between certain dietary variables and incidence of colon cancer. Cox regression analysis was used for adjustment of potential confounding variables:

Quintile[a] of Total Vitamin D Intake (IU/day)	Age-Adjusted Rate Ratio (95% CI)[d]		Multivariate-Adjusted[b] Rate Ratio (95% CI)	
1. (<159)[c]	1.00		1.00	
2. (159–266)	0.71	(0.48–1.07)	0.77	(0.51–1.16)
3. (267–415)	0.76	(0.51–1.13)	0.83	(0.55–1.27)
4. (416–618)	0.78	(0.53–1.17)	0.93	(0.61–1.41)
5. (>618)	0.54	(0.35–0.84)	0.73	(0.45–1.18)
p value for test for linear trend	0.02		0.42	

[a]Quintiles mean that the study population has been divided into five groups of approximately equal size.

[b]Adjusted for age, total energy intake, height, parity, low-fat meat intake, total Vitamin E intake, and a total Vitamin E × age interaction term.

[c]Referent category.

[d]95% confidence interval.

a. What do you conclude about the relation between total Vitamin D intake and colon cancer incidence?

b. What do the rate ratios (and 95% confidence intervals) of 0.54 (0.35–0.84) and 0.73 (0.45–1.18) for quintile 5 mean?

c. What do the tests for trend indicate? Do the age-adjusted and multivariate-adjusted rate ratios show a linear decrease with increased total vitamin D intake?

3. Cox regression analysis is frequently employed in clinical studies where information is gathered prospectively. Collins et al. (1984) used this technique to analyze rates of subsequent pregnancy among couples registered at an infertility clinic. All couples included in the study had had at least a 12-month history of prior infertility. The results for three of the variables examined were as follows:

Variable	Regression Coefficient	Standard Error
Prior pregnancy during this marriage (1 = yes; 0 = no)	0.523	0.119
Duration of infertility (in months)	−0.008	0.003
Length of marriage (in years)	−0.064	0.022

a. Calculate the rate ratio and 95% confidence interval for the association between prior pregnancy during this marriage and subsequent pregnancy. What do the rate ratio and 95% confidence interval mean?

b. Compare the rate of the subsequent pregnancy in couples who have had a duration of infertility of 3 years and who have been married for 10 years with the rate of subsequent pregnancy in couples who have had a duration of infertility of 1 year and who have been married for 2 years.

c. Based on these data, what can be said about the probability that an infertile couple will eventually conceive?

4. In a cohort of male factory workers, 57 deaths from cardiovascular disease are observed over a 5-year period of observation. Based on gender- and age-specific cardiovascular mortality rates for the United States, it is estimated that 83.8 deaths would be expected in this group. Calculate the SMR, construct a confidence interval, and comment on the interpretation of the finding.

5. Milham (1982) reported the following proportionate mortality ratios (observed/expected × 100) (PMRs) for acute leukemia standardized by age and year of death among white males in Washington State between 1950 and 1979. For this report, data were abstracted from death certificates on some 438,000 deaths in 158 cause-of-death groups.

Occupation	No. of Deaths Observed	No. of Deaths Expected	PMR × 100
Electronic technicians	3	1.9	162
Radio and telegraph operators	3	1.3	239
Electricians	23	12.9	178[a]
Power and telephone linemen	6	3.3	183
Television and radio repairmen	4	1.4	291[a]
Power station operators	3	1.1	282
Aluminum workers	11	4.3	258[a]
Welders and flame cutters	4	7.1	56
Motion picture projectionists	1	0.9	111
Electrical engineers	2	2.1	97
Streetcar and subway motormen	0	0.4	0
Total	60	36.7	163[a]

[a] $p < 0.01$.

Reprinted by permission of N Engl J Med 307:249, 1982, Massachusetts Medical Society.

a. What does the PMR of 2.91 in television and radio repairmen mean?

b. What do the data in the table suggest about risk of death from acute leukemia among those occupationally exposed to electrical and magnetic fields?

c. What are some advantages and limitations of these data?

8

Case-Control Studies:
I. Planning and Execution

In a case-control study, persons with a given disease (the cases) and persons without the given disease (the controls) are selected; the proportions of cases and controls who have certain background characteristics or who have been exposed to possible risk factors are then determined and compared. Case-control studies are also sometimes called case-comparison studies, case-referent studies, or retrospective studies. Usually cases enter the study as they are diagnosed over time, and controls enter the study as they are identified. In some studies, however, cases consist of individuals who have been diagnosed with the disease in the past. Such a study is sometimes called a "retrospective case-control study."

Case-control studies are by far the most frequently undertaken type of analytic epidemiologic study. They generally can be carried out in a much shorter period of time than cohort studies, do not require nearly so large a sample size, and consequently are less expensive. For a rare disease, case-control studies are usually the only practical approach to identifying risk factors. Despite their usefulness and wide applicability, certain potential problems and limitations may be associated with case-control studies, and these must be carefully considered before deciding whether a case-control study is appropriate in a given situation. Sackett (1979) and Austin et al. (1994) have listed and discussed a large number of possible sources of bias and error in case-control studies. Among the most common concerns are that (a) accurate information on the potential risk factor may not be available either from records or the people's memories; (b) accurate information on potentially important confounding variables may not be available either from records or the participants' memories; (c) cases may search for a cause for their disease and thereby be more likely to report an exposure than controls (a form of recall bias); (d) the investigator may be unable to determine with certainty whether the agent was likely to have caused the disease or whether the occurrence of the disease was likely to have caused the person to be exposed to the agent; (e) identifying and assembling a case group representative of all cases may be unduly difficult; (f) identifying and assembling an appropriate control group may be unduly difficult; and (g) participation rates may be low.

Because of these potential weaknesses, the case-control study is considered by some to be a type of study that merely provides leads to be followed up by more definitive cohort studies. However, decisions as to preventive actions often must be reached on the basis of information obtained from case-control studies, as when diethylstilbestrol (DES) was removed from the market as an agent to prevent miscarriages after case-control studies had shown that DES exposure during pregnancy was associated with a dramatically elevated risk of cancer of the vagina as well as other genital abnormalities in offspring (Herbst et al., 1971; Greenwald et al., 1974). Results of the first case-control study (Herbst et al., 1971), based on only eight cases and 32 controls, are shown in Table 8–1.

Each case-control study must be evaluated individually because some studies are affected by error and bias to a greater extent than others. For instance, results of a case-control study reporting that stress increases the risk of coronary heart disease would be difficult to interpret because it would probably be impossible to know whether stress caused the coronary heart disease or whether coronary heart disease caused a person to feel stressed or to remember to a greater extent previous stressful events. In contrast, if the study focused on whether blood group O was associated with an increased risk for coronary heart disease, it would not matter whether blood group was determined before or after the disease was diagnosed, unless, of course, survivorship differed according to blood group.

Case-control studies are best suited to the study of diseases for which medical care is usually sought, such as cancers or hip fracture. Otherwise, an expensive community survey would have to be undertaken to identify

Table 8–1. Diethylstilbestrol (DES) Use during Pregnancy in Mothers of Cases of Adenocarcinoma of the Vagina and Matched Controls

Case Number	Use (Y = Yes, N = No)				
	Case	Matched Controls			
		1	2	3	4
1	Y	N	N	N	N
2	Y	N	N	N	N
3	Y	N	N	N	N
4	Y	N	N	N	N
5	N	N	N	N	N
6	Y	N	N	N	N
7	Y	N	N	N	N
8	Y	N	N	N	N
	$p < 0.00001$				

Source: Herbst et al. (1971).

cases, thus canceling out one of the principal advantages of case-control studies, that is, the relatively low cost. Also, case-control studies are most suitable for the study of diseases with a relatively short period between first appearance of symptoms and time of diagnosis and interview, because with a disease of slow onset it becomes difficult to differentiate factors that caused the disease from factors that may have occurred after the disease process began.

Two types of case-control studies are in common use. In *incidence-density* case-control studies, incident cases are sampled as they occur, and controls are sampled over the same time period; note that these controls do not have the disease when selected, but may develop the disease during the course of the study and so become cases as well. Most case-control studies are of the incidence-density type. An example would be a study to determine whether oral contraceptives increase the risk of breast cancer, in which cases are all women with newly diagnosed breast cancer during a specified time period in a certain age range in a defined geographic area, and controls are women in the same age range and geographic area identified through random digit dialing over the same time period as that over which the cases are identified. In *cumulative-incidence* case-control studies, cases occurring over a defined time period are included, but controls are sampled from among persons who at the end of the time period have not developed the disease and therefore are no longer at risk of becoming cases in the study. The cumulative-incidence approach is commonly used in studies of reproductive outcomes and of short-term epidemics (Greenland and Thomas, 1982; Miettinen, 1976; Morgenstern et al., 1980). An example would be a study to identify the source of an outbreak of acute gastroenteritis in which cases are all persons in a specified group (such as those attending a church supper) who developed gastroenteritis over a defined period of time and controls are people in the specified group who at the end of the time period had not developed gastroenteritis. Controls cannot also become cases since they are selected when anyone who could possibly become a case has already been included. The differentiation into incidence-density and cumulative-incidence case-control studies has little effect on most aspects of the design, execution, and interpretation of studies of uncommon diseases, but for common diseases measures of the degree of association between exposure and disease may differ in these two circumstances.

ESTIMATES MADE FROM CASE-CONTROL STUDIES

As was indicated in the description of cohort studies, the investigator should consider what he or she ultimately will want to estimate from the study before planning it. The first quantities an investigator usually calculates in a case-control study are the proportion of cases who were exposed to putative risk factors and the proportion of controls who were exposed. Also, the intensity and lengths of exposure, changes in exposure status over time, and exposures at certain critical time periods (e.g., first month of pregnancy) in cases and controls may be considered. The most frequently used measure of association in case-control studies is the odds ratio, described in earlier chapters. If the disease is uncommon, the odds ratio, rate ratio, and risk ratio are all similar in value in both cumulative-incidence and incidence-density case-control studies. If the study is of the incidence-density type and if neither disease incidence nor the proportion of the population exposed changes over the study period, the odds ratio is a good estimate of the rate ratio, regardless of whether the disease is common.

As in any type of epidemiologic study, it is important to obtain estimates of odds ratios that take into account confounding variables and to determine if exposure to one factor modifies the effect of exposure to another. It is thus important from the outset to collect sufficiently detailed information on exposure, potential confounding variables, and potential effect modifiers to permit these analyses to be done. Although without ancillary information a case-control study cannot provide estimates of actual incidence rates among the exposed and the nonexposed or estimates of incidence rates attributable to a given cause, it can provide estimates of the proportion of disease attributable to a given cause, either in the population as a whole or among the exposed.

SELECTION OF CASES

Cases are usually selected from among persons seeking medical care for the disease(s) under study. Newly diagnosed cases are preferable because if a case has had the disease for a long period of time, it will often be difficult for the case to remember exposures and to distinguish exposures that preceded the disease from those that occurred after the disease had developed; thus, it may be hard to differentiate between cause and effect. Also, use of prevalent cases can lead to an overrepresentation of cases of long duration because those who die of the disease or who are rapidly cured have a lower probability of inclusion. Consequently, it will not be possible to determine to what extent an observed exposure-disease association is due to an association between exposure and incidence or between exposure and duration of disease. Although inclusion of persons with long-term disease increases the number of cases available for study, the possible bias from including them is usually sufficiently great that they should be excluded. However, if the number of persons at risk of becoming cases, the incidence rates, and the survival rates among incident cases remain stable over the period of the study within each level of the covariates of interest, then Begg and Gray (1987) have provided a method of correcting for the potential bias induced by the association of the exposure of interest or covariates with survival.

In most studies, cases are considered incident as of the time they are diagnosed. For a fracture, in which treatment is generally sought rapidly, time of diagnosis is a reasonably good approximation to the time of onset, whereas for many other diseases the actual time of onset is unknown or ill-defined. Therefore, when trying to identify risk factors for a disease, it is important to make sure that the exposure at least preceded the onset of symptoms, because this will render it unlikely that the person changed his or her exposure status as a result of the disease. In studying the possible relationship between diet and colon cancer, for instance, a person may have modified his or her diet as a result of early symptoms of the disease, so that questions should be asked about dietary habits before the first symptoms occurred. Weight loss consequent to ovarian cancer may occur before the cancer comes to medical attention, so that if weight is being considered as a possible risk factor, it is best to consider weight a few years before the cancer was recognized. In studies of diseases with slow onsets, such as multiple sclerosis and sometimes prolapsed intervertebral disc, a question-naire may have to be used to find out when symptoms began; any case in which symptoms began more than one year ago (or some other arbitrary date) can then be excluded (Kelsey and Ostfeld, 1975; Mundt et al., 1993).

As in any epidemiologic study, diagnostic criteria should be established (Lasky and Stolley, 1994). For cancers, the diagnostic criterion generally consists of a pathologist's confirmation of the diagnosis. For other conditions for which no definitive criterion exists that can be applied to all potential cases, various categories of degree of certainty of diagnosis can be established. In a case-control study of prolapsed intervertebral disc (Mundt et al., 1993), cases were classified as "confirmed" if it was recorded on a medical record that the prolapsed disc had been seen at surgery or on CT scan, magnetic resonance imaging, or myelogram; "probable" if the symptoms and signs were strongly consistent with a prolapsed disc but the prolapse had not been confirmed by any of these procedures; and "possible" if the symptoms and signs were suggestive of a prolapsed disc, but not as strongly as for the "probable" cases. When analyzing the data, one can evaluate whether the same variables are risk factors for all categories of cases, and if they are, combine them in the analysis. In the prolapsed disc study, several potential risk factors were more strongly associated with confirmed than with probable or possible cases, providing some evidence for the specificity of the associations with prolapsed disc as opposed to other disorders associated with low back pain. Usually the diagnostic criteria are based on information routinely available in the medical record, such as pathology or radiology reports, but in some studies further information may be obtained by the investigator. In the prolapsed disc study, for instance, symptoms were elicited in a uniform manner by trained interviewers; diagnostic criteria included information from both the interview and from medical records. In a case-control study of preterm delivery, Berkowitz (1981) performed an examination of certain physical and neurological characteristics of the neonates in order to estimate gestational age.

In general the most desirable way of obtaining cases is to include all incident cases in a defined population over a specified period of time. The existence of several population-based tumor registries that are part of the Cancer Surveillance, Epidemiology, and End Results (SEER) program (described in Chapter 3) makes feasible the identification of nearly all newly diagnosed cancer cases in several geographically defined areas of the United States. For instance, a case-control study of the association between oral contraceptives and breast, endometrial, and ovarian cancers (Centers for Disease Control Cancer and Steroid Hormone Study, 1983a,b,c) included cases from nine of the SEER registries in the United States. Studies of adverse reproductive outcomes are also often population-based because the source population of births giving rise to the adverse outcomes generally can be identified readily.

For most diseases and geographic areas, however, registries do not exist, and to identify all cases occurring in residents of a wide area in a timely manner would be prohibitively expensive. The most common way of obtaining cases is therefore to select all incident cases seen at certain hospitals over a specified period of time. The Boston Collaborative Drug Surveillance program, for instance, identifies newly diagnosed cases of a variety of diseases in selected hospitals in the Boston area (Slone et al., 1977). A study designed to determine whether estrogen replacement therapy protects against hip fractures included cases from four hospitals in New Haven and Hartford, Connecticut (Kreiger et al., 1982). Table 8–2 shows that estrogen use of 6 months or longer was greater in each of the two hospital control groups than in the cases, suggesting that indeed estrogen replacement therapy does protect against hip fracture.

For diseases for which hospitalization is not necessarily sought, patients seeking care from office-based physicians should also be included. Kessler (1972a,b) undertook case-control studies of Parkinson's disease both among hospital patients and among patients seen by a panel of 112 private practitioners. The 112 physicians in private practice included all except two neurologists and neurosurgeons and a sample of other practicing physicians in the greater Baltimore area (excluding physicians specializing in anesthe-

Table 8-2. Distribution of Hip Fracture Cases and Controls by Number of Months of Use of Estrogen Replacement Therapy, Connecticut, 1977–1979

No. of Months of Use of Estrogen Replacement Therapy	Cases		Trauma Controls		Nontrauma Controls	
	No.	%	No.	%	No.	%
<6	80	85.1	60	75.0	579	73.1
≥6	14	14.9	20	25.0	213	26.9
Total	94	100.0	80	100.0	792	100.0

Source: Kreiger et al. (1982).

siology, gynecology, obstetrics, ophthalmology, pathology, pediatrics, and psychiatry except neuropsychiatry). In studies of prolapsed intervertebral disc, patients seen in the private offices of orthopedists and neurosurgeons as well as in emergency rooms, clinics, and as hospital inpatients have been included (Kelsey and Ostfeld, 1975; Mundt et al., 1993). Because patients seen in physicians' offices do not expect to be contacted by persons doing research, special procedures may have to be devised to obtain permission to invite them to be in the study, and this process may be unacceptable to some physicians.

Other sources of cases include patients seen at prepaid health plans, schools, places of employment, the military service, and patient service organizations, but the three approaches described above are the ones most commonly used.

Ways of identifying cases at these various facilities (discussed in Chapter 3) depend upon the particular disease being studied. For example, cancer cases would be identified through tumor registries, pathology reports, surgical logs, and admission or discharge diagnoses, whereas hip fracture cases would be identified through radiology logs, surgical logs, and admission or discharge records.

Finally, although typically a case-control study compares one case group with one or more control groups, it may be efficient to compare several case groups with one or more control groups. For instance, several of the same exposures have been considered as possible risk factors for cancers of the breast, endometrium, and ovary, so that in two studies it has been found efficient to study the epidemiology of all three cancers in one case-control investigation. In each study the same questionnaire was administered to the three case groups and one control group (Centers for Disease Control, 1983a,b,c; Hildreth et al., 1981; Kelsey et al., 1981; Kelsey et al., 1982). Also, one case group may be divided into subgroups and compared with one control group, as has been done by subdividing fibrocystic breast disease into its histopathologic components and comparing each subgroup with an overall control group (Pastides et al., 1983). When this is done, the comparability of each of the case groups to the control group with respect to potentially confounding variables must be reconsidered. For instance, the age distribution of some of the case subgroups may be different from that of the control group. If so, age may have to be controlled for in each subgroup analysis, even though the age of all the cases combined is similar to that of the controls.

SELECTION OF CONTROLS

Choice of the most appropriate control group is one of the most difficult and controversial aspects of study design. As Schlesselman (1982) points out, "the control series is intended to provide an estimate of the exposure rate that would be expected to occur in the cases if there were no association between the study disease and exposure." Although different investigators interpret this criterion for a control group in different ways, it is useful to keep in mind this underlying concept when deciding which control groups are most appropriate in any given case-control study. Perhaps the most useful working concept of what a control group should be can be derived from Miettinen (1985): the controls should be selected in an unbiased manner from those individuals who would have been included in the case series, had they developed the disease under study. A series of papers by Wacholder et al. (1992a,b,c) provides a detailed discussion of selection of controls in case-control studies. These authors emphasize that the most difficult issue is the identification of the appropriate study base from which to select controls. The base is the set of persons among whom those developing the disease of interest will become cases in the study; worded slightly differently, the base is the source population from which cases arise during the time period when they are eligible to become cases (Wacholder et al., 1992a).

The three most commonly used control groups are (a) random samples of the population from which the cases came, (b) persons seeking medical care at the same institutions as the cases for conditions believed to be unrelated to the cases' diagnosis, and (c) neighbors of the cases. Other less frequently used control groups are friends, schoolmates, siblings, and fellow workers of the cases. The choice of which control group to use is generally dictated by (a) the source of the cases, (b) the relative costs of obtaining the various types of controls, and (c) the facilities available to the investigator carrying out the study.

Population-based Controls

If cases consist of all individuals developing the disease of interest in a defined population, then the single best control group would generally be a random or probability sample (see Chapter 12) of individuals from the same source population who have not developed the disease. Such a population is usually defined by geographic boundaries; if nearly all residents of a geographic area have telephones, then random-digit dialing may be used to obtain controls from the general population of the area. By selecting random digits instead of using the telephone book, the problem of failure to include people with unlisted numbers is circumvented. When random-digit dialing is used in epidemiologic studies, the method of Waksberg (Waksberg, 1978) is most often employed. The two-stage sampling method described by Waksberg is devised to minimize the chances of calling telephone numbers that are not assigned to households, since such numbers account for about 80% of telephone numbers. Waksberg's method consists of the following steps:

1. Obtain from the telephone company a recent list of all telephone area codes and existing prefix numbers (the first three digits after the area code) within the area.
2. To these, add all possible choices for the next two digits, and thus prepare a list of all the possible first eight digits of the ten digits in telephone numbers. These eight-digit numbers are treated as Primary Sampling Units (PSUs).
3. Randomly select an eight-digit number and also randomly select the final two digits.
4. Dial the number.
5a. If the dialed number is at a residential address, retain the PSU in the sample. Select the additional final two digits at random to be added to the same first eight digits until the desired number of additional residential telephones, k, is reached. Conduct interviews at both the initial number and all the additional randomly selected numbers ($k + 1$ numbers in total).
5b. If the originally dialed number is not residential, reject the PSU.
6. Repeat steps 1–5 until the desired number of PSUs, m, is selected. The total sample size will be m ($k + 1$). The values of m and k are chosen to satisfy criteria for an optimal sampling design.

Waksberg discusses how to handle additional issues, including (a) determining how many household members use the telephone number, (b) asking how many telephone numbers a household has, (c) deciding what to do when no one answers despite repeated calls, (d) the necessity of keeping careful records of all calls, and (e) deciding whether telephone or in-person interviewing should be undertaken once the participants have been selected by random-digit dialing. A recent review by Potthoff (1994) discusses a variety of other issues that have arisen with random digit dialing, including how to deal with technologic advances such as answering machines and call forwarding, and how to select which household member(s) to interview.

When random-digit dialing is used, a simple random sample of the population is occasionally desired, but more often a study is limited to individuals in a certain age range or of a certain gender. A case-control study concerned with hormone replacement therapy as a possible risk factor, for instance, would probably be limited to women of age 45 years and older. Therefore, following a brief introduction, the first step when a residential telephone number is reached may be to take a census of the age, gender, and other characteristics of each household member in order to determine who is eligible for inclusion. If no one at the number is eligible, the interview is terminated. For eligible respondents, either an interview may take place over the telephone or an appointment may be made for a personal interview. Alternatively, a roster of eligible respondents can be prepared and then sampled at a later time as needed.

Random-digit dialing has been used in many case-control studies in the United States, including some in single geographic areas such as King County, Washington (Weiss et al., 1979), and others undertaken in defined geographic areas in several parts of the country (Centers for Disease Control Cancer and Steroid Hormone Study, 1983a,b,c; Hoover and Strasser, 1980). In a case-control study of the possible associations between use of oral contraceptives and cancers of the breast, endometrium, and ovary, it was desired to have a sufficiently large study population that modest increases or decreases in risk could be detected in various subgroups of the population. To obtain sufficiently large numbers of cases, eight of the population-based SEER registries around the United States were included. Because cases came from geographically defined populations, it was decided that controls should be from these same populations. Therefore, random-digit dialing was used. All the random-digit dialing could be done from one central location, thus increasing the efficiency of the study. Once controls were identified from the central location, local interviewers could arrange to administer the questionnaire to them in person. Table 8–3 shows results obtained from this study regarding the association between oral contraceptives and ovarian cancer. A negative association between length of use of oral contraceptives and ovarian cancer is apparent.

In countries or regions with relatively accurate population registries, controls may be selected from the registries. For instance, in a multicenter case-control study of occupations and risk for bladder cancer in Spain (Gonzalez et al., 1989), one of the two control groups used was people selected at random from the same section of the census or municipal registries as that of the case. In a case-control study of diet and endometrial cancer in Shanghai, China, controls were identified through a random selection procedure from resident rosters at the Shanghai Resident Registry (Shu et al., 1993). In a case-control study of the association between use of the injectable contraceptive depot–medroxyprogesterone acetate (DMPA)

Table 8–3. Distribution of Ovarian Cancer Cases and Controls by Duration of Oral Contraceptive Use and Associated Odds Ratio, Centers for Disease Control Cancer and Steroid Hormone Study

Duration of Oral Contraceptive Use	Number of Cases	Number of Controls	Odds Ratio	95% Confidence Interval
Never used[a]	86	683	1.0	—
<3 mo.	16	106	1.0	0.5–1.9
3–11 mo.	13	133	0.7	0.4–1.4
1–2 yr.	32	213	0.8	0.5–1.4
3–4 yr.	12	137	0.6	0.2–1.0
≥5 yr.	17	332	0.4	0.2–0.6

[a]Reference category.

Source: Centers for Disease Control Cancer and Steroid Hormone Study (1983c).

and risk of cervical cancer in Costa Rica (Oberle et al., 1988), controls were randomly sampled from households enumerated in the national census. In a case-control study in Mexico that identified an association between chili pepper consumption and gastric cancer, controls were selected from the households that had been randomly selected for the Mexican National Health Survey (López-Carrillo et al., 1994).

In some instances, cases may be from specified populations other than those defined by geographic boundaries, such as people enrolled in prepaid health care plans, workers at a particular place of employment, or births at selected hospitals. In these instances, the most appropriate control groups would come from other persons enrolled in the prepaid health plan, other workers at the plant, and other births at the same hospitals, respectively.

Patients Seeking Care for Other Conditions as Controls

If cases are individuals whose illness was diagnosed at a few selected medical facilities, it is seldom possible to specify the source population from which the cases arose. Therefore, one seeks to obtain a source of controls subject to the same selective factors as the cases.

The most frequently used source of controls is people seeking care at the same hospitals for other diseases. Because the selective factors may differ by hospital service, the controls are usually chosen from among other persons admitted to the same hospital services as the cases. For instance, case-control studies focusing on breast cancer often use as controls women admitted to the general surgery service for conditions not related to the breast.

Under most circumstances it is desirable to include as controls people with a variety of other conditions, so that no one disease is unduly represented in the control group. When a control group has been assembled, the distribution of controls by diagnosis should be examined. In a hospital-based case-control study of the relationship between use of oral contraceptives and malignant and benign breast diseases (Kelsey et al., 1978), for instance, about one quarter of the controls were found to have been admitted for gallbladder disease. Because some evidence exists that gallbladder disease itself is associated with oral contraceptive use, inclusion of such a high proportion of women with gallbladder disease could bias the findings regarding breast diseases. A more extreme example of this problem would occur if the controls for breast cancer cases were limited to patients with benign breast diseases. Because oral contraceptive use has been found to be negatively associated with benign breast diseases (Kelsey, 1979), such a study might lead to the false conclusion that oral contraceptives increase the risk for breast cancer when in reality they are associated with a reduced risk for benign breast diseases. Similarly, inclusion of a relatively large number of lung cancer patients as controls in a study of the relationship between smoking and bladder cancer would lead to an underestimate of the association between smoking and bladder cancer. Thus, in general, patients with other conditions thought to be related to the exposure of interest should be excluded as controls in the study design.

Another consideration in selection of controls from hospitals is that it may be important to exclude potential controls who have had their disease for a long time because, like the cases, the presence of their disease may have influenced their exposure to possible risk factors. Such characteristics as physical activity, diet, weight, and medication use, for instance, may change as a result of many diseases.

A special problem arises when it is necessary to obtain tissue from a particular organ in both cases and controls. If an investigator wanted to examine laryngeal tissue from cases of cancer of the larynx and from controls for evidence of viral infection, the only feasible control group of living individuals would be patients with benign lesions of the larynx, because it would be unethical to excise tissue from the larynx of individuals who were not having the tissue removed anyway. The investigator would have to have reason to believe that the virus in question was not involved in the etiology of the benign lesions. Sometimes autopsy controls may be the only option. Few patients without lung cancer have lung tissue removed at surgery, so that if an investigator is searching for markers of exposure in lung tissue, the control group would probably have to consist of autopsied individuals, with the appropriate tissue collected as soon as possible after death. When autopsy material is used in this way, not only is one concerned about the nonrepresentativeness of those who are autopsied, but one must also assume that no important changes take place in the tissue after death.

Neighborhood Controls

A third type of control group sometimes used is neighborhood controls. Such controls tend to be employed when the source population from which the cases come cannot be defined and when it is desired to have presumably healthy individuals as controls. The assumption in using such a control group is that neighbors of the cases tend to seek care at the same medical facilities as the cases, and would therefore enter the study as cases if they were to develop the disease of interest. The correctness of this assumption may vary considerably from one setting to another.

Neighborhood controls are usually individually matched to cases by such variables as age and gender. Accordingly, a member of the study team canvasses the neighborhood of the cases by some strict set of rules until a control of the appropriate gender and age group is found. For instance, the study team member might start out by going to the first residence to the right of the case's residence, then the first to the left, then the second to the right, and so on, until an appropriate match is found. Because people who are not at home much of the time are likely to be systematically different from people who usually are at home, it is important to follow the specified algorithm very closely and not to skip households where people are not at home. This means that multiple call-backs are often necessary, thus making studies using neighborhood controls relatively expensive. As a result, random-digit dialing is now more frequently used when controls from the general population are desired. In other words, it is usually less expensive to "let your fingers do the walking." In some areas where telephone exchanges are limited to defined geographic areas, a control in the same general (but not necessarily immediate) neighborhood may be obtained by random-digit dialing within an exchange. Neighborhood controls are almost inevitably somewhat matched to the cases on socioeconomic variables and environmental exposures. If the study is concerned with such variables as potential risk factors, then the use of neighborhood controls may result in some degree of "overmatching" of controls to cases, a phenomenon discussed below.

Other Types of Control Groups

Perhaps the one other type of control group used with a moderate degree of frequency is "friend controls." Most commonly, each case is asked for the name of a friend (or friends) of the same gender and about the same age who does not have the disease of interest. In addition to any intentional matching on such variables as age and gender, friend controls will be matched to cases on many social characteristics as well. Use of friend controls presents various problems. A major one is that, like the cases and neighborhood controls, the cases and friend controls may be overmatched, because they may be more similar in respect to exposures of interest than cases and unmatched population controls would be. If coffee drinking is the exposure of interest, for instance, friends may tend to have similar coffee-drinking habits. Although the estimate of the odds ratio will not be biased provided the matching of controls to cases is accounted for in the analysis, this type of overmatching means that a larger sample size will be needed for the same degree of power to detect an association between the exposure and disease. Second, if the exposure of interest is a determinant of friend-ship, then selection into the control group will depend in part on the exposure, thus creating bias. For instance, in a case-control study con-cerned with occupational exposures, using a friend of each case to compose the control group could create bias because people who work together sometimes become friends. This bias will not be corrected by using a matched analysis (Flanders and Austin, 1986). Third, some cases may not have friends or may not want to give the names of friends to the investiga-tors. Fourth, a case may provide the name of the friend who most likes to talk or who is most sociable; if sociability is related to the exposure of interest, bias will result. Because choosing a friend as a control is not particularly rigorous and may be subject to a variety of biases, friends are generally not the control group of choice (Flanders and Austin, 1986; Robins and Pike, 1990; Wacholder et al., 1992b). Nevertheless, in some instances, such as when cases are identified by mail surveys or from social groups, there may be no other feasible control group. Siblings or spouses are also sometimes used as controls when it is desired to separate genetic and environmental risk factors, but such control groups will not be dis-cussed here.

Strengths and Weaknesses of Commonly Used Control Groups

Each type of control group has its own strengths and weaknesses. Limita-tions of neighborhood and friend controls were discussed above. If hospital controls are used, the controls by definition are different from the cases since they generally have another disease for which they have sought medi-cal care. If smoking is the putative risk factor, for instance, one may be concerned that hospital controls include more than their fair share of smok-ers, because smoking is associated with many diseases that require hospital-ization. If the control group is overrepresented with exposed persons, the odds ratio for the disease of primary interest will be underestimated, where-as if the control group is underrepresented with exposed persons, the odds ratio will be overestimated. One study (Olson et al., 1994) obtained data on characteristics of persons eligible to be hospital controls and on characteristics of persons from the general population of the geographic area in which the hospitals were situated; it was found that odds ratios associated with most of the characteristics considered in that study would be affected very little if hospital controls were used rather than controls from the general population, except for slight bias brought about by the somewhat higher prevalence of obesity and of smoking among hospital controls.

A major concern in studies employing random digit dialing as a means of control selection is that a substantial proportion of potential controls (typically about 30%–40% in otherwise well executed studies) may decline to participate, and it is possible that participants and nonparticipants differ in ways that could affect study results. In the United States, the proportion of nonrespondents has become greater over time; factors contributing to this are the increase in the use of answering machines so that potential respondents often cannot be contacted directly, an increase in the general level of suspicion, and a growing resentment of unsolicited telephone calls. A study (Olson et al., 1992) comparing characteristics of persons successfully selected through random-digit dialing to the characteristics of the general population of the same geographic area found that most odds ratios would be affected only slightly by the 30%–40% refusal to participate. Of the characteristics considered in that study, only the odds ratios associated with previous use of screening tests were likely to be biased because of the greater exposure to screening tests among the persons participating than among the population from which they came. A recent paper by Perneger et al. (1993) provides additional information on the effectiveness of the Waksberg method of random digit dialing for control selection, and concludes that it is indeed an effective method.

In the United States, only about 7% of households do not have telephones, so that in most parts of the country bias from excluding from the control group people without telephones is small. In some localities and population subgroups, however, such as in poor areas of inner cities, this percentage is considerably higher. To prevent possible bias from comparing all cases, regardless of whether they have a telephone, to controls with telephones, cases without telephones can be excluded.

Another problem is that if the study is limited to a certain subgroup of the population, such as a particular racial or ethnic group, the elderly, or individuals in a very narrow age range, a large number of calls will have to be made to identify eligible controls. In such instances, other methods of control selection may be preferred (Wacholder et al., 1992b; also see Chapter 15).

It is also important that the cases and controls be equally likely to report exposure. A person who has developed a disease may think hard and remember exposures that healthy people have forgotten. Although the small amount of empirical evidence of this issue is not entirely consistent (Drews et al., 1990), the potential for "recall bias" is thought to be especially great in case-control studies of congenital malformations, when a mother who has delivered an infant with a malformation tends to search extensively for an explanation. In this instance, a control group consisting of mothers who have delivered infants with other malformations may be the control group of choice. If the association with reported exposure is specific to the malformation of interest, then belief in the validity of the association is enhanced.

If the cases are from selected hospitals rather than all hospitals in a geographic area, then taking a sample of the general population of the entire geographic area as the control group makes little sense because the cases and controls will be from different source populations. Also, if the disease of interest does not generally result in hospitalization, either because those affected do not necessarily seek medical care or because hospitalization is not required for treatment, controls and cases seen at hospitals will be more comparable if controls are chosen from among those also being hospitalized. For instance, autopsy studies show that a significant portion of women with fibrocystic breast disease never have their disease diagnosed (Frantz et al., 1951). In a case-control study to identify risk factors for fibrocystic breast disease in which cases are identified through hospital records, using as controls women who also seek medical care at the same hospitals may reduce bias related to medical-care-seeking behavior. To decrease this potential bias further, additional questions about use of medical care may have to be included in the questionnaire and controlled for in the analysis. If medical care is generally sought for a disease but not necessarily at a hospital, such as for prolapsed intervertebral disc, then controls should come from the same sources as the cases, be it offices of physicians in private practice, clinics, emergency rooms, or hospitals.

Finally, in some situations no single control group is obviously best. In such situations it is helpful if (a) more than one case-control study of an issue of interest is undertaken by different investigators using different types of control groups, and (b) an investigator uses more than one control group with which to compare the cases. Because there tend to be strong feelings for and against various types of control groups by different investigators, an association will have a much greater likelihood of being accepted as valid if it is found when different types of control groups are used. For instance, relatively strong associations between use of estrogen replacement therapy and endometrial cancer have been found in studies in which cases have been compared to controls obtained by random-digit dialing (Weiss et al., 1979) and several types of hospital controls (Kelsey et al., 1982). However, a study using controls admitted to hospital for dilatation and curettage

Table 8–4. Endometrial Cancer Cases and Three Control Groups by Duration of Estrogen Use and Associated Age-Adjusted Odds Ratios, North Carolina, 1970–1976

Duration of Use (Years)	No. of Cases	D and C		Gynecology		Community	
		No.	Odds Ratio	No.	Odds Ratio	No.	Odds Ratio
Never used[a]	125	136	1.0	118	1.0	172	1.0
<0.5	8	13	0.7	12	0.7	20	0.8
0.5–3.4	9	14	0.7	9	0.9	21	0.7
3.5–6.4	9	16	0.8	1 ⎫	3.8	7	1.7
6.5–9.4	9	11	1.2	2 ⎭		5	2.5
≥9.5	19	10	2.0	2	5.1	4	5.5
Unknown	7	8		9		7	

[a]Reference group.

Source: Hulka et al. (1980).

(D and C) did not show such a strong association (Horwitz and Feinstein, 1979), and the authors of this study put forward the argument that the controls used in the studies showing positive results were inappropriate because of "detection bias" among the cases but not the controls. That is, a certain proportion of the endometrial cancer cases in these studies were purported to have come to medical attention only because they used estrogen, which induced bleeding and brought them to medical attention so that the cancer could be diagnosed. Therefore, a study using three different types of control groups simultaneously (hospital controls, community controls, D and C controls) was undertaken (Hulka et al., 1980) in order to shed more light on the reasons for the discrepancies in the different studies. The findings of the study, shown in Table 8–4, have added to the general belief that estrogen replacement therapy is indeed causally related to endometrial cancer because it was found that (a) there was a strong association with length of use when gynecology or community controls but not D and C controls were used and (b) among the D and C controls but not among the cases or the gynecology controls, there was an association between bleeding and estrogen use. Thus, only among the D and C controls did estrogen use appear to bring women to medical attention because of bleeding, indicating that this control group, and not the case group, was overrepresented with exposed women. Detailed examination of the reason for discrepant results when different control groups are used, as was done by Hulka et al. (1980), is indeed useful.

Other Considerations

Occasionally, different control groups are needed to examine the effects of different risk factors in the same study. For instance, in a case-control study of Hodgkin's disease in São Paulo, Brazil, most case-control comparisons used as controls (a) age- and gender-matched patients from the same hospitals as the cases who had cancers of nonlymphatic tissue and (b) siblings of the cases. Identification of controls by random-digit dialing or by neighborhood was not feasible because the patients came from a wide geographic area, much of it rural or low-income and without telephones (Kirchoff et al., 1980). A different set of controls was used to study antibodies to the Epstein-Barr virus because various diseases and associated therapies can alter these levels. Hospital controls for these comparisons consisted of blood donors, postpartum women, and patients on the orthopedic service (Evans et al., 1980).

Another situation in which the choice of a control group is not clear is when a certain proportion of cases have died before they can be contacted. When this occurs, information on exposure and other relevant variables for the deceased cases is generally obtained from relatives or from records. Gordis (1982) has raised and discussed the question of whether cases and controls should be matched according to dead versus alive status or whether the controls should be selected without regard to vital status. On the one hand, if some cases are dead and all controls are alive, the quality and quantity of information obtained may differ systematically, although, as Gordis points out, (a) this may not be a problem for some variables, and (b) it is difficult to predict in what direction such bias might operate. On the other hand, dead controls are overrepresented with individuals with characteristics associated with early mortality, such as cigarette smoking. Thus, when a certain proportion of cases has died, the choice of a control group should depend in part on the nature of the putative risk factors of interest, and, again, use of more than one control group may be desirable if no one group is clearly preferable.

ASCERTAINMENT OF EXPOSURE TO RISK FACTORS

Information on exposure to putative risk factors may be obtained in several ways, depending on the nature of the exposure. Exposure data are most commonly obtained by means of personal interview of cases and controls. For instance, the best way to find out about a person's smoking history is to ask the person. Existing records may sometimes be used to find out about exposures. Hospital records or birth certificates would be appropriate places to find out about birthweight. Physical measurements or laboratory tests on sera or other tissue drawn from cases and controls may also be used.

Issues involved in making measurements in these ways have been reviewed by Correa et al. (1994) and will be covered in detail in this book in

Chapters 14 and 15. However, it should be emphasized that no matter which method is used, ensuring that ascertainment of exposure status is comparable in cases and controls is of the utmost importance. Accordingly, if personal interviewing is used to obtain the data on exposure, all cases and controls should be asked exactly the same questions in exactly the same manner. Although it is of course desirable that the interviewer not know whether he or she is interviewing a case or control, such "blindness" is not always possible because often the case will say at the outset something like "you're interviewing me because I have cancer" or controls will ask for an explanation of why they have been invited to be in the study. It may help if at least the interviewer does not know the major hypothesis being tested in the study so that the possibility of interviewer bias is reduced.

If record abstraction is being used to obtain exposure information, it is likewise important that the abstractor not know the main purpose of the study because it may be tempting for the abstractor to look harder for certain pieces of information on some records than others. When considering record abstraction as a means of obtaining information on cases and controls, it is also important to determine whether the information is equally likely to have been recorded for cases and controls. A person admitted to a hospital for lung cancer is much more likely to be asked about smoking habits than a person admitted for emergency surgery on a fractured hip or for an appendectomy. Accordingly, in most hospitals, the vast majority of lung cancer patients will have smoking data recorded whereas the majority of hip fracture or appendicitis patients will not, and when the information is not recorded, the investigator has no way of knowing whether the person smoked.

Thus, unless the information of interest is routinely recorded on medical records, the records should not be used to obtain it. Only a few non-medical variables, such as age, gender, race, and method of payment, are routinely recorded. Similarly, if a participant is unlikely to know about or remember exposure to a possible risk factor, then there is no point in asking. For instance, there is little point in asking people about constituents of the water they drank ten years ago.

Sometimes measurement may be made of the physical environment, such as of pollutants in the ambient air, constituents of drinking water, or exposures in the workplace. Unless past measurements are available, it has to be assumed that the exposure incurred at the time of the study is the same as the exposure at the time the disease process began; this assumption is frequently not valid.

A variety of physical measurements, such as blood pressure, may be made directly on the cases and controls. Again, careful consideration must be given to whether the level measured at the time the disease is diagnosed is the same as when the disease developed.

The same general reservations apply to measurements made on sera or other tissue taken around the time of diagnosis; that is, the measurements made after diagnosis may not reflect levels at the time the disease developed. Many studies have measured concentrations of estrogens and other hormones in the sera of breast cancer cases and controls. For the most part, little difference has been found in hormone levels of cases and controls. However, the crucial period of exposure to hormones may be decades before the disease is diagnosed, so the findings at the time of diagnosis may have little meaning. In such instances, banks of sera that have been frozen and stored for many years are of particular value. If sera from large enough numbers of people have been properly stored, if no degradation has occurred in the serum constituents of interest, and if most of these people can be traced and their disease status determined, then nested case-control studies using stored sera to determine exposure status can be employed. Such studies were described in Chapter 5.

Obtaining evidence of prior exposure to infectious diseases by questionnaire is fraught with error unless several conditions are present. First, the clinical disease should be highly characteristic and not mimicked by any other common condition, and subclinical disease should be absent or very rare. Measles, for example, has a characteristic clinical picture, with its Koplik spots in the mouth, respiratory involvement, and seasonal pattern; almost all infections with measles virus are clinically manifested and have these typical features. Second, it is important that the diagnosis have been recorded by a competent physician. Third, laboratory tests should have been performed and recorded to verify the diagnosis. Finally, belief that the disease actually occurred is enhanced if there is a characteristic residual of the disease, such as the flaccid paralysis of poliomyelitis or the typical scars of smallpox. Without these features, a history of an infectious disease must be accepted with great caution. Determining prior immunization by questionnaire is subject to even greater error unless some unique aspect of administration exists that will be distinctly remembered, unless scarification methods (a set of small, superficial incisions or punctures in the skin) are used, such as in some programs of smallpox and Bacillus Calmette-Guérin (BCG) vaccinations, or unless residual scars are left by a successful take of the vaccines themselves.

Serologic studies have documented the lack of accuracy in reporting the previous occurrence of certain infectious diseases and immunizations against them (Carvalho et al., 1976; Comstock et al., 1973; Evans, 1980; Evans et al., 1979). The reliability of a history of each disease or immunization must be judged individually. In two studies (Comstock et al., 1973; Evans et al., 1979) concerned with immunity to poliomyelitis, for instance, 79.0% and 90.5% of those with a history of immunization or disease had polio type-3 antibody, and 20.0% and 72.2% had antibodies with a negative history of immunization or disease. This discrepancy in percentage having antibodies but a negative history in the two studies probably occurred because the first study (Comstock et al., 1973) was carried out in Maryland, United States, where clinical and subclinical poliomyelitis are uncommon, and the latter (Evans et al., 1979) was undertaken in Barbados, where subclinical infection at an early age occurs frequently. These observations emphasize the need for laboratory confirmation of historical data in case-control studies of infectious diseases.

EXCLUSIONS

In many case-control studies, it is necessary to exclude certain potential participants. Although excluding potential cases and controls limits generalizability, the validity of the comparison between cases and controls and efficiency of the study must take high priority. The general principle that the same exclusion criteria should be applied to cases and controls should be maintained whenever possible. If cases are restricted to a certain gender or age range, controls should be similarly restricted. If cases with certain medical conditions are excluded, then controls with those conditions should also be excluded. If the disease for which the cases are admitted affects an organ that may have been removed from some members of the population, then controls without the organ should generally be excluded. Also, under most circumstances, cases and controls with essentially zero likelihood of exposure to the putative risk factors of primary interest should be excluded, since they usually add no useful information to the case-control comparison. Inclusion of males, for instance, would add nothing to a study focusing on oral contraceptive use.[1]

Another common exclusion is cases and controls who have had their disease for more than a certain period of time, such as 6 months or a year, because, as discussed previously, it is important to have incident cases and controls. If questionnaires are to be used, cases and controls who do not speak English fluently are sometimes excluded because it is doubtful that comparable information can be obtained using an English-language questionnaire from people who do and people who do not speak English well. However, in areas where substantial numbers of people speak another language, it will generally be worth translating a questionnaire to the other language(s), then back-translating it into English to check on the reliability of the translation, and, after making any necessary modifications, to use it. The effect of questionnaire language on measures of association can be considered in the analysis in much the same way that the effects of self-respondents versus proxy respondents are considered (see Chapter 15).

ASCERTAINMENT OF EXPOSURE TO CONFOUNDING VARIABLES

The same procedures that are used to determine exposure to putative risk factors are also used to ascertain exposure to confounding variables. In some instances, questionnaires are the best method; less often, existing records contain the desired information, while physical measurements or laboratory assays may occasionally be needed. Not infrequently one hears an investigator say that the quality of measurement of a variable does not matter because it is "only a potentially confounding variable." Quite to the contrary, accurate measurement of a confounding variable *is* important, or else it cannot be taken into account adequately in the analysis. This will be discussed in greater detail in Chapter 13.

Occasionally data may be obtained on all cases and controls for some variables, but on only a sample of cases and controls for other variables because of cost or logistic considerations. Assuming that the cases and controls for whom complete information is available are representative of all cases and controls, the methods of Cain and Breslow (1988) can be used to analyze such data.

REFERENCES

Austin H, Hill HA, Flanders P, Greenberg RS. 1994. Limitations in the application of case-control methodology. *Epidemiol Rev* 16:65–76.

Begg CB, Gray RJ. 1987. Methodology for case-control studies with prevalent cases. *Biometrika* 74:191–195.

Berkowitz GS. 1981. An epidemiologic study of preterm delivery. *Am J Epidemiol* 113:81–92.

Cain KC, Breslow NE. 1988. Logistic regression analysis and efficient design for two-stage studies. *Am J Epidemiol* 128:1198–1206.

Carvalho RPS, Evans AS, Grossman L, Pannuti CS. 1976. Anticorpos para os virus da rubeola, do sarampo e da caxumba em criancas de Sao Paulo, Brasil. *Rev Saude Publica* 10:279–284.

Centers for Disease Control Cancer and Steroid Hormone Study. 1983a. Long-term oral contraceptive use and the risk of breast cancer. *JAMA* 249:1591–1595.

Centers for Disease Control Cancer and Steroid Hormone Study. 1983b. Oral contraceptive use and the risk of endometrial cancer. *JAMA* 249:1600–1604.

Centers for Disease Control Cancer and Steroid Hormone Study. 1983c. Oral contraceptive use and the risk of ovarian cancer. *JAMA* 249:1596–1599.

Comstock GW, Brownlow WJ, Joseph JM, Garber HG. 1973. Validity of interview information in estimating community immunization levels. *Health Serv Rep* 88:750–757.

Correa A, Stewart WF, Yeh H-C, Santos-Burgoa C. 1994. Exposure measurement in case-control studies: reported methods and recommendations. *Epidemiol Rev* 16:18–31.

Drews CD, Kraus JF, Greenland S. 1990. Recall bias in a case-control study of Sudden Infant Death Syndrome. *Int J Epidemiol* 19:405–411.

Evans AS. 1980. The need for serologic evaluation of immunization programs. *Am J Epidemiol* 112:725–731.

Evans AS, Kirchhoff LV, Pannuti CS, Carvalho RPS, McClelland KE. 1980. A case-control study of Hodgkin's disease in Brazil. II. Seroepidemologic studies in cases and family members. *Am J Epidemiol* 112:609–618.

Evans AS, Wells AV, Ramsay F, Drabkin P, Palmer K. 1979. Poliomyelitis, rubella, and dengue antibody survey in Barbados. A follow-up study. *Int J Epidemiol* 8:235–241.

Flanders WD, Austin H. 1986. Possibility of selection bias in matched case-control studies using friend controls. *Am J Epidemiol* 124:150–153.

Frantz VIC, Pickren JW, Melcher GW, Auchincloss H Jr. 1951. Incidence of chronic cystic disease in so-called "normal breasts": a study based on 225 postmortem examinations. *Cancer* 4:762–783.

Gonzalez CA, Lopez-Abente G, Errezola M, Escolar A, Riboli E, Izarzugaza I, Nebot M. 1989. Occupation and bladder cancer in Spain: a multi-centre case-control study. *Int J Epidemiol* 18:569–577.

Gordis L. 1982. Should dead cases be matched to dead controls? *Am J Epidemiol* 115:1–5.

Greenland S, Thomas DC. 1982. On the need for the rare disease assumption in case-control studies. *Am J Epidemiol* 116:547–553.

Greenwald P, Barlow JJ, Nasca PC, Burnett WS. 1974. Vaginal cancer after maternal treatment with synthetic hormones. *N Eng J Med* 285:390–392.

Herbst AL, Ulfelder H, Poskanzer DC. 1971. Adenocarcinoma of the vagina: association of maternal stilbestrol therapy with tumor appearance in young women. *N Engl J Med* 284:878–881.

Hildreth NG, Kelsey JL, LiVolsi VA, Fischer DB, Holford TR, Mostow ED, Schwartz PE, White C. 1981. An epidemiologic study of epithelial carcinoma of the ovary. *Am J Epidemiol* 114:398–405.

Hoover RN, Strasser PH. 1980. Artificial sweeteners and human bladder cancer. *Lancet* 1:837–840.

Horwitz RI, Feinstein AR. 1979. Alternative analytic methods for case-control studies of estrogens and endometrial cancer. *N Engl J Med* 299:1089–1094.

Hulka BS, Grimson RC, Greenberg BG, Kaufman DG, Fowler WC Jr, Hogue CJR, Gerger GS, Pulliam CC. 1980. "Alternative" controls in a case-control study of endometrial cancer and exogenous estrogens. *Am J Epidemiol* 112:376–387.

Kelsey JL. 1979. A review of the epidemiology of human breast cancer. *Epidemiol Rev* 1:74–109.

Kelsey JL, Fischer DB, Holford TR, LiVolsi VA, Mostow ED, Goldenberg IS,

White C. 1981. Exogenous estrogens and other factors in the epidemiology of breast cancer. *J Natl Cancer Inst* 67:327–333.

Kelsey JL, Holford TR, White C, Mayer ES, Kilty SE, Acheson RM. 1978. Oral contraceptives and breast disease: an epidemiological study. *Am J Epidemiol* 107:236–244.

Kelsey JL, LiVolsi VA, Holford TR, Fischer DB, Schwartz PE, O'Connor T, White C. 1982. A case-control study of endometrial cancer. *Am J Epidemiol* 116:333–342.

Kelsey JL, Ostfeld AM. 1975. Demographic characteristics of persons with acute herniated lumbar intervertebral disc. *J Chron Dis* 28:37–50.

Kessler II. 1972a. Epidemiologic studies of Parkinson's disease. II. A hospital-based survey. *Am J Epidemiol* 95:308–318.

Kessler II. 1972b. Epidemiologic studies of Parkinson's disease. III. A community-based survey. *Am J Epidemiol* 96:242–254.

Kirchoff L, Evans AS, McClelland KE, Carvalho RPS, Pannuti CS. 1980. A case-control study of Hodgkin's disease in Brazil: epidemiologic aspects. *Am J Epidemiol* 112:595–608.

Kreiger N, Kelsey JL, Holford TR, O'Connor T. 1982. An epidemiologic study of hip fracture in postmenopausal women. *Am J Epidemiol* 116:141–148.

Lasky T, Stolley PD 1994. Selection of cases and controls. *Epidemiol Rev* 16:6–17.

López-Carrillo L, Hernandez Avila M, Dubrow R. 1994. Chili pepper consumption and gastric cancer in Mexico: a case-control study. *Am J Epidemiol* 139:263–271.

Miettinen OS. 1985. The "case-control" study: valid selection of subjects. *J Chron Dis* 38:543–548.

Miettinen OS. 1976. Estimability and estimation in case-referent studies. *Am J Epidemiol* 103:226–235.

Morgenstern H, Kleinbaum DG, Kupper LL. 1980. Measures of disease incidence used in epidemiologic research. *Int J Epidemiol* 9:97–104.

Mundt DL, Kelsey JL, Golden AL, Pastides H, Berg AT, Sklar J, Hosea T, Panjabi MM. 1993. An epidemiologic study of non-occupational lifting as a risk factor for herniated lumber intervertebral disc. The Northeast Collaborative Group on Low Back Pain. *Spine* 18:595–602.

Oberle MW, Rosero-Bixby L, Irwin KL, Fortney JA, Lee NC, Whatley AS, Bonhomme MG. 1988. Cervical cancer risk and use of depot-medroxyprogesterone acetate in Costa Rica. *Int J Epidemiol* 17:718–723.

Olson SH, Kelsey JL, Pearson TA, Levin B. 1992. Evaluation of random-digit dialing as a method of control selection in case-control studies. *Am J Epidemiol* 135:210–222.

Olson SH, Kelsey JL, Pearson TA, Levin B. 1994. Characteristics of a hypothetical group of hospital controls for a case-control study. *Am J Epidemiol* 139:302–311.

Pastides H, Kelsey JL, LiVolsi VA, Holford TR, Fischer DB, Goldenberg IS. 1983. Oral contraceptive use and fibrocystic breast disease with special reference to its histopathology. *J Natl Cancer Inst* 71:5–9.

Perneger TV, Myers TL, Klag MJ, Whelton PK. 1993. Effectiveness of the Waksberg telephone sampling method for the selection of population controls. *Am J Epidemiol* 138:574–584.

Poole C. 1986. Exposure opportunity in case-control studies. *Am J Epidemiol* 123:352–358.

Potthoff RF. 1994. Telephone sampling in epidemiologic research: to reap the benefits, avoid the pitfalls. *Am J Epidemiol* 139:967–978.

Robins J, Pike M. 1990. The validity of case-control studies with nonrandom selection of controls. *Epidemiology* 1:273–284.

Sackett DL. 1979. Bias in analytic research. *J Chron Dis* 32:51–68.

Schlesselman JJ. 1982. Case-Control Studies. New York, Oxford University Press.

Schlesselman JJ, Stadel BV. 1987. Exposure opportunity in epidemiologic studies. *Am J Epidemiol* 125:174–178.

Shu XO, Zheng W, Potischman N, Brinton LA, Hatch MC, Gao Y-T, Fraumeni JF Jr. 1993. A population-based case-control study of dietary factors and endometrial cancer in Shanghai, People's Republic of China. *Am J Epidemiol* 137:155–165.

Slone D, Shapiro S, Miettinen OS. 1977. Case-control surveillance of serious illnesses attributable to ambulatory drug use. In: Epidemiological Evaluation of Drugs. Amsterdam, Elsevier North Holland Biomedical Press, pp 59–70.

Wacholder S, McLaughlin JK, Silverman DT, Mandel JS. 1992a. Selection of controls in case-control studies. I. Principles, *Am J Epidemiol* 135:1019–1028.

Wacholder S, Silverman DT, McLaughlin JK, Mandel JS. 1992b. Selection of controls in case-control studies. II. Types of controls. *Am J Epidemiol* 135:1029–1041.

Wacholder S, Silverman DT, McLaughlin JK, Mandel JS. 1992c. Selection of controls in case-control studies. III. Design options. *Am J Epidemiol* 135:1042–1050.

Waksberg J. 1978. Sampling methods for random digit dialing. *J Am Stat Assoc* 73:40–46.

Weiss NS, Szekely DR, English DR, Schweid AI. 1979. Endometrial cancer in relation to patterns of menopausal estrogen use. *JAMA* 242:261–265.

Exercises

1. Design one of the following case-control studies:

a. A study to identify risk factors for epithelial carcinoma of the ovary. Possible risk factors of interest include parity; age at menarche and age at menopause; age at first pregnancy and at first full-term delivery; a history of mumps, measles, and chicken pox; exposure to talc and asbestos; use of oral contraceptives and estrogen replacement therapy; body build. Your study may focus on one or several of these risk factors.

b. A study to identify risk factors for cancer of larynx. Possible risk factors of interest include smoking habits; alcohol consumption; use of gargles and mouth-washes; occupational exposures to asbestos, cutting oils, nickel, and wood dust; use of hair dyes.

NOTE

1. The increase in precision of estimates of association between risk factor and disease that could result from the greater sample size obtained when those at zero

risk of exposure are included has been described by Poole (1986). However, if cases and controls with zero likelihood of exposure were to be included, such as males in a study of the association between oral contraceptive use and bladder cancer, then the investigator would have to be certain that the reason for being at zero risk of exposure (i.e., being a male) is not related to another imperfectly measured risk factor for the disease under study. In this example, males would be more likely than females to have smoked cigarettes and to have had various occupational exposures that are associated with risk for bladder cancer; it is unlikely that these exposures could be measured accurately enough to be controlled for completely in the analysis. Males would therefore have to be placed in a separate stratum that would provide no useful information because no male cases and no male controls would have been exposed to oral contraceptives. For this reason, and because one does not in any event want to generalize to males, it would be unwise to include males in such a study (Schlesselman and Stadel, 1987). In fact it is rare that the investigator could be sure that the reason for no exposure among a subgroup was not related to risk of disease.

9

Case-Control Studies: II. Further Design Considerations and Analysis

This chapter is concerned mainly with control of confounding in case-control studies. When controlling for potential confounding variables in a case-control study, the investigator often has the options of (a) matching controls to cases on potential confounding variables at the time they are selected and using methods of statistical analysis appropriate for matched studies; (b) not matching controls to cases on any potential confounding variables at the time they are selected, but rather controlling for all potential confounding variables in the analysis, using statistical procedures appropriate for unmatched designs; and (c) using a combination of matching at the time cases and controls are selected and controlling for confounding variables in the analysis, using methods of analysis that take into account the matching. Combining the approaches may involve matching controls to cases on some potential confounding variables, not matching on others, and controlling for them all appropriately in the analysis. It may also entail matching loosely on certain potential confounding variables and controlling for them more tightly in the analysis. Although matching on potential confounding variables has considerable intuitive appeal, it also has limitations, and should be used only when its advantages outweigh its disadvantages. The first section of this chapter considers the advantages and disadvantages of matching as a means of controlling for confounding variables. Guidelines are presented as to which variables to match on, if matching is to be employed. The second part of the chapter describes methods of statistical analysis appropriate for unmatched and for matched designs. More detailed descriptions of methods of analysis of case-control studies are given by Breslow and Day (1980), Hosmer and Lemeshow (1989), and Clayton and Hills (1993).

ADVANTAGES AND DISADVANTAGES OF MATCHING CONTROLS TO CASES

The procedure of matching controls to cases as a part of a strategy for controlling for the effects of confounding variables is intuitively appealing in part because even people with little background in statistics appear to understand its use. If a case is a 43-year-old black male, then in principle it is straightforward to select a matched control who is also 43 years old, black, and male. In addition to its intuitive appeal, matching in case-control studies can have other logistical advantages.

First, matching may eliminate the need to assemble a comprehensive list of all eligible controls. In a hospital-based study, matched selection of the next eligible admission following the admission of each case circumvents the costly and time-consuming task of enumerating all admissions and then selecting controls randomly.

A second advantage is that matched selection of controls may make it feasible to obtain an appropriate nonhospitalized control group for comparison with hospitalized cases when an appropriate unmatched control group cannot be specified. Because of the complexity of referral patterns, it may not be possible to specify precisely the geographic region from which cases are drawn. Consequently, one would be unable to define the appropriate area from which to select an unmatched group of nonhospitalized controls. Identification of persons living in the same neighborhoods as the cases provides a control group that to some extent can be compared with cases. It may be necessary to measure and then control on potential confounding variables related to referral patterns more finely in the statistical analysis, but the matching by neighborhood is often a useful first step.

Third, matching controls to cases may make it possible to control to some extent for confounding variables that are difficult to measure directly and therefore cannot be adjusted for in an unmatched study. One example is the use of siblings as matched controls, a procedure that ensures a certain degree of comparability of cases and controls on a number of genetic and environmental factors.

The main statistical consideration in matching controls to cases is the possible gain or loss in precision in estimating the odds ratio (Karon and Kupper, 1982; Kupper et al., 1981; Samuels, 1981; Thompson et al., 1982). Precision can be gained by matching because one can prevent the occurrence of very small numbers of controls in some of the strata of the confounding variables. In an unmatched study, little overlap may occur between cases and controls in the distribution of the confounding variables. If a confounding variable is a strong risk factor for the disease, then the matching process will result in the controls having a distribution for the confounding variable that differs markedly from the distribution of the confounding variable that would be obtained if an unmatched group of controls were used instead.

For instance, Table 9–1 presents a hypothetical unmatched case-control study of the relation between an indicator of frailty and risk for hip fracture. Because age is strongly related to risk of hip fracture as well as to frailty, it must be taken into account as a confounding variable. For purposes of this example, we will assume there are two categories of frailty, two categories of age, 100 cases of hip fracture, and a control-to-case ratio of 2:1. Note that most of the cases are in the older stratum, whereas most of the controls are in the younger stratum. Because of this imbalance in the ratio of controls to cases, the estimates of the odds ratios within levels tend to be less than optimally precise, and this imprecision carries over to the summary measure of the odds ratio as well. Using methods to be described later in this chapter, the variance of the summary log odds ratio for the example is calculated to be 0.123. Table 9–2 gives the expected sample outcome for the corresponding matched study. Because the same ratio of controls to cases is imposed within each level of the confounding variable, greater precision of estimation is attained. The variance of the summary log odds ratio is in this instance only 0.081, which is appreciably smaller than the variance calculated for an unmatched design. The ratio of variances for an unmatched versus matched design is in this instance 1.51, indicating that in

Table 9–1. Hypothetical Example of an Unmatched Case-Control Study of the Relation between Frailty and Hip Fracture, Adjusting for Age in the Analysis by the Mantel-Haenszel Procedure

Confounding variable:
  stratum 1: age ≥70 years

		Hip fracture	Control	
Exposure	Frail	72	20	
	Not frail	18	20	
	Total	90	40	$N_1 = 130$

Confounding variable:
  stratum 2: age <70 years

		Hip fracture	Control	
Exposure	Frail	5	32	
	Not frail	5	128	
	Total	10	160	$N_2 = 170$

Summary odds ratio adjusted for age = 4.00
Variance of summary log odds ratio = 0.12264

Table 9-2. Hypothetical Example of a Case-Control Study of the Relation between Frailty and Hip Fracture, With Cases and Control Matched on Age in the Study Design

Confounding variable:
stratum 1: age ≥70 years

		Hip fracture	Control	
Exposure	Frail	72	90	
	Not frail	18	90	
	Total	90	180	$N_1 = 270$

stratum 2: age <70 years

		Hip fracture	Control	
Exposure	Frail	5	4	
	Not frail	5	16	
	Total	10	20	$N_2 = 30$

Summary odds ratio adjusted for age = 4.00
Variance of summary log odds ratio = 0.08138

order for an unmatched study to provide the same precision of estimation as a matched study with 100 cases and 200 controls, the sample size would have to be increased by about 50% to 151 cases and 302 controls.

Matching on a covariate is generally most advantageous as a means of increasing statistical efficiency when the covariate is fairly strongly related to both the disease and the exposure; in other words, when there is substantial confounding, as in Table 9-1 (Thompson et al., 1982; Thomas and Greenland, 1983). If the disease and covariate are strongly related, but the exposure and covariate are associated only weakly or not at all, the precision of the estimate of the odds ratio will usually not vary greatly between a matched and unmatched design. When a covariate is unrelated to the disease but strongly related to the exposure, a sizable loss of precision can result from matching on that variable (Miettinen, 1970a; Samuels, 1981; Smith and Day, 1981; Thomas and Greenland, 1983).

Tables 9-3 and 9-4 illustrate this loss in precision. Table 9-3 gives hypothetical data for an unmatched study in which a covariate (e.g., coffee drinking) is strongly related to exposure (e.g., cigarette smoking) but not related to the outcome (e.g., delivery of a low-birthweight infant) in either the exposed or the unexposed group. In the next section we shall see that the Mantel-Haenszel estimate of the summary odds ratio for the association between the exposure and the disease while controlling for the covariate in the unmatched study can be calculated to be 2.33. If in the unmatched study the two strata are combined and the covariate is ignored, then the

Table 9–3. Hypothetical Example of an Unmatched Case-Control Study in which the Covariate (Coffee Consumption) Is Unrelated to the Outcome (Delivery of a Low Birth Weight Infant) among Exposed (Smoker) and Unexposed (Nonsmoker) Individuals

Covariate:
  stratum 1: coffee drinker

		Case	Control	
Exposure	Smoker	504	324	
	Nonsmoker	40	60	
	Total	544	384	$N_1 = 928$

Covariate:
  stratum 2: non-coffee drinker

		Case	Control	
Exposure	Smoker	56	36	
	Nonsmoker	360	540	
	Total	416	576	$N_2 = 992$

Both strata combined:

		Case	Control	
Exposure	Smoker	560	360	
	Nonsmoker	400	600	
	Total	960	960	$N = 1920$

Odds ratio = 2.33
Variance of log odds ratio = 0.00873

crude odds ratio estimate is still 2.33 because the covariate is unrelated to the disease; neither matching nor adjustment in the analysis for the covariate would be needed in order to obtain a valid estimate of the odds ratio. Table 9–4 illustrates the consequences of unnecessary matching for this example. It is no longer valid to combine the two strata because the resulting estimate of the odds ratio would be $(560 \times 475)/(400 \times 485) = 1.37$ rather than the stratified estimate of 2.33. The variance of the summary log odds ratio for a matched design (0.024) is in this instance nearly three times greater than the variance of the crude log odds ratio for an unmatched design (0.009). Consequently, matching on a variable related to the exposure of interest but not the disease has resulted in a substantial loss in the precision of estimation. Matching in such situations should usually be avoided (Kalish, 1986).

To a lesser extent, other characteristics of the population have also been found to influence the magnitude of the difference in precision for matched versus unmatched designs (Kupper et al., 1981; Samuels, 1981; Smith and

Table 9–4. Hypothetical Example of a Matched Case-Control Study in which the Covariate (Coffee Consumption) Is Unrelated to the Outcome (Delivery of a Low Birth Weight Infant) among Exposed (Smoker) and among Unexposed (Nonsmoker) Individuals and in Which Cases and Controls Are Matched on the Covariate

Covariate:
stratum 1: coffee drinker

		Case	Control	
Exposure	Smoker	504	459	
	Nonsmoker	40	85	
	Total	544	544	$N_1 = 1088$

Covariate:
stratum 2: non-coffee drinker

		Case	Control	
Exposure	Smoker	56	26	
	Nonsmoker	360	390	
	Total	416	416	$N_2 = 832$

Summary odds ratio adjusted for coffee drinking status = 2.33
Variance of summary log odds ratio = 0.02422

Both strata combined[a] (analyzed without regard for the matching variable):

		Case	Control	
Exposure	Smoker	560	485	
	Nonsmoker	400	475	
	Total	960	960	$N = 1920$

[a]This table yields an invalid estimate of the odds ratio.

Day, 1981; Thompson et al., 1982; Thomas and Greenland, 1983). These characteristics include (a) the magnitude of the exposure-disease association, with a matched design being more clearly preferable when the exposure is related only weakly to the disease; and (b) the prevalence of exposure in the population, with matching being particularly advantageous when the exposure is fairly infrequent.

Monetary costs of matching also need to be taken into account. In order to select a matched group of controls, information on the matching variables must be obtained for a group of potential controls that is generally much larger than the final matched group included in the study. For instance, it would be expected that approximately 900 potential controls would have to be examined in order to obtain the 200 matched controls for the example given in Table 9–2. This extra effort required for a matched study may have the effect of reducing the number of cases and controls that can be studied within a limited research budget. If obtaining information on the matching variables for potential controls is costly, such as when an interview is required, then there will be a substantial reduction in the number of cases and controls that can be studied for fixed study costs. It has been found that if obtaining information on the matching variables for a potential control costs as much as 10% of the cost of actually including the person as a control, then any potential gains in precision as a result of the matching process are likely to be lost. Under such circumstances, an unmatched design generally permits greater precision of estimation than a matched one, for a fixed total cost (Thompson et al., 1982). Matching is therefore clearly preferable only when the information on the matching variables for potential controls is available at essentially no cost to the investigator.

Matching on more than a very few variables quickly becomes unwieldy. If a matched design is to be employed, then it is usually important to identify a limited number of matching variables that meet the following criteria:

1. Related both to the exposure and the disease, so that they are in fact confounders and therefore will need to be controlled in some manner;
2. Fairly strongly related to the disease, so that matching will have the potential for increasing the precision of estimation materially;
3. Readily available at little or no cost to the investigator, so that it will be feasible to include as many cases and controls as could be included in an unmatched study.

Ideally, all of these criteria should be fulfilled if matching is to be employed, but in practice under certain circumstances one or two of them may tip the scales in favor of matching.

It is generally desirable to avoid matching on any variable whose relation to the disease might be of interest in its own right and for which the distribution in the population is unknown. For example, matching controls to cases on smoking history would usually preclude study of associations between tobacco consumption and disease. If the distribution of smoking habits in the population from which the controls are selected is known, however, then odds ratios can be estimated taking this distribution into account (Benichou and Wacholder, 1994).

In conclusion, despite its intuitive appeal, matching on a variable should not be done routinely, but only after careful consideration of its appropriateness for the particular problem at hand.

TYPES OF MATCHING

Two general types of matched selection are commonly used in case-control studies. One is *individual matching*, which entails selecting one or more controls for each individual case. The second major type is *frequency match-ing,* which requires first knowing or estimating the expected number of cases within each level of the confounding variable or variables, such as white females aged 20–24, white females aged 25–29, and so forth. The appropriate number of controls for each stratum is then selected from the pool of potential controls until the number needed in each stratum is achieved.

In individual matching, when controls are matched to cases within broad categories of quantitative variables, the term *category matching* is used. For instance, a male case in the age range 40–49 might be matched to a male control in the age range 40–49. In *caliper matching* a case would be matched to a control within a specified distance (e.g., two years of age) for a quantitative variable. For example, a 49-year-old male case might be matched to a male control between the ages of $49 - 2 = 47$ and $49 + 2 = 51$ years. If the overall control-to-case ratio is to be 1:1, then one such man would be selected. For an overall ratio of 2:1, two such men would be selected. Particularly when several matching variables are used, it may be difficult or impossible to find controls who match the cases exactly. Conse-quently, less stringent matching criteria are usually specified, such as matching on age within five or ten years, but the looser the matching criteria become, the less certain can the investigator be of the comparability of the two groups. However, any residual differences can generally be han-dled adequately through statistical adjustment in the analysis. The breadth of the intervals within which cases and controls are matched depends large-ly on feasibility. The investigator might start with relatively narrow intervals and in a pilot study discover that these have to be made wider.

ANALYSIS OF UNMATCHED OR FREQUENCY MATCHED DATA BY HAND OR CALCULATOR

Because in a case-control study diseased and nondiseased individuals are generally selected concurrently over a limited time interval, the complex-ities arising from variable periods of observation do not affect the analysis of case-control studies as they do the analysis of cohort studies. In particu-lar, the time of case occurrence can often be ignored when case-control studies are analyzed.

There is another respect in which the interpretation of case-control data differs from that of cohort data. Because the relative numbers of cases and controls in the sample are determined by the investigator and not by the incidence of disease in the population, it is not possible to calculate abso-lute rates or risks for a person with a particular set of values for the predic-tor variables, unless external information on the absolute rate or risk of

Table 9–5. Breast Cancer Cases and Controls According to Menopausal Status[a]

	Case	Control	
Premenopausal	887	868	
Menopausal	1979	2273	
	2866	3141	$N = 6007$

$$\text{Odds ratio} = \frac{887 \times 2273}{868 \times 1979} = 1.17$$

[a]Data from Brinton et al. (1988).

disease is available. All that can be obtained directly from the study results is the *relative magnitude* of the rate or risk of disease for individuals having various sets of values for the predictor variables.

If matching of controls to cases has been employed, such that the investigator has determined the relative number of cases and controls within strata defined by the matching variable(s), then the matching must be taken into account in the analysis. This is done by including the strata used for matching as covariates in the analysis.

A case-control study of 2866 breast cancer cases and 3141 controls derived from a nationwide screening program can be used to illustrate analysis of a case-control study by hand or calculator. In this study, Brinton et al. (1988) examined the relationship between menopausal status and risk for breast cancer. From this study, the 2 × 2 table in Table 9–5 can be obtained. The odds that a breast cancer case is premenopausal are 887/1979 = 0.448, and the odds that a control is premenopausal are 868/2273 = 0.382. Thus, the odds ratio relating the menopausal status of cases to that of controls is 0.448/0.382 = 1.17, meaning that the odds of a case being premenopausal are 1.17 times the odds of a control being premenopausal. It was shown in Chapter 2 that the ratio of odds of exposure among cases to odds of exposure among controls is identical to the ratio of odds of disease among exposed to odds of disease among unexposed. This latter odds ratio approximates the rate ratio for the two menopausal groups. So, approximately, the data in Table 9–5 suggest that premenopausal women have about 1.17 times the breast cancer rate of menopausal women.

Having estimated the odds ratio relating menopausal status to breast cancer risk, we now need confidence intervals for it. Because the confidence intervals are based on the assumption that the estimate is normally distributed, and because the sampling distribution of the natural logarithm of the odds ratio is more nearly normally distributed than that of the odds ratio itself, more accurate confidence intervals are obtained by working with the log odds ratio. The approximate variance of the latter is the sum of the reciprocals of the four counts in the table:

$$\frac{1}{887} + \frac{1}{868} + \frac{1}{1979} + \frac{1}{2273} = 0.0032,$$

and the standard error is $\sqrt{.0032} = 0.0568$. The 95% confidence interval for the log odds ratio is then

$$\text{Lower limit} = \ln(1.1737) - (1.96 \times .0568) = 0.0488$$

and

$$\text{Upper limit} = \ln(1.1737) + (1.96 \times .0568) = 0.2715.$$

Exponentiation of these two values gives values of $e^{0.0488} = 1.05$ and $e^{0.2715} = 1.31$ for the confidence interval around the odds ratio itself.

The breast cancer cases and controls in Table 9–5 were actually frequency matched on age, so that one should compute a summary odds ratio adjusted for age. For stratified case-control data, such as those in Tables 9–2, 9–3, and 9–4, Mantel and Haenszel (1959) proposed an easily computed estimate of the summary odds ratio. Table 9–6 gives the general setup for arranging the case and control data into K 2×2 tables, where K is the number of strata of the covariates. The Mantel-Haenszel estimate for such data is defined as

$$\text{OR}_{\text{MH}} = \frac{a_1 d_1/N_1 + a_2 d_2/N_2 + \ldots + a_K d_K/N_K}{b_1 c_1/N_1 + b_2 c_2/N_2 + \ldots + b_K c_K/N_K}. \tag{9.1}$$

For the data in Table 9–3 for example, there are $K = 2$ strata, and the Mantel-Haenszel estimate is $\text{OR}_{\text{MH}} = (504 \times 60/928 + 56 \times 540/992)/(40 \times 324/928 + 360 \times 36/992) = 63.07/27.03 = 2.33$.

Notice that the Mantel-Haenszel estimate of a summary odds ratio given by equation (9.1) is similar to the Mantel-Haenszel estimate of a summary rate ratio given by equation (6.5) in Chapter 6.

When cases and controls in the study of Brinton et al. (1988) were divided into four age groups, the following table was obtained (Table 9–7). The Mantel-Haenszel summary odds ratio for the data of Table 9–7 is computed as

$$\frac{\dfrac{(278)(83)}{740} + \dfrac{(334)(197)}{1003} + \dfrac{(240)(467)}{1291} + \dfrac{(35)(1526)}{2973}}{\dfrac{(314)(65)}{740} + \dfrac{(323)(149)}{1003} + \dfrac{(193)(391)}{1291} + \dfrac{(38)(1374)}{2973}} = 1.33,$$

which is close to the value 1.17 obtained from the unstratified analysis. Thus, confounding by age does not explain the elevation in risk among women still menstruating compared to those who are not. In fact, because

Table 9–6. Notation for Classifying Cases and Controls into Two Exposure Categories and K Levels of One or More Covariates

Confounding variable:
   level 1

		Case	Control
Exposure	Yes	a_1	b_1
	No	c_1	d_1

N_1

Confounding variable:
   level 2

		Case	Control
Exposure	Yes	a_2	b_2
	No	c_2	d_2

N_2

. . . . .

Confounding variable:
   level k

		Case	Control
Exposure	Yes	a_k	b_k
	No	c_k	d_k

N_k

. . . . .

Confounding variable:
   level K

		Case	Control
Exposure	Yes	a_K	b_K
	No	c_K	d_K

N_K

they tend to be younger than the postmenopausal women and because breast cancer risk increases with age, the summary odds ratio is somewhat higher than the crude odds ratio.

Confidence intervals for the Mantel-Haenszel summary odds ratio may be obtained by the method of Robins et al. (1986). To estimate the variance of the logarithm of the summary odds ratio, the following five sums are first calculated:

$$S_1 = a_1 d_1 / N_1 + \ldots + a_K d_K / N_K$$

$$S_2 = b_1 c_1 / N_1 + \ldots + b_K c_K / N_K$$

Table 9–7. Age-Stratified Data from the Case-Control Study in Table 9–5ᵃ

Age <45

	Case	Control	
Premenopausal	278	314	odds ratio
Menopausal	65	83	= 1.13
Total	343	392	N_1 = 740

Age 45–49

	Case	Control	
Premenopausal	334	323	odds ratio
Menopausal	149	197	= 1.37
Total	483	520	N_2 = 1003

Age 50–54

	Case	Control	
Premenopausal	240	193	odds ratio
Menopausal	391	467	= 1.49
Total	631	660	N_3 = 1291

Age ≥55

	Case	Control	
Premenopausal	35	38	odds ratio
Menopausal	1374	1526	= 1.02
Total	1409	1564	N_4 = 2973

ᵃData from Brinton et al. (1988).

$$S_3 = (a_1 + d_1)a_1 d_1/N_1^2 + \ldots + (a_K + d_K)a_K d_K/N_K^2$$
$$S_4 = (b_1 + c_1)b_1 c_1/N_1^2 + \ldots + (b_K + c_K)b_K c_K/N_K^2$$
$$S_5 = [(a_1 + d_1)b_1 c_1 + (b_1 + c_1)a_1 d_1]/N_1^2 + \ldots + [(a_K + d_K)b_K c_K + (b_K + c_K)a_K d_K]/N_K^2.$$

For example, the five sums for the data in Table 9–6 are

$$S_1 = \frac{(278)(83)}{740} + \ldots + \frac{(35)(1526)}{2973} = 201.5637,$$

$$S_2 = \frac{(314)(65)}{740} + \ldots + \frac{(38)(1374)}{2973} = 151.5793,$$

$$S_3 = \frac{(278 + 83)(278)(83)}{740^2} + \ldots + \frac{(35 + 1526)(35)(1526)}{2973^2} = 106.9180,$$

$$S_4 = \frac{(314 + 65)(314)(65)}{740^2} + \ldots + \frac{(38 + 1374)(38)(1374)}{2973^2} = 71.4892,$$

$$S_5 = \frac{[(278 + 83)(314)(65) + (314 + 65)(278)(83)]}{740^2} + \ldots$$

$$+ \frac{[(35 + 1526)(38)(1374) + (38 + 1374)(35)(1526)]}{2973^2} = 174.7359.$$

The approximate variance of the logarithm of the summary odds ratio is then

$$\frac{S_3}{2S_1^2} + \frac{S_5}{2S_1 S_2} + \frac{S_4}{2S_2^2}.$$

For the breast cancer data, this gives

$$\frac{106.9180}{2(201.5637)^2} + \frac{174.7359}{2(201.5637)(151.5793)} + \frac{71.4892}{2(151.5793)^2} = 0.0057.$$

The 95% confidence limits for the logarithm of the summary odds ratio are then:

$$\text{Lower limit} = \ln(1.3298) - (1.96 \times \sqrt{0.0057}) = 0.1366$$

$$\text{Upper limit} = \ln(1.3298) + (1.96 \times \sqrt{0.0057}) = 0.4334.$$

For the summary odds ratio itself, the 95% confidence limits are $e^{0.1366} = 1.15$ and $e^{0.4334} = 1.54$.

LOGISTIC REGRESSION OF UNMATCHED OR FREQUENCY MATCHED DATA BY THE METHOD OF MAXIMUM LIKELIHOOD

We have seen that the Mantel-Haenszel summary odds ratio can be used for the analysis of K simple 2×2 tables. For more complex analyses, however, logistic regression is the method of choice. Logistic regression is a useful tool for estimating odds ratios associating a disease with one or more risk factors and potential confounding variables, for taking into account variables for which frequency matching was employed, and for the systematic appraisal of effect modification. As in earlier chapters, we use the term *predictor variables* to denote the risk factors of interest, the potential confounding variables, and any variables that may modify the effects of the risk factors. Let $x_1, \ldots, x_r$ denote a particular person's values for the r predictor variables to be examined in a logistic regression model. The model specifies that the person's log odds of disease is

$$\ln\left[\frac{P(D)}{1 - P(D)}\right] = a + b_1 x_1 + \ldots + b_r x_r, \tag{9.2}$$

where $P(D)$ is the probability of disease and $a, b_1, \ldots, b_r$ are constants estimated from the data. A logistic model always yields values for the probability of disease that are between zero and one. The logistic model is often referred to as a multiplicative model because it incorporates the assumption that an individual variable in the model multiplies the odds of disease by an amount that is the same regardless of the values for the other variables.

The relationship between the log odds of disease and the probability of disease is shown in Figure 9–1. If the regression coefficient b_i for the ith variable is close to zero, then variation in that variable will not contribute much to the variation in the log odds of disease as calculated from equation (9.2). On the other hand, if the coefficient is a large number (either positive or negative), then that variable will contribute substantially to the magnitude of the log odds of disease as calculated from the equation.

The specific values of the intercept, a, and of the regression coefficients, $b_1, \ldots, b_r$, are estimated by the method of maximum likelihood. The details of the statistical techniques used to obtain the maximum likelihood estimates of the intercept and the regression coefficients will not be presented here. Instead, the interpretation of the results of logistic regression analysis will be illustrated in the context of a specific example of an unmatched case-control study of ovarian cancer. The study was conducted at six Connecticut hospitals (Hildreth et al., 1981). Cases were women between the ages of 45 and 74 years who were newly diagnosed with epithelial cancer of the ovary between 1977 and 1979. Controls were women in the same age range who were admitted to surgical services other than gynecology. Information on risk factors was obtained from in-person interviews of 62 cases and 1068 unmatched controls. (The reason for the large number of controls is that other more common cancers were also included as case groups.)

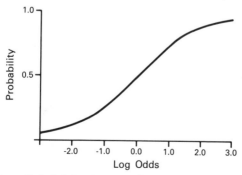

Figure 9–1. Relation between log odds and probability.

We shall consider results from logistic regression analyses that include age (a continuous variable, whose values x_1 were coded in years), number of childbirths (a count variable), and history of oral contraceptive use (for purposes of this example, a categorical variable with categories: ever, never). Our interest focuses on ovarian cancer risk in relation to parity and prior oral contraceptive use. Because age is related to ovarian cancer risk and may also be related to parity and prior oral contraceptive use, age is a potential confounding variable. Notice that if we include age in the regression model as a continuous variable, b_1 represents the change in log odds of cancer associated with an increase in age of one year, which is assumed (implicitly) to be the same for women of all ages.

Similarly, if we represent parity in the logistic model as an ordinal variable x_2, we assume implicitly that each additional childbirth is associated with the same change in the log odds of cancer, regardless how many childbirths preceded it. Thus, the log odds ratio for a uniparous woman relative to a nulliparous one would be b_2, and the log odds ratio for a woman with two children relative to a uniparous one also would be b_2, and so forth. To avoid this assumption and yet to keep the model parsimonious (i.e., with few parameters), we could classify women into a few categories (e.g., nulliparous women, uniparous women, women with two or three childbirths, and women with four or more childbirths) and estimate a separate odds ratio for each category. Formation of such categories should be done thoughtfully, since the assumption is being made that categorization in this way reflects relative homogeneity within categories. (See Greenland [1995] for a discussion of this issue.)

Specifically, in model 1 we include age as a continuous variable x_1, and we use three predictor variables x_2, x_3 and x_4 to code the four categories: $x_2 = 1$ if a woman had one birth and 0 otherwise, $x_3 = 1$ if a woman had two or three births and 0 otherwise, and $x_4 = 1$ if a woman had four or more births and 0 otherwise. Thus, parity for a nulliparous woman is coded $x_2 = x_3 = x_4 = 0$, and parity for a uniparous woman is coded as $x_2 = 1, x_3 = x_4 = 0$. From equation (9–2) we see that the log odds ratio for disease risk in a uniparous woman relative to a nulliparous woman with the same values of all the other predictors is $(a + b_1 x_1 + b_2 \cdot 1 + b_3 \cdot 0 + \cdots + b_r \cdot 0) - (a + b_1 x_1 + b_2 \cdot 0 + b_3 \cdot 0 + \cdots + b_r \cdot 0) = b_2$. Similarly, b_3 represents the log odds ratio for a woman with two or three childbirths relative to that for a nulliparous woman, and b_4 is the corresponding log odds ratio for a woman with four or more births. We use this same scheme to code the variable x_5 for oral contraceptive use as $x_5 = 1$ for ever use and $x_5 = 0$ for never use, so that b_5 represents the log odds ratio for ever users relative to never users. This coding is summarized in the upper part of Table 9–8. Predictor variables such as x_2, x_3, x_4, x_5 that are given the value 1 when the participant belongs to a certain category and are given the value 0 otherwise, are called

Table 9–8. Coded Values of Predictor Variables for a Case-Control Study of Ovarian Cancer and Examples of How the Values of Predictor Variables for Certain Women Are Coded

Variable		Type	Unit	
x_1	age	continuous	one year	
x_2	parity	indicator	1	one childbirth
			0	otherwise
x_3	parity	indicator	1	2–3 childbirths
			0	otherwise
x_4	parity	indicator	1	4+ childbirths
			0	otherwise
x_5	ever use of OCs[a]	indicator	1	ever use
			0	never use

Description of Participant	Predictor Variable				
	x_1	x_2	x_3	x_4	x_5
Nulliparous woman aged 43 years, who used OCs	43	0	0	0	1
Woman with 5 childbirths, aged 67, who never used OCs	67	0	0	1	0
Uniparous woman, aged 56, who used OCs	56	1	0	0	1

[a]OCs = oral contraceptives.

indicator variables. The lower part of Table 9–8 gives values of the predictor variables $x_1, \ldots, x_5$ for various types of study participants.

The columns headed Model 1 in Table 9–9 give the corresponding regression coefficients $b_1, \ldots, b_5$, their standard errors, their exponentiated values (that is, the odds ratio estimates), 95% confidence intervals for the odds ratios, and p values for the likelihood ratio tests of the null hypothesis that the regression coefficient is zero. The odds ratios were computed by exponentiating the logistic regression coefficients. The 95% confidence intervals were obtained by exponentiating the values of the lower and upper confidence limits for the regression coefficients. Thus, the regression coefficient $b_5 = -.604$ for x_5 (the indicator for ever use of oral contraceptives) suggests that, after adjustment for the other variables in the model, the odds of ovarian cancer for a woman with a history of oral contraceptive use are $e^{-.604} = 0.55$ times the corresponding odds for a woman without a history of oral contraceptive use. In other words, the odds of being a case are reduced by $1 - .55 = 45\%$ among women with a history of oral contraceptive use. The lower confidence limit is $e^{-0.604-1.96(0.623)} = e^{-1.82} = 0.16$, and the upper confidence limit $= e^{-0.604+1.96(0.623)} = e^{0.62} = 1.86$. The 95% confidence intervals for all of the odds ratios are wide because of the small number of cases ($N = 62$) enrolled in the study.

The odds ratio of 1.02 for age in Model 1 indicates that in this study

Table 9-9. Logistic Regression Analyses of a Case-Control Study of Ovarian Cancer[a]

Predictor Variable	Regression Coefficient (Standard Error)		Adjusted Odds Ratio[b] (95% Confidence Interval)		p Value[c]	
	Model 1	Model 2	Model 1	Model 2	Model 1	Model 2
Age (yrs)	.016 (.017)		1.02		.35	
Age (yrs)						
<40		0		1.0		
40–49		.45 (.51)		1.6 (.58–4.3)		.38
50–59		.50 (.52)		1.6 (.59–4.6)		.34
60+		.27 (.60)		1.3 (.40–4.2)		.66
Parity						
0	0	0	1.0	1.0		
1	−.057 (.425)	−.045 (.425)	.94 (.41–2.2)	.96 (.42–2.2)	.89	.91
2–3	−.343 (.335)	−.366 (.335)	.71 (.37–1.4)	.69 (.36–1.3)	.31	.27
4+	−.583 (.445)	−.635 (.444)	.56 (.23–1.3)	.53 (.22–1.3)	.19	.15
OC use						
never	0	0	1.0	1.0		
ever	−.604 (.623)	−.630 (.622)	.55 (.16–1.9)	.53 (.16–1.8)	.33	.31

[a]Data from study reported by Hildreth et al. (1981).

[b]Adjusted odds ratio is obtained by exponentiating the corresponding regression coefficient.

[c]Significance level of a two-tailed test of the null hypothesis that the regression coefficient is zero.

with this particular control group, the odds of a woman being a case increase by about 2% for each increase of one year in age. If one wanted to know the odds ratio associated with an increase of 10 years in age, the regression coefficient of 0.016 would be multiplied by 10 ($0.016 \times 10 = 0.160$). Exponentiating the resulting number ($e^{0.160} = 1.17$) gives the odds ratio associated with a 10-year increase in age. The 95% confidence limits corresponding to this estimate would be formed by multiplying the standard error for 1 year by 10 ($0.017 \times 10 = 0.170$), multiplying this figure by 1.96 ($0.170 \times 1.96 = 0.3332$), subtracting this from the coefficient of 0.160 ($0.160 - 0.3332 = -0.1732$) and exponentiating for the lower confidence limit ($e^{-0.1732} = 0.84$). Similarly, we would add 0.3332 to the coefficient of 0.160 ($0.160 + 0.3332 = 0.4932$) and exponentiate for the upper confidence limit ($e^{0.4932} = 1.64$).

It is good practice to evaluate the robustness of estimated odds ratios to changes in the choice of predictor variables included in the model and in the way that the predictor variables are coded. We have seen that by entering age in Model 1 as a continuous variable we have implicitly assumed that the log odds associated with an increase in age of one year is the same for women of all ages. An alternative modeling strategy for controlling the effects of age is to form age strata, which are coded using indicator variables. Because of sparse numbers of cases, we consider only four strata: 45–49 years, 50–59 years, 60–69 years, and 70–74 years. The distribution of cases and controls according to the $4 \times 4 \times 2 = 32$ joint categories of age, parity, and oral contraceptive use are shown in Table 9–10. The columns headed Model 2 in Table 9–9 give the regression coefficients for parity and oral contraceptive use when age is coded as a categorical variable, i.e., with indicator variables for the four strata. Comparison of the columns headed Model 1 and Model 2 shows that the way age is coded in the analyses has very little effect on the magnitudes of the odds ratios relating risk of ovarian cancer to parity and oral contraceptive use.

Just as the deviance is useful for hypothesis testing and model criticism for cohort data (see Chapters 6 and 7), it can be applied usefully to a series of nested logistic regression models. The deviance for a nested pair of logistic regression models is twice the logarithm of the ratio of the likelihood of the data under the large model to the likelihood under the small model. Most computer programs for logistic regression provide as standard output the value of the logarithm of the maximized likelihood under a given model (i.e., the "log-likelihood"). These "log-likelihoods" for large and small models can be subtracted and the result multiplied by 2 to obtain the deviance.

To illustrate, the log-likelihood for Model 2 (large model) is given by the SAS output as -236.79. The small model, obtained by equating to zero

Table 9–10. Distribution of Ovarian Cancer Cases and Controls According to Parity and Oral Contraceptive (OC) Use

Age (yrs)	Parity	Case OC Use Never	Case OC Use Ever	Control OC Use Never	Control OC Use Ever
<50	0	0	0	7	5
	1	1	1	11	1
	2–3	2	1	53	27
	4+	0	0	38	12
50–59	0	5	0	54	7
	1	2	0	39	0
	2–3	15	0	178	35
	4+	2	1	101	21
60–69	0	8	0	75	0
	1	3	0	52	1
	2–3	8	0	166	2
	4+	5	0	44	2
70+	0	2	0	37	0
	1	3	0	25	0
	2–3	2	0	64	0
	4+	1	0	11	0

Source: Hildreth et al. (1981).

the regression coefficient for oral contraceptive use, has log-likelihood -237.39. The deviance between large and small models is thus $2[-236.79 - (-237.39)] = 1.20$. The number of degrees of freedom associated with this deviance is the difference between the number of parameters in large and small models. Because the small model has one less parameter than the large one (the regression coefficient for oral contraceptive use), there is one degree of freedom associated with this deviance of 1.20. This value is not large when compared to a χ^2 statistic on one degree of freedom ($p = 0.28$). Therefore, we conclude that although this study is consistent with others in suggesting a protective effect of oral contraceptives against ovarian cancer, the association is not statistically significant in this study, perhaps because of the small number of cases.

ANALYSIS OF MATCHED DATA BY HAND OR CALCULATOR

The analysis of matched case-control studies must employ statistical techniques that make explicit provision for the matched nature of the data. As was mentioned above, for frequency matched data the same techniques may be applied as are used for unmatched data, with the strata used for matching included as covariates in the analysis. Analyzing matched data as if they were unmatched will generally lead to biased estimates of the odds ratio (Seigel and Greenhouse, 1973). Table 9–4 provided an example of this type of bias. Although matching on the covariate ensured that the ratio of cases to controls was identical in each of the two strata, ignoring the covariate in the analysis would lead to a value of 1.37 for the odds ratio. This value differs markedly from the value of 2.33 within levels of the covariate.

For studies employing individual matching of controls to cases, two approaches may be taken. If several cases have the same matching criteria (e.g., gender, age group, year of diagnosis in a hospital-based study), then the matched pairs may be reduced to matched sets or strata in which a stratum consists of all cases and controls with exactly the same matching factors. Then the Mantel-Haenszel procedures or logistic regression as described in the previous section may be used to obtain a summary estimate of and confidence limits for the odds ratio. (See Brookmeyer et al. [1986] for discussion.)

When cases and controls are matched quite closely and data within strata used for matching are sparse because there are at most a few pairs with the same matching criteria, then other methods appropriate for individually matched studies should be used (Miettinen, 1970b; Holford et al., 1978; Breslow et al., 1978; Breslow and Day, 1980). The analysis of individually matched studies illustrated here uses data from a case-control study of risk factors for acute prolapsed lumbar intervertebral disc (Kelsey and Hardy, 1975).

Cases for this study had newly diagnosed prolapsed lumbar intervertebral disc, and controls were matched individually to cases on gender, age, and hospital service or radiologist's office. A 1:1 control-to-case ratio was used, and a total of 217 matched pairs was included. One of the risk factors examined by the authors was driving a motor vehicle. Table 9–11 gives the results comparing cases and controls on this factor. Note that although the data are arranged in a 2 × 2 table, this table is different from the 2 × 2 table that would be used to present the results of an unmatched study; for a

Table 9–11. Number of Case-Control Pairs from a Pair-Matched Case-Control Study of Prolapsed Lumbar Disc, According to Whether or Not the Case or Control Drives a Motor Vehicle

| | | Control | |
		Does drive	Does not drive
Case	Does drive	144	41
	Does not drive	19	13

Odds ratio $= \dfrac{41}{19} = 2.16$

Source: Kelsey and Hardy (1975).

matched study, each *pair* contributes one observation to the table. The rows designate the exposure status of the case member of the pair, whereas the columns denote the exposure status of the control member of the pair. Estimation of the odds ratio for matched pairs is based on the discordant pairs only, that is, only on those pairs for which one member is exposed and the other is not. Pairs in which both members are exposed or both are unexposed provide no information as to whether the cases are more or less likely than controls to be exposed.

It can be shown (Kraus, 1960) that the odds ratio relating exposure to the disease or condition of interest is the ratio of the number of pairs for which the case is exposed and not the control to the number of pairs for which the control is exposed and not the case. The estimate of the odds ratio for driving a motor vehicle as it relates to the incidence of prolapsed disc is thus $41/19 = 2.16$, indicating that the incidence of prolapsed disc is more than twice as great among people who drive than among people who do not.

Methods of calculating odds ratios and approximate confidence intervals when controls are matched to cases are described in detail by Clayton and Hills (1993), Breslow and Day (1980), and Hosmer and Lemeshow (1989). Most of these methods require the use of a computer.

LOGISTIC REGRESSION OF MATCHED DATA BY COMPUTER

For the previous example, we have seen that the estimate of the odds ratio for driving a motor vehicle in relation to the incidence of prolapsed disc is 2.16. This estimate is adjusted for the matching variables of age, gender, and hospital service or radiologist's office. Nevertheless, it is possible that variables other than the matching variables confound the association between driving and prolapsed disc. One such variable considered by the authors was living in the suburbs as opposed to the city. Living in the suburbs was found to be strongly related to whether controls drove a car, in that 65% of those who drove lived in the suburbs, as opposed to only 13% of those who did not drive. Table 9–12 gives the 4 × 4 classification of the 217 pairs according to the place of residence and the driving status of the case and control members of the matched pairs.

To evaluate the combined effects of driving and place of residence while each variable is adjusted for the effect of the other, we use conditional logistic regression. Conditional logistic regression is a method for combining all the information in Table 9–12 to obtain a good estimate of the effect of, say, driving, with adjustment for place of residence. Using maximum likelihood estimation, the conditional likelihood that is maxi-

Table 9–12. Number of Case-Control Pairs from a Pair-Matched Case-Control Study of Prolapsed Lumbar Disc According to Place of Residence and Whether or Not the Case or Control Drives a Motor Vehicle

		Control			
		Suburban residence		City residence	
		Does drive	Does not drive	Does drive	Does not drive
	Suburban residence — Does drive	63	4	32	22
	Does not drive	1	2	1	2
Case	City residence — Does drive	29	1	20	14
	Does not drive	7	0	10	9

Source: Kelsey and Hardy (1975).

mized is very similar to the Cox partial likelihood discussed in Chapter 7 for nested case-control studies. In the terminology of that chapter, each case-control pair forms a risk set. Pairs that are concordant for both exposures do not contribute to the analysis. Conditional logistic regression analysis yields parameter estimates and standard errors that have the same interpretation as they do when a logistic regression analysis is performed using unmatched data.

Table 9–13 gives results from the output of a conditional logistic regression program using maximum likelihood estimation conducted using SAS software (SAS Language, 1990). Model 1 gives results that are not adjusted for type of residence, which agree well with the simple matched pair analysis of the preceding section. Model 2 gives regression coefficients and odds ratios for both variables, each adjusted for the other. As seen in the table, the regression coefficients for driving and suburban residence, each adjusted for the other, are 0.658 and 0.255, respectively. Exponentiation leads to estimates of 1.93 and 1.29 for the odds ratios relating each factor to the disease while adjusting for the other factor. Standard errors of the corresponding log odds ratios are 0.294 and 0.226, giving 95% confidence intervals of 1.09 to 3.44 and 0.83 to 2.01, respectively. Thus, statistical analysis suggests a significant effect of driving with adjustment for residence but not of residence with adjustment for driving.

These estimates were obtained using a model that specifies the log odds of prolapsed disc as the sum of a term for driving and a term for suburban residence, as shown in equation (9–2). By exponentiating, we see that the odds of prolapsed disc is assumed to be the product of two factors, one for driving and one for type of residence. Thus, we call this model a multiplicative model. Stated differently, the logistic model assumes that the odds ratio

Table 9–13. Conditional Logistic Regression Analyses of a Pair-Matched Case-Control Study of Prolapsed Lumbar Disc

Predictor Variable	Regression Coefficient (Standard Error)		Adjusted Odds Ratio (95% Confidence Interval)		p Value	
	Model 1	Model 2	Model 1	Model 2	Model 1	Model 2
Driving a motor vehicle						
No	0	0	1.0	1.0		
Yes	.769 (.277)	.658 (.294)	2.2 (1.3–3.7)	1.9 (1.1–3.4)	.006	.025
Residence						
Urban		0		1.0		
Suburban		.255 (.226)		1.3 (.83–2.0)		.258

Source: Kelsey and Hardy (1975).

relating prolapsed disc to driving is the same for those in suburban and in urban areas.

We can test the logistic model for the odds ratio by allowing a separate odds ratio for each type of residence. This can be achieved by using three indicator variables in equation (9–2). For example, we might let x_1 assume the value 1 if a participant was a suburban nondriver and zero otherwise; let x_2 assume the value 1 if the participant was an urban driver and 0 otherwise; and let x_3 assume the value 1 if the participant was a suburban driver and 0 otherwise. Notice that urban nondrivers, for whom $x_1 = x_2 = x_3 = 0$, form the referent group. To determine whether we need this more complicated model, we can examine deviances.

Figure 9–2 shows a series of nested models for the prolapsed disc data, and the deviances between them. Model 5, the most general model, allows for interaction (on the logistic scale) between driving and type of residence. Model 4 is the logistic model that we fit in Table 9–13. Because Model 5 has 3 parameters and Model 4 has 2 parameters, the deviance has approximately a chi-squared distribution on $3 - 2 = 1$ degree of freedom, when Model 4 (the small model) adequately describes the data. We see in Figure 9–2 that the deviance between Model 5 and Model 4 is only 0.08, not at all large compared to a chi-squared variable on one degree of freedom ($p = 0.79$). Thus, the logistic Model 4 appears to fit the data well.

As noted in Chapter 6, the deviance between a pair of nested models (large and small) is twice the difference in the log-likelihoods for the models, with unknown constants in the log-likelihood function replaced by their maximum likelihood estimates. The log-likelihood for a model is part of the standard output of all commercial regression software. For example, the SAS output gives the values -145.64 and -146.28 for the log-likelihood under, respectively, Model 4, which allows for both driving a motor vehicle and type of residence (large model), and Model 3, which allows only for driving a motor vehicle (small model). Thus, the deviance comparing Model 3 and Model 4 is twice the difference between these two log-likelihoods, i.e., $\chi^2_{DEV} = 2[-145.64 - (-146.28)] = 1.28$. The deviance has one degree of freedom (the difference between two and one parameters in Models 4 and 3, respectively). The value 1.28 is not large when compared to a table of values of a chi-squared statistic on one degree of freedom ($p = 0.25$). Thus, the deviance comparing Models 3 and 4 provides further support for the inference that driving a motor vehicle is a risk factor for prolapsed disc, and that after controlling for this factor, type of residence is unrelated to the incidence of this condition.

Notice in Figure 9–2 that the deviance comparing Model 1 (no effect of driving or of residence) with Model 2 (effect of residence but not of driving) shows that Model 2 fits the data significantly better (deviance = 4.29

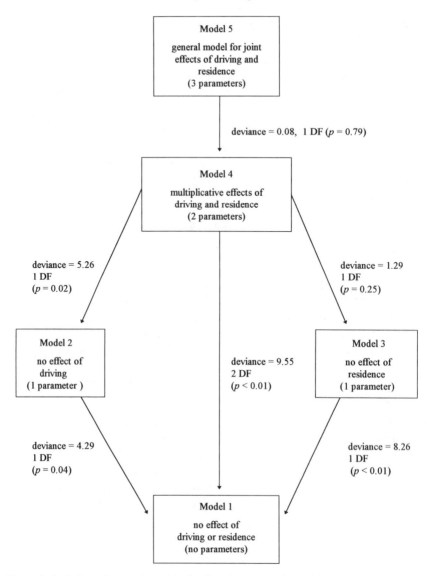

Figure 9–2. Series of nested models for the data on prolapsed lumbar disc, shown in Tables 9–11 and 9–12.

on one degree of freedom, $p = 0.04$). This comparison, which is unadjusted for driving status, contrasts with the comparison of Model 4 with Model 3, which showed no improvement in fit by allowing for residence after adjusting for driving status. Thus, examination of these deviances again supports the inference that type of residence is not a risk factor for prolapsed disc, after adjusting for driving status.

In summary, this example shows that the availability of multivariate methods for the analysis of matched case-control studies makes it feasible to control for readily available confounding variables through matching, while deferring the control of other confounders until the analysis. Also, coarse matching may be used in the study design and then the matching variables can be controlled more finely in the analysis. Comparable methods are also available for studies in which two or more controls are matched to each case (Breslow and Day, 1980; Breslow et al., 1978). Although some investigators still analyze matched studies as if they were unmatched, the goal of obtaining the most valid estimates possible dictates that the matched nature of the data be reflected in the choice of statistical methods.

CALCULATION OF RATES FROM CASE-CONTROL STUDIES

Although rate ratios can be estimated from case-control studies, actual incidence rates for specific subgroups of the population cannot be estimated unless ancillary information is available. If exposure is related to disease, then the incidence rate for the total population is a composite of the incidence rates for exposed and nonexposed individuals. Provided that an estimate of this overall incidence rate is available from some other source, the results of a case-control study of a rare disease can be used to estimate incidence rates for exposed and for nonexposed individuals. The incidence rate for the total population may be written as:

Incidence rate in population =
[(Proportion exposed) × (Incidence rate for the exposed)]
+ [(Proportion nonexposed) × (Incidence rate for the nonexposed)]

After noting that the incidence rate among the exposed is the product of the rate ratio and the incidence rate among the nonexposed and after solving for the incidence rate in the population as a whole, the following expression is obtained for the incidence rate among the nonexposed:

Incidence rate among nonexposed =

$$\frac{\text{Incidence rate in total population}}{[(\text{Proportion exposed}) \times (\text{Rate ratio})] + (\text{Proportion nonexposed})}.$$

The incidence rate among the exposed is then obtained by multiplying this result by the rate ratio. The proportion of the population exposed can generally be estimated from the control group of an unmatched case-control study.

Suppose, for example, that an unmatched case-control study yields an odds ratio of 2.00 as an estimate of the rate ratio. Suppose also that 40% of the control group is found to be exposed. If from ancillary information it is known that the annual incidence rate is 15.0 per 100,000, then an estimate of the incidence rate among the nonexposed may be obtained as follows:

$$\frac{15 \text{ per } 100,000}{[(0.4) \times (2.0)] + (0.6)} = 10.7 \text{ per } 100,000 \text{ per year.}$$

The estimate of incidence rate for exposed individuals is then $(10.7) \times (2.0) = 21.4$ per 100,000 per year. More extensive discussions of the estimation of rates from case-control studies are available elsewhere (Greenland, 1981; Neutra and Drolette, 1978; Cornfield, 1951; Benichou and Wacholder, 1994; Greenland, 1987).

Although ancillary information on incidence rates is needed in order to estimate exposure-specific incidence rates from case-control studies, most other important measures can be estimated directly. These include the attributable fraction for the exposed and for the population (see Chapter 2), as well as the rate ratio itself.

REFERENCES

Benichou J, Wacholder S. 1994. A comparison of three approaches to estimate exposure-specific incidence rates from population-based case-control data. *Stat Med* 13:651–661.

Breslow NE, Day NE. 1980. Statistical Methods in Cancer Research. Volume 1: The Analysis of Case-Control Studies. Lyon, International Agency for Research on Cancer. IARC Scientific Publications No. 32.

Breslow NE, Day NE, Halvorsen KT, Prentice RL, Sabai C. 1978. Estimation of multiple relative risk functions in matched case-control studies. *Am J Epidemiol* 108:299–307.

Brinton LA, Schairer C, Hoover RN, Fraumeni JF Jr. 1988. Menstrual factors and breast cancer. *Cancer Invest* 6:245–254.

Brookmeyer R, Liang KY, Linet M. 1986. Matched case-control designs and over-matched analyses. *Am J Epidemiol* 124:693–701.

Clayton D, Hills M. 1993. Statistical Models in Epidemiology. Oxford, Oxford University Press.

Cornfield J. 1951. A method of estimating comparative rates from clinical data. Applications to cancer of the lung, breast, and cervix. *J Natl Cancer Inst* 11:1269–1275.

Greenland S. 1981. Multivariate estimation of exposure-specific incidence from case-control studies. *J Chron Dis* 34:445–453.

Greenland S. 1987. Estimation of exposure-specific rates from sparse case-control data. *J Chron Dis* 40:1087–1094.

Greenland S. 1995. Dose-response and trend analysis in epidemiology: Alternatives to categorical analysis. *Epidemiology* 6:356–365.

Hildreth NG, Kelsey JL, LiVolsi VA, Fischer DB, Holford TR, Mostow ED, Schwartz PE, White C. 1981. An epidemiologic study of epithelial carcinoma of the ovary. *Am J Epidemiol* 114:398–405.

Holford TR, White C, Kelsey JL. 1978. Multivariate analysis for matched case-control studies. *Am J Epidemiol* 107:245–256.

Hosmer DW, Lemeshow S. 1989. Applied Logistic Regression. New York, John Wiley.

Kalish LA. 1986. Matching on a non-risk factor in the design of case-control studies does not always result in an efficiency loss. *Am J Epidemiol* 123:551–554.

Karon JM, Kupper LL. 1982. In defense of matching. *Am J Epidemiol* 116:852–866.

Kelsey JL, Fischer DB, Holford TR, LiVolsi VA, Mostow ED, Goldenberg IS, White C. 1981. Exogenous estrogens and other factors in the epidemiology of breast cancer. *J Natl Cancer Inst* 67:327–333.

Kelsey JL, Hardy RJ. 1975. Driving of motor vehicles as a risk factor for acute herniated lumbar intervertebral disc. *Am J Epidemiol* 102:63–73.

Kraus AS. 1960. Comparison of a group with a disease and a control group from the same families, in search for possible etiologic factors. *Am J Public Health* 50:303–311.

Kupper LL, Karon JM, Kleinbaum DG, Morgenstern H, Lewis DK. 1981. Matching in epidemiologic studies: validity and efficiency considerations. *Biometrics* 37:271–291.

Mantel N, Haenszel W. 1959. Statistical aspects of the analysis of data from retrospective studies of disease. *J Natl Cancer Inst* 22:719–748.

Miettinen OS. 1970a. Matching and design efficiency in retrospective studies. *Am J Epidemiol* 91:111–118.

Miettinen OS. 1970b. Estimation of relative risk from individually matched series. *Biometrics* 26:75–86.

Neutra RR, Drolette ME. 1978. Estimating exposure-specific disease rates from case-control studies using Bayes' theorem. *Am J Epidemiol* 108:214–222.

Robins J, Breslow N, Greenland S. 1986. Estimators of the Mantel-Haenszel variance consistent in both sparse data and large-strata limiting models. *Biometrics* 42:311–323.

Samuels ML. 1981. Matching and design efficiency in epidemiologic studies. *Biometrika* 68:577–588.

SAS Language. 1990. Version 6.x. First Edition. Cary, NC, SAS Institute Inc.

Seigel CG, Greenhouse SW. 1973. Validity in estimating relative risk in case-control studies. *J Chron Dis* 26:219–225.

Smith PC, Day NE. 1981. Matching and confounding in the design and analysis of epidemiological case-control studies. In: Bithell J F, Copp R. Perspectives in Medical Statistics. New York, Academic Press, pp 39–64.

Thomas DC, Greenland S. 1983. The relative efficiencies of matched and independent sample designs for case-control studies. *J Chron Dis* 10:685–697.

Thompson WD, Kelsey JL, Walter SD. 1982. Cost and efficiency in the choice of matched and unmatched case-control studies. *Am J Epidemiol* 116:840–851.

EXERCISES

1. Cite an example of a case-control study of a specific exposure-disease association for which a matched design would be preferable to an unmatched one. Explain your reasoning.

2. The table below presents results from a logistic regression analysis of breast cancer cases (N = 322) and unmatched controls (N = 1353) (Kelsey et al., 1981) from the same study as the ovarian cancer cases and controls (Hildreth et al., 1981) described in this chapter. The age distributions of cases and controls were similar, so that age does not appear as a variable in this table. The age range of cases and controls was 45–74 years.

   a. What do the odds ratio (and 95% confidence interval) of 1.87 (1.26–2.78) for the association of breast cancer with a history of breast cancer in a sister or mother mean?

   b. What do the odds ratio (and 95% confidence interval) of 1.34 (1.00–1.81) for the association of breast cancer with age at first birth mean?

   c. How much more likely to develop breast cancer is a woman whose menopause occurs at age 55 than a woman who is similar in other respects but whose menopause occurs at age 45? Calculate a confidence interval for your estimate.

   d. What does the statistically significant interaction of weight with time since last menstrual period mean?

Logistic Regression Analysis of a Case-Control Study of Breast Cancer

Variable	Unit	Regression Coefficient	Standard Error	Adjusted Odds Ratio[a]	95% Confidence Interval	P
Quantitative variables						
Oral contraceptive use	1 year of use	-0.127	0.056	0.88	0.78–0.99	0.02
Estrogen-replacement therapy use	1 year of use	-0.030	0.022	0.97	0.93–1.01	0.17
Age at first birth	10-year increase	0.294	0.149	1.34	1.00–1.81	0.05
Age at menarche	5-year increase	-0.437	0.204	0.65	0.43–0.97	0.03
Age at menopause	5-year increase	0.257	0.063	1.29	1.14–1.47	<0.001
Categorized variables						
Religion	Jewish:all other	0.419	0.235	1.52	0.95–2.43	0.08
Place of birth	Europe:all other	0.525	0.222	1.69	1.08–2.64	0.02
History of benign breast disease	Yes:no	0.485	0.167	1.62	1.16–2.27	0.004
Breast cancer in sister or mother	Yes:no	0.625	0.198	1.87	1.26–2.78	0.002
History of clots in veins	Yes:no	-0.559	0.218	0.57	0.37–0.88	0.01
Ever used a vaginal hormone	Yes:no	-0.819	0.420	0.44	0.19–1.02	0.05
Postmenopausal vs. premenopausal or perimenopausal		2.687	0.718	Indicator variable		<0.001
Ever had a live birth	Yes:no	-1.136	0.416	Indicator variable		0.06
Variables involved in interaction						
Interaction of weight with grouped time since last menstrual period[b]						0.04
Weight	10-pound increase	-0.145	0.076			0.06
Grouped time since last menstrual period[b]						0.05

[a]For quantitative variables, increase in adjusted odds ratio and 95% confidence intervals for given change in level of risk factor; for categorical variables, adjusted odds ratio and 95% confidence intervals around adjusted odds ratios. Each odds ratio is adjusted for all other variables in the table.

[b]Years since last menstrual period is considered in three groups: premenopausal, last menstrual period >3 months ago but no more than 5 years ago, and last menstrual period >5 years ago. Therefore, the comparisons have two degrees of freedom, and Wald's classification statistic (W^2) rather than Z is used to test for statistical significance. $W^2 = 6.37$ ($P = 0.04$) for the interaction of weight with grouped time since last menstrual period and $W^2 = 5.82$ ($P = 0.05$) for time since last menstrual period.

Source: Kelsey et al. (1981).

10

Cross-Sectional and Other Types of Studies

CROSS-SECTIONAL (PREVALENCE) STUDIES

In a cross-sectional, or prevalence, study, exposure status and disease status are measured at one time or over a short period of time in the participants. Prevalence rates[1] among those with and without the exposure or at varying levels of exposure are then determined and compared. Prevalence studies are often employed for public health planning, but it is their use in studies of etiology that will be considered here.

Prevalence studies concerned with disease etiology are most often carried out to learn about risk factors for diseases of slow onset and long duration for which medical care is often not sought until the disease has progressed to a relatively advanced stage. Such diseases as osteoarthritis, chronic bronchitis, and various mental disorders fall into this category. Because medical care is generally not sought at the outset, case-control studies, which usually identify newly diagnosed cases at the time medical care is first obtained, would for the most part be impractical or at best difficult to interpret because the case group would consist mostly of persons with relatively advanced disease. Cohort studies of these diseases are also difficult to conduct because of the usual problems of large sample size and long period of follow-up. Also, it is difficult to say exactly when people have these diseases and when they do not. In other words, it would be difficult in a cohort study to define incident cases of these diseases, although progression of symptoms or signs could be monitored. A disease of short duration would generally not be suitable for a cross-sectional study because very few people would have the disease at any one time.

Cross-sectional studies have one major advantage over many case-control studies in that they are often based on a sample of the general population, not just on people seeking medical care. Thus, their generalizability may be considered a strength. One major advantage over cohort studies is that they tend to be carried out over a relatively short time period, thus greatly reducing costs.

Cross-sectional studies also suffer from two major limitations. First, it is often difficult to separate cause and effect because if measurement of exposure and disease are made at the same time, it may be impossible to determine which came first. It has been found repeatedly, for instance, that people in low social classes have higher prevalence rates of many mental illnesses than do people of higher social classes. Do people in low social classes have a greater tendency to develop mental illness than those in upper social classes, or do people migrate down the social class scale once they become mentally ill and are therefore found in the lower social classes at the time a study is done? This issue remains controversial. In England, it was found that people who developed severe chronic bronchitis had difficulty holding a job because of their frequent sickness absence, and consequently they tended to take jobs of lower social status or to lose their jobs entirely (Meadows, 1961). Thus, the higher prevalence rates of chronic bronchitis in low social classes in England were probably in part a consequence of the disease itself. In the United States, people with severe chronic bronchitis have tended to move away from areas with high levels of air pollution to areas with low pollution levels; accordingly, prevalence rates of severe chronic respiratory disease may actually be higher in the less polluted areas than in the more polluted areas (Anderson et al., 1964; Kelsey et al., 1968; Winkelstein and Kantor, 1969). However, current place of residence does not reflect the levels in the locality where people developed the disease. More generally, it is important to keep in mind that a person's exposure status at the time he or she is included in a cross-sectional study may have little to do with his or her exposure status at the time the disease process began.

The second major disadvantage of cross-sectional studies is that a series of prevalent cases will have a higher proportion of cases with disease of long duration than a series of incident cases. People who either recover from or die of a disease quickly have less of a chance of being included in the disease group. If characteristics of persons whose disease is either of short duration or rapidly fatal are different from those whose disease is of long duration, then the exposure-disease association observed in a cross-sectional study will misrepresent the association of exposure with incidence. An additional problem with cross-sectional studies is that for diseases with periods of exacerbations and remissions, a person whose disease is in remission may be falsely classified as not having the disease. Also, the question of how to handle treated cases must be addressed. Persons under treatment may not present evidence of the disease at the time of the prevalence study, but if they were not under treatment, most of them probably would be classified as diseased. How to classify such persons depends on the purpose of the study, but during the course of the study they must at least be identified so that they can be classified appropriately in the analysis.

Choice of Study Population

Given that a cross-sectional study is to be done, the question arises as to who should be included as participants. The groups to be compared are sometimes selected on the basis of exposure status, particularly if the exposure can be identified readily. For instance, if the exposure of interest is whether or not a person belonged to the Maori ethnic group and the condition of interest is elevated serum uric acid levels (a correlate of gout), one could take a sample of Maoris and measure their prevalence rate of elevated serum uric acid levels and compare this to the prevalence rate of elevated serum uric acid levels in a sample of non-Maoris (Brauer and Prior, 1978). If one wanted to compare the prevalence of mental disorders in different geographic areas of New York City, one could sample people from the different areas and compare prevalence rates by geographic area. If an occupational exposure was of interest, prevalence rates in a plant with the exposure could be compared to prevalence rates in a plant without the exposure, or prevalence rates in one part of a plant could be compared with prevalence rates in another part of the plant. If relatively small numbers are involved, an entire population can be included; if including the entire population is not practical or is prohibitively expensive, a sample of the exposed and unexposed groups may be taken.

Often, however, the investigator does not actually measure exposure status until the sample is taken. In this instance, one approach is to take a sample of people or households or some other unit in a defined geographic area. In a study examining the relationship between air pollution and chronic respiratory disease in Buffalo, New York (Winkelstein and Kantor, 1969), a random sample of households in Buffalo was chosen and all the household members within a certain age range were included. Their status regarding exposure to air pollution was assigned according to where they lived, and a questionnaire was used to determine the occurrence of respiratory symptoms. Other studies have used more complex sampling schemes. In a study of the relationship between air pollution and chronic respiratory disease in England and Wales (Lambert and Reid, 1970), geographic areas of the country were first stratified according to degree of urbanization (and hence to presumed levels of air pollution), and samples of the population within a certain age range were taken from each stratum; these sampling procedures were employed to ensure sufficient representation from places with differing levels of air pollution. In a study of air pollution and chronic respiratory disease in Berlin, New Hampshire (Ferris and Anderson, 1962), part of the strategy was to include a higher proportion of people in the age range 55–74 years than in the age range 25–54 years because disease prevalence was expected to be higher in the 55–74 year group. In the New Haven Survey of Joint Diseases (Acheson, 1966), census tracts were stratified by social class, and one census tract from each social class was selected, again to ensure representation from each class.

The sampling procedures to be described in Chapter 12 play a major role in cross-sectional studies by enabling the investigator to obtain the most efficient study design possible. Once the sample is selected, consideration must be given to measurement of the exposure status (if it is not known in advance), disease occurrence, and potential confounding variables.

Measurement of Exposure

The methods for measuring exposure status are in general similar to those used in cohort and case-control studies, that is, by questionnaires, records, laboratory tests, physical measurements, and special procedures. For instance, cross-sectional studies examining the relationship between cigarette smoking and prevalence of chronic bronchitis measure smoking status by means of questionnaires. Studies of the relationship between HLA antigens and arthritic disorders measure HLA antigens by laboratory tests. Studies of the relationship between air pollution and chronic bronchitis usually involve measurements of the levels of pollutants in the ambient air.

Finding out for how long and when exposures to these various agents took place is often important. For instance, an investigator might like to determine if prevalence rates of disease increase with longer duration of smoking. It is helpful if the time of exposure can be related to the time of onset of the disease. As mentioned above, the current level of air pollution to which a person is exposed may give little indication of the level at the time the disease developed. Therefore, taking a complete residential history is advisable, so that an estimate can be made of previous exposure levels; this requires that records of air pollution levels be available from the previous places of residence at the time the study participants lived there. If one wants to know whether obesity predisposes to osteoarthritis of the hip, in a strictly cross-sectional approach it would be impossible to know whether a positive association meant that obesity predisposes to arthritis or whether people who develop arthritis exercise less and put on weight. In such a study, previous weight of participants should be ascertained through records or, if records are not available, by asking participants what their weight was before the symptoms developed. In many instances, such re-cords are not available and people do not remember or never knew their exposure status. Lack of information on past exposures is one of the major problems of cross-sectional studies. Therefore, they are best suited to the study of factors that do not change as a result of the disease, such as ABO blood groups or HLA antigens.

Measurement of Occurrence of Disease

The issues in measurement of disease occurrence are similar to those in other types of studies concerned with disease etiology. Usually, disease status is determined by questionnaire, such as when questions on symp-toms are asked for evidence of chronic respiratory disease; by physical examination, such as when joints are examined for evidence of arthritis; or by special procedures, such as when x-rays are taken for evidence of arthri-tis and tests of respiratory function are administered for evidence of chronic respiratory disease. Frequently some combination of these procedures is used. Time of onset of first symptoms of disease should be determined whenever possible, although in many instances a person will not remember, will find it difficult to pinpoint because of the gradual onset, or will not even know the disease is present until it is detected in the prevalence survey.

For diseases with periods of exacerbation and remission, it is important to ask people without signs or symptoms at the time of the study whether they have had such symptoms in the past. Although the investigator may not be able to determine definitively whether they have the disease, they can at least be considered as possibly affected and analyzed separately.

Diagnostic criteria need to be established in advance. For instance, Table 10–1 shows a set of diagnostic criteria for rheumatoid arthritis, re-vised by the American Rheumatism Association in 1987 (Arnett et al., 1988). Application of these criteria requires collection of data from ques-tionnaires, physical examinations, and laboratory tests. The use of standard criteria such as these permits comparisons of prevalence rates from one geographic area to another. However, it is important to employ some re-liability testing to make sure that the criteria are being applied in the same way in all areas.

Statistical Analysis and Control of Confounding Variables

In cross-sectional studies, fourfold tables may be constructed and preva-lence rates in exposed and nonexposed persons compared. For instance, an investigator studying the relation between obesity and osteoarthritis of the hip in a sample of 600 people from a community might obtain the results shown in Table 10–2.

Table 10–1. Summary of 1987 Revised Diagnostic Criteria for Rheumatoid Arthritis. Rheumatoid Arthritis Is Defined by the Presence of Four or More Criteria:

Criterion	Definition
1. Morning stiffness	Morning stiffness in and around the joints, lasting at least 1 hour before maximal improvement
2. Arthritis of three or more joint areas	Soft tissue swelling (arthritis) of three or more joint areas observed by a physician
3. Arthritis of hand joints	Swelling of the proximal interphalangeal, metacarpophalangeal, or wrist joints
4. Symmetric arthritis	Simultaneous involvement of the same joint areas on both sides of the body
5. Rheumatoid nodules	Subcutaneous nodules, over bony prominences, or extensor surfaces, or in juxtaarticular regions, observed by a physician
6. Serum rheumatoid factor	Demonstration of abnormal amounts of serum rheumatoid factor
7. Radiographic changes	Radiographic erosions and/or periarticular osteopenia in hand and/or wrist joints

Criteria 1 through 4 must have been present for at least 6 weeks.

Source: Arnett et al. (1988)

The investigator could then compare the prevalence rate of osteoarthritis in the obese (20%) to the prevalence rate in the non-obese (10%), and a χ_1^2 test of significance could be applied. An odds ratio could be calculated as $20 \times 450/80 \times 50 = 2.25$, but it must be recognized that this ratio is concerned with having the disease, not developing incident disease. As emphasized previously, it would be impossible to determine from this cross-sectional study whether obesity predisposes to osteoarthritis, whether osteoarthritis leads to obesity, or whether both phenomenon to some extent occur.

Confounding is just as important a source of potential bias in cross-sectional studies as in other types of observational studies of disease etiology. Available methods of controlling for confounding variables in cross-sectional studies are the ones discussed in earlier chapters, namely, match-

Table 10–2. Results from a Hypothetical Cross-Sectional Study of the Association between Obesity and Osteoarthritis of the Hip

		Osteoarthritis Yes	Osteoarthritis No	Total
Obese	Yes	20	80	100
	No	50	450	500
	Total	70	530	600

ing in the study design or adjustment in the analysis of the data. Matching, however, is seldom used in cross-sectional studies for two reasons. First, because such studies are often conducted in general population groups, information on potentially confounding variables for individual participants is usually not available prior to data collection. Second, information on the level of exposure is also frequently unavailable at the outset of a cross-sectional study, so that it is not feasible to divide potential participants into exposed and unexposed groups for purposes of matching. Consequently, control in the analysis is typically the only feasible method available for removing the effects of potentially confounding variables in cross-sectional studies.

When controlling for confounding, many of the multivariate statistical techniques used to analyze other types of studies are also appropriate for the analysis of cross-sectional studies. When the outcome of interest is the presence or absence of prevalent disease, then stratified analysis of cross-sectional data can be performed using the Mantel-Haenszel procedure as described in Chapter 9. Logistic regression techniques are equally well suited to cross-sectional studies as to case-control studies and to cohort studies in which there is a uniform period of follow-up (see Chapter 9). To avoid repetition, these techniques will not be illustrated here. In a cross-sectional study, the dependent variable in the Mantel-Haenszel procedure or in logistic regression analysis is the odds of having the disease at the time the study is conducted, rather than of developing new disease. It is important to bear in mind that the problems of interpretation of studies based on prevalence data rather than incidence data persist regardless of how the data are analyzed. Because by definition cross-sectional studies involve no follow-up, methods developed for the analysis of observations with varying lengths of follow-up (e.g., the Kaplan-Meier estimator and the Poisson and Cox regression methods discussed in Chapters 6 and 7) are not applied in such studies.

When the outcome of interest is not the presence or absence of a disease but instead a continuously distributed variable such as blood pressure (Ueshima et al., 1984) or bone mineral density (Edelstein and Barrett-Connor, 1993), simple linear regression (if there are no covariates to take into account), or multiple linear regression (if there are covariates to control for) are frequently used (Kleinbaum and Kupper, 1988; Glantz and Slinker, 1990). In simple linear regression, a linear relationship between an independent, or predictor, variable (x) and a dependent, or outcome, variable (y) is expressed as $y = a + bx$, where a and b are constants estimated from the data. Multiple linear regression analysis entails expressing the continuously distributed outcome variable as a linear function of a number of predictor variables, which may be either binary or continuous. More specifically, if y denotes the dependent variable, then its relationship to the predictor variables in the population from which the sample was drawn is described as follows:

$$y = a + b_1x_1 + \ldots + b_r x_r$$

where r denotes the number of predictor variables included in the model, where $a, b_1, \ldots, b_r$ are constants (coefficients) estimated from the data, and where $x_1, \ldots, x_r$ are a particular person's set of values for the regressor variables.

As in logistic regression, the coefficients $b_1, \ldots, b_r$ are estimated in such a way that the prediction equation obtained is maximally descriptive of the direction and magnitude of the relationships of the predictor variables to the dependent variable in the data being analyzed. The coefficients represent the magnitude of the increase (or, if negative, the decrease) in the value of the dependent variable resulting from an increase of one unit for the relevant predictor variable, while holding constant all other predictor variables in the model.

Table 10–3 gives selected results from a cross-sectional study of the relationship between current alcohol consumption (an independent variable) and systolic blood pressure (the dependent variable) among Japanese men between the ages of 40 and 69 years (Ueshima et al., 1984). Because several other factors are thought to be related to blood pressure, the following variables were considered for inclusion in the model: age, smoking,

Table 10–3. Stepwise Multiple Regression[a] of Systolic Blood Pressure on Current Daily Alcohol Intake, Ponderal Index, Cholesterol, Triglycerides, Hemoglobin, Uric Acid, Smoking and Age, Men Aged 40–69 Years, Osaka and Akita, 1975–1977

Variable	Regression Coefficient	ΔR^2	Standard Error
Osaka (487 men)			
Age (yr)	0.7187	0.0918	0.09608
Daily alcohol intake[b]	2.4704	0.0465	0.54582
Ponderosity index[c]	1.8275	0.0328	0.47979
Uric acid (mg/dl)	1.4627	0.0059	0.78953
Akita (365 men)			
Age	0.8208	0.0596	0.14395
Daily alcohol intake[b]	3.1268	0.0528	0.67293
Ponderosity index[c]	1.2090	0.0135	0.75454
Triglycerides (mg/dl)	0.0327	0.0080	0.01842
Hemoglobin (g/dl)	1.5488	0.0053	0.92881
Cholesterol (mg/dl)	−0.0665	0.0065	0.04075

R^2 for Osaka and Akita are 0.1771 and 0.1458, respectively.

[a]The selection criterion is $F = 2$. See statistical text for definition of F.

[b]See text for a description of this measure.

[c]Ponderosity index = weight kg/height cm$^3 \times 10^6$.

Source: Ueshima et al. (1984).

ponderal index, hemoglobin, uric acid, cholesterol, and triglycerides. Smoking was measured on a five-point scale that was treated as a continuous variable in the analysis, and the remaining factors were all continuous. Alcohol intake, the exposure variable of primary interest, was measured on a six-point scale ranging from total abstention to consumption of more than 83 grams of alcohol per day. Variables were added to the model in a stepwise fashion, beginning with the variable that was most strongly related to blood pressure. The stepwise procedure then added to the model the variable that, once the strongest predictor was included in the equation, correlated most strongly with the dependent variable. This procedure was repeated until all important variables (as determined by some a priori criterion) were added to the model. Other methods of variable selection are also available, and are discussed in many standard statistics textbooks.

Results of a stepwise multiple regression analysis for two areas of Japan (Osaka and Akita) are shown in Table 10–3. In both areas age was the strongest predictor of systolic blood pressure. For Osaka, the coefficient for age was 0.7187, indicating that a man one year older than another man on the average would have a blood pressure that is about 0.7 mm Hg higher, provided that the two have equal values for the remaining variables in the model. Although this difference in blood pressure is rather trivial from a biologic point of view, one year of age is also a rather small difference. For a 20-year difference in age, the difference in systolic blood pressure would be $20 \times 0.7187 = 14.4$ mm Hg. A 95% confidence interval for this estimate may be constructed from its standard error of 0.09608 as follows:

Lower limit = $(20 \times 0.7187) - (1.96 \times 20 \times 0.09608) = 10.6$ mm Hg

and

Upper limit = $(20 \times 0.7187) + (1.96 \times 20 \times 0.09608) = 18.1$ mm Hg

The positive sign of the coefficient indicates that blood pressure increases with alcohol intake. A negative coefficient, such as the one for cholesterol in the Akita group, indicates a decrease in blood pressure with higher values of cholesterol.

The variable of primary interest to the investigators, daily alcohol intake, was determined in the stepwise regression procedure to be the second strongest predictor of systolic blood pressure in both areas. It was therefore the second variable to enter the equations. A difference of one unit on the alcohol intake scale was associated with an average difference of 2.5 mm Hg in Osaka and 3.1 mm Hg in Akita. Looking at the extremes of the alcohol intake scale, men in Osaka who drank more than 83 grams per day had systolic blood pressures that averaged $5 \times 2.4704 = 12.3$ mm Hg higher than that of men in Osaka who abstained from alcohol but who were otherwise similar. The 95% confidence interval for this estimate is 7.0–17.7 mm Hg. The corresponding point estimate and 95% confidence interval for Akita is 15.6 mm Hg and 9.0–22.2 mm Hg.

In Table 10–3, a quantity denoted $\triangle R^2$ is listed in addition to the regression coefficients and their standard errors. This quantity denotes the proportion of the total variance in systolic blood pressure that is explained or accounted for by each of the variables in the regression equation. For the Osaka men, age alone accounts for about 9% of the variance in systolic blood pressure. Alcohol intake accounts for an additional 5% of the variance in systolic blood pressure, and so on. When the ponderal index and uric acid are included in the equation, the percentage of the variance in systolic blood pressure accounted for by the four variables together is about 18% ($R^2 = 0.1771$). This rather low percentage indicates that most of the variability in systolic blood pressure cannot be accounted for by the variables selected for possible inclusion in the multiple regression equation. Less than perfect measurement of the variables may have contributed to the low percentage of variance explained, but it also seems likely that important determinants of systolic blood pressure were not measured at all.

Although R^2 is a frequently reported measure, it is important to note that its value depends not only on the biologic relationship between the predictor and the outcome of interest but also on the amount of variance in the risk factors in the particular population studied. Therefore, the quantities that can be most readily interpreted in many epidemiologic contexts are the regression coefficients themselves (Greenland et al., 1986; Greenland et al., 1991).

The finding of an association between alcohol intake and systolic blood pressure in the study by Ueshima et al. (1984) must be considered in light of the cross-sectional nature of the study design. Because both of these variables were measured at the same time, the possibility exists that blood pressure in some way influences drinking behavior or the reporting of that behavior. However, because these data are consistent with prospective studies of non-Japanese men, the authors favor an interpretation of a causal effect of alcohol on blood pressure. Of course, regardless of what observational study design is used, the possibility of unmeasured or inadequately measured confounding variables remains a possible alternative explanation of the results.

Although multiple linear regression has been illustrated in the context of cross-sectional studies, the technique is equally useful for cohort studies in which the length of follow-up is constant and in which the outcome is a continuously distributed variable.

Prevalence Studies Measuring Serologic Profiles

Another use of cross-sectional studies arises when serologic techniques are employed to measure various components in samples of blood drawn from individuals from the general population or from a specific target population such as military recruits or college students. Serologic tests can determine the presence (and level) or absence of antigen type, antibodies, immune complexes, various biochemical components, or genetic characteristics such as blood group and HLA antigens at the time the blood sample is obtained. Most serologic tests can be performed on sera frozen at -20 to $-70°C$. Unlike diagnostic tests, which are usually applied to individual patients with some evidence of disease, seroepidemiologic tests are applied to population groups, usually healthy persons, to determine current and past patterns of infection and disease as reflected in tests carried out on the blood samples. The results of the serologic tests are correlated with other characteristics of the participants using data obtained from questionnaire and records (Paul and White, 1973). Seroepidemiologic data may also be used in determining the medical care needs of a community and in evaluating immunization programs. These and other uses of serologic epidemiologic surveys are listed in Table 10–4.

The term *antibody prevalence*, although referring to the number of persons possessing a given antibody at the time that the blood sample was taken, actually reflects the cumulative experience of the population regarding infection. If the antibody tested is of the IgG type, which often lasts a lifetime, then the prevalence pattern will reflect infections from the time of

Table 10–4. Examples of Uses of Seroepidemiology

Use	Examples
Determination of prevalence	Presence of antibody, antigen, chemical, hormone, or other component in blood at the time of procurement
Determination of incidence	The appearance of or increase in some blood component in blood samples obtained at the second of two points in time
Diagnostic serology	Identification of the various causes of a clinical syndrome or of the spectrum of disease associated with a single causal agent or risk factor
Identifying an association between an agent and a disease	Finding the disease or condition associated with a certain component noted in the blood
Identifying an association between two or more markers	Finding the relationship of genetic markers, antibody levels, or markers of chronic disease in blood samples

birth to the time of sampling. If it is of the IgM type, which is of short duration, then the presence of antibody indicates that the person was infected within the past few months. The absence of an antibody or other marker of a chronic disease (high blood glucose, high cholesterol, high uric acid) in the first sample of blood and its appearance, or increase, in a second sample taken at a later date indicates that infection, or the development of a pathologic process, has occurred in the interval between the time the two samples were taken. The appearance of the new serologic marker does measure an incident event, but it does not necessarily indicate clinical disease, because the change in the marker may or may not be accompanied by actual illness.

Because of the high cost of collecting and testing large numbers of blood samples, multiple tests are often carried out on the same sample so that the study can serve multiple purposes (World Health Organization, 1970). These surveys provide guidance for immunization and control programs. Examples of a multipurpose survey involving a single targeted population are cross-sectional studies carried out on entering military recruits in Argentina (Evans et al., 1971), Brazil (Florey et al., 1967; Niederman et al., 1967), and Colombia (Evans et al., 1969). Although such populations are highly select in that they are all male, young adults, and in presumed good health, they offer the advantages of wide geographic representation and reduced cost since they use part of the blood from samples taken routinely on entry into the service. The nationwide survey of military recruits in Brazil (Niederman et al., 1967) showed that yellow fever–neutralizing antibodies, used as an index of previous infection, were common in recruits from most areas of the country. Measles and mumps antibodies were highly prevalent in all areas, but prevalence rates were higher in urban than rural areas. Most recruits (92%–94%) had detectable antibodies to one or more types of poliovirus, even though few had been vaccinated. In general, there were 10 times as many arbovirus infections in Brazilian military recruits in 1964 as there had been in recruits in the United States in 1962.

Examples of serologic surveys undertaken in more general populations are those done in St. Lucia (Evans et al., 1979) and Barbados (Evans et al., 1974). Among the findings of these surveys was that no persons under age 11 years in Barbados had rubella antibody, indicating that the rubella virus had not been circulating there for the previous decade. In contrast, rubella antibody was evident in all age groups in St. Lucia, including children aged 1–5 years, thus demonstrating continuing rubella activity. Why rubella should be active on one island and not another was not clear. In some remote areas of Brazil, rubella activity is essentially absent, indicating that the virus has not been introduced from the outside into those tribes (Black et al., 1974).

Cross-sectional studies have also been undertaken to determine the epidemiologic features of some newly discovered agent by measuring antibody prevalence in various geographic, age, and occupational groups. Such studies have focused on the hepatitis A and B viruses, Epstein-Barr virus, *Legionella pneumophilia,* the rotaviruses, and most recently the retroviruses associated with leukemia (human T-cell leukemia virus type 1 [HTLV-1]) and with AIDS (HIV-1). For instance, seroepidemiologic testing for antibodies to HTLV-1 showed that HTLV-1 infection is prevalent in geographic areas where there are virus-associated leukemia clusters, and that the prevalence of antibodies varies by country, region within a country, age, and possibly race and gender. These findings are consistent with other evidence suggesting that HTLV-1 is etiologically linked to a specific subtype of mature T-cell malignancy. For instance, this virus has been isolated from patients with T-cell malignancies (Blattner et al., 1983). Similar surveys for HIV-1 antibody have indicated not only the presence of antibody in AIDS patients but also high prevalence of antibodies in high-risk populations in the United States (homosexual males, IV drug users, and hemophiliacs) as well as in healthy adults in Zaire and other African countries.

In order to encourage the use of serologic surveys, three WHO Reference Serum Banks were set up in 1960 (in the Institute of Epidemiology and Microbiology, Prague, Czechoslovakia; the Department of Epidemiology and Public Health, Yale University School of Medicine, New Haven, Connecticut; and the South African Institute of Medical Research in Johannesburg, South Africa). A fourth was added in Japan in 1971 at the National Institute of Health. These banks contain large collections of sera from various population groups; the sera can be obtained for seroepidemiologic studies by other investigators, who are also encouraged to store their own collections there. The International Agency for Cancer Research has compiled a list of these and other serum banks available in other institutions.

Most seroepidemiologic studies require the testing of a large number of blood samples, so the test procedures should be simple, rapid, reliable, economical, safe, and adaptable to microtechniques using microtiter plates. The reagents should be readily available. Automated techniques for both the performance and reading of the tests are desirable. For antibody, antigen, and many biologic and biochemical tests, the microtiter procedure is used; this procedure employs disposable flat plates containing 96 small wells to hold the serum antigen, conjugate, and other test ingredients. They are widely used for hemagglutination inhibition, complement fixation, neutralization, and the enzyme-linked immunosorbent assay (ELISA) tests measuring antibody levels.

The laboratory tests should be reproducible both when the same sample is retested in the same laboratory and when the same sample is tested in other laboratories. It should be specific (with few false positives) and sensitive (with few false negatives). Good laboratory practice requires that in each run, samples be included from standard sources known to be positive and known to be negative, and also that the test sera be coded and tested blindly by the technician. Some samples should be subdivided and tested separately by the technician without the technician knowing which samples are the duplicates. The accuracy of the technician's readings of the standard samples and the reliability of the technician's readings on two halves of the same sample can be tested by the methods to be presented in Chapter 13.

PANEL STUDIES

Panel studies can be considered a type of prospective cohort study in which information is sought from the same participants (the panel) on exposure and disease (or symptom) occurrence at multiple intervals of time. Unlike traditional cohort studies, however, study participants need not be free of disease at the outset of the study. A panel study may also be thought of as a series of cross-sectional studies done on the same participants at various intervals of time; unlike conventional cross-sectional studies, longitudinal measurements on individuals are made. This permits changes in one variable to be related to changes in another variable. For instance, in a study undertaken among students of seven California universities, measurements of meteorological variables and air pollution levels over time were related to the occurrence of respiratory symptoms over the same time period (Durham, 1974). In a study of the development and progression of scoliosis (lateral curvature of the spine) in adolescents, changes in the height and weight of growing adolescents can be related to changes in the degree of curvature in their spines over the same period of time. Stressful life events recorded at monthly intervals can be related to onsets of illness during the same or subsequent months. As defined here, panel studies include those in which the temporal relationships among the various events of interest can be determined, as well as those simply correlating changes in one characteristic with changes in another, without knowing which came first. The ability to determine the correct temporal ordering of course depends in large part on how frequently the measurements of various events are made.

In some panel studies, participants are asked to keep daily diaries, in some they are interviewed at frequent intervals (either in person or by telephone) regarding events that occurred since the last interview, and in others objective measurements are made at predetermined intervals, such as once a day or once a month. In many panel studies, combinations of these methods are used. In general, diaries are better than interviews for obtaining incident events, but not for prevalent events (Verbrugge, 1980). In other words, people are likely to record new events or changes in circumstances in diaries. Accordingly, diaries appear to be especially advantageous for determining the occurrence of acute conditions and changes in symptomatology of chronic conditions during the study period. An interview with extensive questions about chronic conditions will generally provide the most complete information about chronic conditions in which the symptomatology is not changing over time. Interviews obtaining information retrospectively are especially likely to miss illnesses that did not result in activity restriction and in which medical care was not sought.

In panel studies, participants are not required to remember events over long periods of time, thus increasing the likelihood that their reports are accurate. Furthermore, making measurements in the same individuals over time almost always enables the investigator to monitor these changes with greater precision than if independent samples are taken at each interval and to study characteristics of people who change, rather than just the total change. If the temporal ordering of events can be determined, differentiation of cause from effect is facilitated. Also, the nature of the temporal relationship can be addressed more precisely. For instance, do respiratory symptoms increase in frequency at the same time as air pollution levels, or is there a lag time of a day or two?

Practical problems in carrying out panel studies are in many ways similar to the problems encountered in undertaking other prospective cohort studies. Unless the outcome of interest is common, large sample sizes will be needed. Recruiting people willing to be included in a study requiring continued participation over a period of time may be difficult. Some participants will drop out, decreasing the sample size and possibly creating bias. When panel members are asked the same questions over time they may give more accurate responses, or, on the other hand, they may become fatigued and sloppy. Trends can appear in the data that are in reality attributable to such "conditioning effects."

As in other types of prospective cohort studies, interpretation of the nature of a causal relationship may not always be straightforward (Link and Shrout, 1992). For instance, it might appear that rapid growth leads to scoliosis when it is some hormonal factor that is causing both the growth spurt and the curvature of the spine. Some underlying psychological state could predispose a person to the tendency both to experience stressful life events and to develop disease. Recognition and accurate measurement of these other contributing variables along with analysis of the effects of the variables of primary interest are necessary to sort out these possibilities.

Statistical techniques for analyzing panel studies are complex (Kessler and Greenberg, 1982) and will not be covered here.

ECOLOGICAL STUDIES

In most epidemiologic studies, the unit of analysis is an individual person, who is classified in terms of exposure status and disease status. Occasionally, however, studies are conducted in which the unit of analysis is some aggregate of individuals. Such studies are called *ecological studies,* a term that derives from the frequent use of geographic areas as the basis for defining aggregates for analysis. A second commonly used unit for defining aggregates is time period. In an ecological study, a summary measure of the frequency of exposure and a second summary measure of the frequency of disease are obtained within each ecological unit. The analysis centers on determining whether those ecological units with a high frequency of occurrence of the exposure tend also to be the units with a high (or low) frequency of occurrence of disease. An example of results from an ecological study is given in Figure 10–1, in which mortality from cancer of the rectum is plotted as a function of per capita consumption of beer for several countries around the world (Breslow and Enstrom, 1974).

The distinction between ecological studies and studies that use the individual as the unit of analysis can perhaps be clarified by considering the series of 2 × 2 tables in Table 10–5. In an ecological study, the numbers of individuals having specific combinations of exposure status and disease status (cells *a, b, c, d*) are not known. Instead, the only information avail-

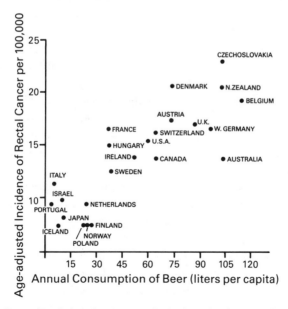

Figure 10–1. Example of data from an ecological study (from Breslow and Enstrom, 1974).

Table 10–5. Data Employed for Ecological Studies of Exposure-Disease Associations

Area 1

		Disease		Total
		Present	Absent	
Exposure	Present	$a_1 = ?$	$b_1 = ?$	$a_1 + b_1$
	Absent	$c_1 = ?$	$d_1 = ?$	$c_1 + d_1$
	Total	$a_1 + c_1$	$b_1 + d_1$	$a_1 + b_1 + c_1 + d_1$

Area 2

		Disease		Total
		Present	Absent	
Exposure	Present	$a_2 = ?$	$b_2 = ?$	$a_2 + b_2$
	Absent	$c_2 = ?$	$d_2 = ?$	$c_2 + d_2$
	Total	$a_2 + c_2$	$b_2 + d_2$	$a_2 + b_2 + c_2 + d_2$

Comparison made:

If $\dfrac{a_1 + b_1}{a_1 + b_1 + c_1 + d_1}$ is greater (or less) than $\dfrac{a_2 + b_2}{a_2 + b_2 + c_2 + d_2}$, then is

$\dfrac{a_1 + c_1}{a_1 + b_1 + c_1 + d_1}$ also greater (or less) than $\dfrac{a_2 + c_2}{a_2 + b_2 + c_2 + d_2}$?

able is the total numbers of exposed and unexposed individuals and the total numbers of diseased and nondiseased individuals, that is, the totals $a + b, c + d, a + c, b + d$, respectively.

The principal reason that only these totals may be available is that data on exposure and disease are collected separately, often for rather different purposes. For example, incidence and mortality rates used in ecological studies are usually from data routinely collected by health agencies for countries, states, counties, municipalities, or other geographic units. Aggregate information on the proportion of workers in each geographic area who are employed in a specific industry may be compiled by other agencies. Because each of the two sets of statistics is compiled independently of the other, information is not available concerning the numbers of individuals with various combinations of exposure status and disease status. In other words, it is not known whether the individuals employed in the industry are the ones who develop the disease.

One example of an ecological study is an analysis by Robertson and Zador (1978) of the relationship between driver education and the incidence of fatal automobile accidents involving teenage drivers. Information was not available at the individual level, in that teenage drivers who had taken driver education could not be compared directly to other teenage drivers regarding their involvement in fatal automobile accidents. Instead, data were employed that had been compiled for each of 27 states. Information on the participation in driver education courses of students in public and private high schools had been compiled for certain years by the Insurance Institute for Highway Safety and the National Safety Council. Information on involvement in fatal automobile accidents was obtained from reports of state police and motor vehicle administrations in the 27 states. The specific indices used in the analysis were the proportion of licensed teenage drivers in the state who had taken driver education and the number of fatal crashes involving teenage drivers per 10,000 licensed teenage drivers in the state. Statistical analyses were then performed to assess whether these two measures were associated when examined across the 27 states, each of which had 2 to 5 years of available data.

As in other types of studies, it is important to consider potentially confounding variables when analyzing and interpreting the results of an ecological study. In their evaluation of driver education, Robertson and Zador included in the analysis the total number of motor vehicle deaths per 10,000 licensed drivers of all ages. Inclusion of this variable would help to control partially for such regional differences as road safety, traffic patterns, speed limits, and the average amount of time people spend driving. Although the authors found no relationship between driver education and the frequency of fatal crashes per 10,000 teenage drivers when they controlled for this potentially confounding variable, they did note a substantial positive association between driver education and the number of teenage drivers on the road. They then examined the association between (a) driver education and (b) the frequency of fatal crashes involving teenagers divided by the size of the total teenage population of the state rather than by the size of the population of teenage drivers. A positive association was found when controlling in the analysis for the potentially confounding variable of the total frequency of fatal crashes in all age groups. Thus, the results suggest that the net effect of driver education is to put more teenagers on the road and thereby to increase rather than reduce the number of fatal crashes involving drivers in that age group. This example is a relatively unusual one in that most ecological studies do not yield this sort of insight into what appears to be a causal chain.

Control of confounding variables at the aggregate level may help to improve the validity of ecological studies, but just because an association is found at the ecological level does not guarantee that the association will also hold if a subsequent study of individuals is conducted. Referring to Table 10–5, note that the mere fact that both the proportion exposed and the proportion diseased may be higher in Area 1 than in Area 2 does not *necessarily* imply that within areas there is an association between exposure

Table 10-6. Hypothetical Example of a Strong Ecological Correlation when the Risk Ratio at the Individual Level Is Only 1.25[a]

Area	Proportion Exposed	Proportion Developing the Disease
1	0.20	$(0.20)(0.10) + (1 - 0.20)(0.08) = 0.084$
2	0.40	$(0.40)(0.10) + (1 - 0.40)(0.08) = 0.088$
3	0.60	$(0.60)(0.10) + (1 - 0.60)(0.08) = 0.092$
4	0.80	$(0.80)(0.10) + (1 - 0.80)(0.08) = 0.096$

[a]The proportion of exposed individuals developing the disease is assumed to be 0.10, as opposed to 0.08 for the unexposed. It is also assumed that there is no confounding at the aggregate level.

and disease for individuals. Inappropriate conclusions regarding relationships at the individual level based on ecological data are frequently referred to as the *ecological fallacy* (Selvin, 1958).

Even when there is an association between exposure and disease at the individual level, it is often difficult to assess the magnitude of that relationship on the basis of ecological data. Consider, for example, the hypothetical data for the four areas shown in Table 10-6. It is assumed that among the exposed individuals the proportion developing the disease is 0.10 and that the corresponding proportion among the unexposed individuals is 0.08 within each area, for a risk ratio of 1.25. If the proportion exposed is assumed to vary from 0.20 to 0.40 to 0.60 to 0.80 across the areas, then in the absence of any confounding at the aggregate level, the proportions of the total populations of the areas who develop the disease are as given in the final column of the table. These risks increase in a linear fashion as a function of the proportion exposed in the four areas.

When examined closely, these hypothetical ecological data do provide some indication that the association may not be strong at the individual level, because a fourfold differential in the proportion exposed corresponds to only a 1.14-fold differential across areas in the risk of disease. Nevertheless, in many ecological studies, only a crude ranking of areas regarding exposure level is possible, and because in this example the rankings for the two variables of interest are identical, it might be tempting to conclude inappropriately that the association is likely to be strong at the individual level.

In fact, it has been shown that in ecological studies with nondifferential misclassification of exposure (misclassification of exposure unrelated to disease status), large overestimates may be obtained of the magnitude of associations at the individual level (Brenner et al., 1992; Greenland and Robins, 1994). Another problem is that bias in summary ecological estimates can result from effect modification by another variable, even if the variable does not appear to be a confounder at the ecological or individual levels. Bias can also result when the relationship between exposure and disease or between a confounder and disease is assumed to be linear when in fact the relationship is nonlinear (Richardson et al., 1987; Greenland, 1992; Greenland and Robins, 1994). Control of such effect modifiers and variables having nonlinear effects in an ecological statistical analysis is generally insufficient to remove the bias and can sometimes worsen the bias, even if no measurement error exists (Greenland and Morgenstern, 1989). Using multiple summary measures of the confounder can under some circumstances (Greenland and Robins, 1994) reduce such bias in ecological studies, but several different measures are usually not available.

In summary, associations derived from ecological studies under various circumstances can be overestimates, underestimates, or even in the opposite direction from associations at the individual level. Thus, particular caution is needed in interpreting associations found in ecological studies.

Additional problems of interpretation arise because of the difficulties in distinguishing cause and effect in ecological studies. For instance, an early ecological study was performed to assess the relationship between social class and serious forms of mental illness (Faris and Dunham, 1939). Various social and economic indicators for census tracts in an urban area were correlated with rates of psychiatric hospitalization in those census tracts. Although the results suggested that people living in areas of low socioeconomic status were at elevated risk, it may have been that there was no causal role for socioeconomic status, but that because of the lowered social functioning of mentally ill persons, they drift into the lower socioeconomic areas. Cohort data on individuals would be needed in order to determine whether the social drift hypothesis is the correct explanation for the observed association.

Despite their considerable problems of interpretation, ecological studies can serve a useful purpose in the generation of initial leads for pursuit in more definitive studies, as was illustrated in Chapter 1. Additionally, there are some problems for which the ecological approach may be the most reasonable one. If broad social or cultural processes are of interest, then the individual may not be the most appropriate unit of analysis, because inferences are to be drawn about whole societies rather than about individuals. Nevertheless, in most epidemiologic contexts as opposed to sociologic or anthropologic contexts, one is interested in drawing inferences about disease etiology in individual persons. Consequently, the collection of extensive data at the individual level is nearly always required before a cause-effect relationship can be inferred, although occasionally an ecological study can provide fairly compelling evidence for a causal relationship, as in the example involving driver education. More detailed discussions of ecological studies are available elsewhere (Firebaugh, 1978; Morgenstern,

1982; Richardson et al., 1987; Brenner et al., 1992; Greenland and Mor-genstern, 1989; Greenland et al., 1991; Greenland, 1992; Greenland and Robins, 1994).

REFERENCES

Acheson RM. 1966. The New Haven Survey of Joint Disease: selection of the study population. *Proceedings of the Third International Symposium on Population Studies of the Rheumatic Diseases.* New York, Excerpta Medica International Congress Series No. 148, pp 490–498.

Anderson DO, Ferris BG Jr, Zickmantel R. 1964. Levels of air pollution and respiratory disease in Berlin, New Hampshire. *Am Rev Respir Dis* 90:877–887.

Arnett FC, Edworthy SM, Bloch DA, McShane DJ, Fries JF, Cooper NS, Healey LA, Kaplan SR, Liang MH, Luthra HS, Medsger TA Jr, Mitchell DM, Neustadt DH, Pinals RS, Schaller JG, Sharp JT, Wilder RL, Hunder GG. 1988. The American Rheumatism Association 1987 revised criteria for the classification of rheumatoid arthritis. *Arth Rheum* 31:315–324.

Black FL, Hierholzer WJ, Pinheiro F deP, Evans AS, Woodall JP, Opton EM, Emmons JE, West BS, Edsall G, Downs WG, Wallace GD. 1974. Evidence for persistence of infectious agents in isolated human populations. *Am J Epidemiol* 100:230–250.

Blattner WA, Blayney DW, Robert-Guroff M, Sarngadharan MG, Kalyanaraman VS, Sarin PS, Jaffe ES, Gallo RC. 1983. Epidemiology of human T-cell leukemia/lymphoma virus. *J Infect Dis* 147:406–416.

Brauer GW, Prior IAM. 1978. A prospective study of gout in New Zealand and Maoris. *Ann Rheum Dis* 37:466–472.

Brenner H, Savitz DA, Jöckel K-H, Greenland S. 1992. Effects of nondifferential exposure misclassification in ecologic studies. *Am J Epidemiol* 135:85–95.

Breslow NE, Enstrom JE. 1974. Geographic correlations between cancer mortality rates and alcohol-tobacco consumption in the United States. *J Natl Cancer Inst* 53:631–639.

Durham WH. 1974. Air pollution and student health. *Arch Environ Health* 16:853–861.

Edelstein SL, Barrett-Connor E. 1993. Relation between body size and bone mineral density in elderly men and women. *Am J Epidemiol* 138:160–169.

Evans AS, Casals J, Opton EM, Borman EK, Levine L, Caudrado R. 1969. A nationwide serum survey of Colombian military recruits, 1966. I. Description of sample and antibody patterns with arboviruses, polioviruses, respiratory viruses, tetanus, and treponematosis. *Am J Epidemiol* 90:292–303.

Evans AS, Casals J, Opton EM, Borman EK, Levine L, Caudrado R. 1971. A nationwide serum survey of Argentinean military recruits, 1965–1966. I. Description of sample and antibody patterns with arboviruses, polioviruses, respiratory viruses, tetanus and treponematosis. *Am J Epidemiol* 93:111–121.

Evans AS, Cook JA, Kapikian AZ, Nankervis G, Smith AL, West B. 1979. A serological survey of St. Lucia. *Int J Epidemiol* 8:327–332.

Evans AS, Cox F, Nankervis G, Opton E, Shope R, Wells AV, West B. 1974. A health and seroepidemiological survey of a community in Barbados. *Int J Epidemiol* 3:167–175.

Faris RE, Dunham HW. 1939. Mental Disorders in Urban Areas: An Ecological Study of Schizophrenia and Other Psychoses. Chicago, University of Chicago Press.

Ferris BG, Anderson DO. 1962. The prevalence of chronic respiratory disease in a New Hampshire town. *Am Rev Respir Dis* 86:165–177.

Firebaugh G. 1978. A rule for inferring individual-level relationships from aggregate data. *Am Sociol Rev* 43:557–572.

Florey C duV, Cuadrado R, Henderson JR, de Goes PA. 1967. A nationwide serum survey of Brazilian military recruits, 1964. I. Methods and sampling results. *Am J Epidemiol* 86:314–318.

Glantz SA, Slinker BK. 1990. Primer of Applied Regression and Analysis of Variance. New York, McGraw-Hill.

Greenland S. 1992. Divergent biases in ecologic and individual-level studies. *Stat Med* 11:1209–1223.

Greenland S, Maclure M, Schesselman JJ, Poole C, Morgenstern H. 1991. Standardized regression coefficients: a further critique and review of some alternatives. *Epidemiology* 2:387–392.

Greenland S, Morgenstern H. 1989. Ecologic bias, confounding, and effect modification. *Int J Epidemiol* 18:269–274.

Greenland S, Robins J. 1994. Invited commentary: Ecologic studies—biases, misconceptions, and counterexamples. *Am J Epidemiol* 139:747–760.

Greenland S, Schesselman JJ, Criqui MH. 1986. The fallacy of employing standardized regression coefficients and correlations as measures of effect. *Am J Epidemiol* 123:203–208.

Kelsey JL, Mood EW, Acheson RM. 1968. Population mobility and the epidemiology of chronic bronchitis in Connecticut. *Arch Environ Health* 16:853–861.

Kessler R, Greenberg D. 1982. Linear Panel Analysis: Models of Quantitative Change. New York, Academic Press.

Kleinbaum DG, Kupper LL. 1988. Applied Regression Analysis and Other Multivariable Methods. Boston, PWS-Kent Publishing Company.

Lambert PM, Reid DD. 1970. Smoking, air pollution, and bronchitis in Britain. *Lancet* 1:853–857.

Last JM, Editor. 1995. A Dictionary of Epidemiology. Third Edition. New York: Oxford University Press.

Link BG, Shrout PE. 1992. Spurious associations in longitudinal research. *Res Commun Mental Health* 7:301–321.

Meadows SH. 1961. Social class migration and chronic bronchitis. *Br J Prevent Soc Med* 15:171–175.

Morgenstern H. 1982. Uses of ecologic analysis in epidemiologic research. *Am J Public Health* 72:1336–1344.

Niederman JC, Henderson JR, Opton EM, Black FL, Skvrnova K. 1967. A nationwide serum survey of Brazilian military recruits, 1964. II. Antibody patterns with arboviruses, polioviruses, measles, and mumps. *Am J Epidemiol* 86:319–329.

Paul JR, White C, Eds. 1973. Serological Epidemiology. New York, Academic Press.

Richardson S, Stücker I, Hémon D. 1987. Comparison of relative risks obtained in individual and ecological studies: Some methodological considerations. *Int J Epidemiol* 16:111–120.

Robertson LS, Zador PL. 1978. Driver education and fatal crash involvement of teenage drivers. *Am J Public Health* 68:959–965.

Selvin HC. 1958. Durkheim's *Suicide* and problems of empirical research. *Am J Sociol* 63:607–619.

Ueshima H, Shimamoto T, Iida M, Konishi M, Tanigaki M, Doi M, Tsujioka K, Nagano E, Tsuda C, Ozawa H, Kojima S, Komachi Y. 1984. Alcohol intake and hypertension among urban and rural Japanese populations. *J Chron Dis* 37:585–592.

Verbrugge LM. 1980. Health diaries. *Med Care* 18:73–95.

Winkelstein W Jr, Kantor S. 1969. Respiratory symptoms and air pollution in an urban population of northeastern United States. *Arch Environ Health* 18:760–767.

World Health Organization. 1970. Multipurpose Serological Surveys and WHO Serum Reference Banks. Geneva, WHO Technical Report No. 454.

EXERCISES

1. List the potential problems in interpretation if a prevalence (cross-sectional) study (as opposed to other types of observational studies) is used to test each of the following hypotheses.

　　a. Low calcium intake increases the risk of osteoporosis.

　　b. Pet ownership decreases the risk of high blood pressure.

　　c. Obesity increases the risk of cerebrovascular accidents (strokes).

　　d. Females are at greater risk for high blood pressure than males among persons aged 65 years and older.

　　e. Risk of peptic ulcers varies according to ABO blood group.

2. Design a panel study to test one of the following hypotheses. Discuss the strengths and weaknesses of your proposed study.

　　a. Fluctuations in levels of particulate air pollution affect the frequency of coughing among people with chronic bronchitis.

　　b. Stressful life events increase the risk for falls in the elderly.

　　c. Rapid fluctuations in ambient air temperature affect the risk of developing the common cold.

3. In their cross-sectional study of blood pressure in Japan, Ueshima et al. (1984) obtained the following regression coefficients for their Akita sample when diastolic blood pressure was employed rather than systolic blood pressure as the dependent variable:

Variable	Regression Coefficient	ΔR^2	Standard Error
Daily alcohol intake[a]	1.7329	0.0491	0.3800
Hemoglobin (g/dl)	1.2234	0.0277	0.5215
Ponderosity index (weight/height^3 × 10^6)	0.8256	0.0145	0.4259
Triglycerides (mg/dl)	0.0209	0.0087	0.0010
Age (yr)	0.1293	0.0064	0.0814

[a]See text for description of this measure.

a. Compare the results for alcohol to those reported for the Akita sample in Table 10–3.

b. What is the interpretation of the coefficient for hemoglobin?

c. Construct a 95% confidence interval for the coefficient for the relationship of age to diastolic blood pressure.

4. Describe the sources of data that might be used to conduct ecological studies of the following relationships:

a. Climate (e.g., temperature, humidity, rainfall) and multiple sclerosis.

b. Use of oral contraceptives and the incidence of stroke.

c. Sunlight and cutaneous melanoma, a form of skin cancer.

NOTE

1. The term *prevalence rate* is used here as in *A Dictionary of Epidemiology* (Last, 1995), because this definition is in common use even though it does not meet the strict definition of a "rate" (see Chapter 2).

11

Epidemic Investigation

This book has considered studies that are prospective and retrospective from the standpoint of the observer, studies that require observation of a cohort of persons, and studies that involve comparisons of cases with controls. The placement of epidemic investigations in this scheme is difficult because the methods of study vary considerably, depending on the circumstances, and may involve different approaches at different times, or even several approaches during a single outbreak.

DEFINITION OF AN EPIDEMIC

One definition of an epidemic is (Last, 1995)

> the occurrence in a community or region of cases of an illness, specific health-related behavior, or other health-related events clearly in excess of normal expectancy. The community or region, and the period in which the cases occur are specified precisely. The number of cases indicating the presence of an epidemic varies according to the agent, size and type of population exposed, previous experience or lack of exposure to the disease, and time and place of occurrence. Epidemicity is thus relative to usual frequency of the disease in the same area, among the specified population, at the same season of the year. A single case of a communicable disease long absent from a population or first invasion by a disease not previously recognized in that area requires immediate reporting and full field investigation; two cases of such a disease associated in time and place may be sufficient evidence to be considered an epidemic.

An epidemic may then be considered an increase in the number of cases over past experience for a given population, time, and place. This time period may be either short or long so that both acute and chronic illnesses, irrespective of the incubation or induction period, may occur in epidemics. The agent may be infectious or noninfectious. It should be emphasized that at the same time as clinical cases occur, there are usually many inapparent infections and "subclinical" cases of diseases of both infectious and noninfectious etiology. The term *endemic* is used to reflect the occurrence of a disease or condition at a relatively constant level in a given setting. *Pandemic* refers to an epidemic occurring over a very wide area and usually affecting a large proportion of the population.

ESSENTIAL INGREDIENTS OF AN EPIDEMIC

The term *pathogen* will be used to indicate both infectious and noninfectious substances (agents) that are capable, acting either alone or in combination with other agents, of producing tissue damage or initiating a pathologic process that can lead to disease. The three common conditions for the occurrence of an outbreak or epidemic are usually:

1. The introduction of a new pathogen, or the increased amount of or a change in the virulence of a known pathogen, from an infected human, animal, bird, or arthropod vector, or from air, water, food, soil, drug, or other environmental source.
2. An adequate number of exposed and susceptible persons. The proportion susceptible needed for an epidemic to occur will depend on the communicability of the agent. Measles can result in an outbreak when 90% or more of the population is already immune (Agocs et al., 1992), whereas levels of 50%–60% immune will prevent the spread of less infectious organisms such as typhoid bacillus.
3. An effective means of transmission between the source of the pathogen and the susceptible persons.

Recent reports illustrate these essential ingredients of an epidemic. Outbreaks of eosinophilia-myalgia syndrome from the ingestion of tryptophan-containing products provide an example of epidemics resulting from a new agent. This was first recognized in 1989 (Varga et al., 1992), and will be discussed later in this chapter. The appearance of a new type of Hanta virus pulmonary syndrome in the southwestern United States represents an emerging virus infection, newly introduced into this country (Centers for Disease Control, 1993b). An example of a change in an old agent is the emergence of antibiotic-resistant strains of *Mycobacterium tuberculosis* in patients with AIDS and in tuberculosis patients who interrupt their therapy; these strains may then be spread to other persons. Outbreaks attributable to an increased number of susceptibles are illustrated by the spread of influenza in nursing homes among elderly who have lost their immunity or fail to respond to vaccination (Centers for Disease Control, 1992). The enhanced spread of an infection because of a changing environment is exemplified by the rapid transmission of tuberculosis in crowded shelters for the homeless (Centers for Disease Control, 1991).

COMMON CIRCUMSTANCES FOR AN EPIDEMIC

Keeping in mind these essential ingredients, some common circumstances for an epidemic are then (a) the introduction of susceptibles into an endemic area where a pathogen new to them exists, such as when people travel to the rainforests of Africa or Brazil, when military forces were sent to the Persian Gulf or Haiti, or when explorations into new ecological settings take place; (b) a recent change in dosage or virulence of a known organism, such as occurred in the massive water-borne outbreak of cryptosporidium in the public water supply in Milwaukee (MacKenzie et al., 1994); (c) the introduction of a pathogen into a setting where it has not been before, such as the introduction of the Hanta virus into the southwestern United States (Centers for Disease Control, 1993b) and the introduction of an Ebola-like virus into a monkey colony in Reston, Virginia, with exposure of animal handlers (Centers for Disease Control, 1990a, 1990b); (d) an enhanced method of transmission so that more susceptibles are exposed, such as when E. coli was transmitted in undercooked hamburgers in 19 states from a fast food chain (Centers for Disease Control, 1993c); (e) a change in the susceptibility of the host response to infection or cancer, as exemplified by

Table 11–1. Common Circumstances of an Epidemic as Dependent on Three Different Groups of Factors

Pathogen factors
  Introduction of new pathogen
  Change in old pathogen
  Old pathogens with new means of entry into host
  Increased dosage
  Increased virulence
  Longer exposure to old pathogen
  Multiple pathogens

Transmission of factors in environment
  New growth media, either man-made or in nature (e.g., cooling towers, home humidifiers)
  New methods of dispersion (e.g., intravenous flasks, air conditioners)
  Specialized facilities (e.g., intensive care units, day-care centers)
  Invasive procedures
  New sexual practices
  Intravenous drug abuse
  Migration of infected persons, animals, birds, insects
  Exposure to new environments

Host factors
  Highly susceptible subgroups (e.g., newborns, nonimmunized)
  Travel of susceptibles to endemic area
  Increased susceptibility (e.g., from immunosuppressive drugs, natural immunodeficiency)
  Cultural or behavioral factors

the increased incidence of certain cancers in patients with AIDS (Biggar, 1990); and (f) social, cultural, sexual, or behavioral factors that increase exposure or involve introduction through new portals of entry, such as the transmission of HIV-1 and hepatitis B and C by intravenous drug abusers. Some of the factors related to the pathogen, the modes of transmission, and the host are summarized in Table 11–1. Some overlap in these categories exists because it may not always be clear if the method of transmission or the pathogen has changed, if new portals of entry into the human host are involved, or if the response of the host to the same pathogen has been modified. Sometimes all three factors are important. For example, the occurrence of various opportunistic infections, Kaposi's sarcoma, and EBV-related lymphomas in AIDS patients involved both new and old pathogens, new portals of entry for old pathogens, increased dosage and repeated exposure, and an altered host response as indicated by the development of abnormalities in the immune system. In addition, high-risk activities took place in new environments, such as the transmission of HIV-1 in urban bathhouses used for sexual activity by homosexual men and the "shooting gallery" involving shared hypodermic needles by IV drug users.

TYPES OF EPIDEMICS

Epidemics can be classified as to the nature and length of exposure to the pathogen, the means of spread or propagation, and the duration of the epidemic.

Common source outbreaks refer to the exposure of a susceptible population or group to a common source of a pathogen often at the same time, such as at a church picnic or neighborhood restaurant. However, the commercial distribution of foodstuffs or other vehicles of contamination through many states or through a chain of stores has created a new form of common source epidemic in which the time and pattern of delivery, purchase, and consumption in a local area define the nature of the epidemic. This has added a new component to the epidemiology of food-borne disease (Hedberg et al., 1994). It is also possible that a single object is contaminated, and exposure to it occurs at different times. Such contaminated objects could include packaged foods, bottled beverages, or drugs; when contamination occurs in this way, the place and time of exposure can vary widely. Thus, the nature and duration of the contamination, the distribution pattern to the public, and the nature and duration of exposure of the individuals are important determinants of the patterns of epidemics. *Point epidemics* are common source outbreaks in which a group of susceptibles is exposed at the same time to a common source of the pathogen, usually in a single exposure; these most frequently result in a short, sharp epidemic curve, the shape of which depends on the dosage and pathogenicity of the agent, the duration of the exposure, and variations in host response. If the agent is transmissible to others by person-to-person contact, then secondary peaks may occur.

Propagative, or *progressive*, *epidemics* involve the transfer of the pathogen from one host to another. This usually entails multiplication and excretion of an infectious agent in the host and sometimes includes intermediate animal/human or arthropod/human multiplication cycles in the spread of the organism. Most noninfectious or nonmultiplying causes do not behave this way, although under certain circumstances they may simulate this pattern. The spread of illness associated with the use of addictive and narcotic drugs in young adult populations may lead to epidemic curves suggestive of person-to-person propagation. Propagative spread of an infectious agent may involve several mechanisms. For example, a person infected by hepatitis B or HIV-1 from a blood transfusion or from intravenous drug use may spread it to a sexual partner, and, in the case of hepatitis B, intrafamilial propagation may also occur.

Mixed epidemics involve both a single, common exposure to an infectious agent and secondary, propagative spread to other individuals, usually by person-to-person transmission. Examples include many food-borne pathogens (*E. coli, Salmonella,* typhoid, hepatitis A) and airborne organisms (*Mycobacterium tuberculosis*).

TEMPORAL ASPECTS

Epidemics may vary in duration from hours to years, depending on the nature of the pathogen, its incubation period (time from first exposure to onset of clinical symptoms), the length of time required for effective contact between the source of the pathogen and the exposed populations, and the number of susceptibles. Table 11–2 shows the varying incubation periods for several diseases. The temporal aspects become more complex when two pathogens acting simultaneously are needed to produce disease, such as *Haemophilus influenzae* and influenza virus to produce swine influenza, or when two agents in succession, one acting as the "initiator" and the other as the "promoter," are needed, as postulated for the role of the Epstein-Barr virus (EBV) and malaria in African Burkitt's lymphoma. Marked variations may occur in incubation periods of the same disease depending on dosage, route of inoculation, host susceptibility, age at the time of infection, and the particular clinical manifestation that appears first. In AIDS, the incubation period is shorter following transfusions of HIV-1–containing blood or after

Table 11-2. Examples of Epidemics According to the Incubation Period

Time Frame	Examples
1. Hours	a. Acute food poisoning: toxins, *Staphylococci, Clostridium perfringens* b. Heavy metal exposures: cadmium, copper, zinc c. Certain other poisonings: monosodium glutamate, mushroom, shellfish toxins
2. Days	a. Some food poisonings: *Salmonella* (1–2 days), *Vibrio cholera, Campylobacter jejuni* b. Bacterial infections: Legionnaires' disease, *Mycoplasma pneumoniae* c. Viral infections: influenza (1–3 days), adenovirus (1–5 days), enteroviral infections (5–6 days)
3. Weeks	a. Common childhood diseases: measles, mumps, rubella (2–3 weeks) b. Hepatitis A (2–6 weeks)
4. Months	a. Hepatitis B (2–6 months) b. Rabies (0.5–12 months)
5. Years	a. Radiation-induced leukemia after atomic bomb (peak after 6 years) b. Kuru (1–27 years) c. Bladder cancer in dyestuff workers (1–40 years)

transmission to an infant from an infected mother than when it is spread through sexual contact. The longest known incubation period for an infectious agent is for kuru, which is transmitted by ingestion of infected human brain at funeral feasts and in which the incubation period can be 25 years or more (Klitzman et al., 1984).

Cessation of an outbreak usually occurs when one or more of the following four events takes place:

1. The source of contamination is eliminated or modified, or the pathogen is rendered nonpathogenic, as when a water supply is chlorinated.
2. The mode of transmission is interrupted or eliminated.
3. The number of exposed and susceptible persons is markedly reduced or exhausted. This can occur by their removal from the source of infection, by development of the disease, by active or passive immunization to the infectious agent, by chemoprophylaxis against a sensitive infectious agent, or by some other modification of the pattern of host response.
4. Some other pathogen that is in the causal pathway or that modifies the effect of the primary pathogen is modified or eliminated. For example, reduction of malaria infection in hyperendemic regions by antimalarial drugs or by mosquito control might reduce the occurrence of EBV-related African Burkitt's lymphoma (see Chapter 1).

An *epidemic curve* is a graph of the distribution of cases according to time of onset. The nature of the epidemic curve varies with the pathogen, its generation time (time from entry to maximum excretion of infectious particles), the method of transmission, and the type and duration of exposure. The epidemic curve also depends on the length and variability of the incubation period and the number of susceptible individuals who are exposed.

A single defined peak suggests an almost simultaneous exposure of a group of persons to a single source of the pathogen. The shape of the epidemic curve depends on the incubation period as well as the variability of the host response. Figure 11–1 depicts an acute outbreak of viral gastroenteritis in Maryland from a single contaminated source, in this instance, oysters. As in most common-source outbreaks, it is characterized by a relatively sharp peak (that is somewhat extended in Fig. 11–1 because the consumption of oysters was not simultaneous), short duration, and, in this instance, a small number of secondary cases. The epidemic in Maryland was part of multistate epidemic that occurred in 23 clusters in four states. The source of contamination was identified in an oyster bed off the Louisiana coast (Centers for Disease Control, 1993a).

Some common-source point outbreaks may show variation in the incubation period and in the pattern of the epidemic curve. For instance, an epidemic of hepatitis resulted from contamination of a yellow fever vaccine lot with human serum containing hepatitis B virus. This one lot was admin-

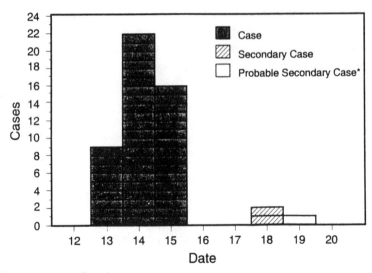

*Not laboratory confirmed.

Figure 11–1. Cases of gastroenteritis associated with oyster consumption, Maryland, November 13–19, 1993 (from Centers for Disease Control, 1993a).

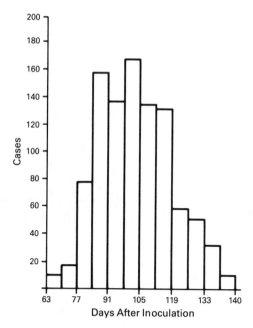

Figure 11–2. Demonstration of variability of incubation period in soldiers developing viral hepatitis following injection of yellow fever vaccine contaminated with hepatitis B virus and given in the same amount into the arm of young adult healthy males on the same day at Fort Polk (from Parr, 1945).

istered subcutaneously on the same day to approximately 5000 healthy soldiers of about the same age at Fort Polk on February 27, 1942 (Parr, 1945). Figure 11–2 shows that despite the similarity of the doses of the hepatitis B virus present in the vaccine and of the hosts receiving it, great variation in the incubation period occurred. Only 20% of the 5000 soldiers receiving the vaccine showed evidence of jaundice, and the incubation period to the development of jaundice ranged from 15 to 147 days with a mean of 96.4 days.

Exposure to a common source, be it an infected person, an environmental vehicle (food, water, air), or a contaminated drug, medical apparatus, or solution, can result in exposure all at once, over a continuous time period, or at intermittent points in time. If exposure occurs at different times, the epidemic curve may spread out considerably. Drawn-out epidemic curves may also be seen if the incubation period is long and the dosage of the pathogen is low, as might occur in the contamination of a public water supply with certain pathogens such as viral hepatitis or cholera. Figure 11–3 shows the epidemic curve from a massive outbreak of diarrhea from contamination of the public water supply in Milwaukee by cryptosporidium. In this epidemic, over 403,000 persons fell ill (MacKenzie et

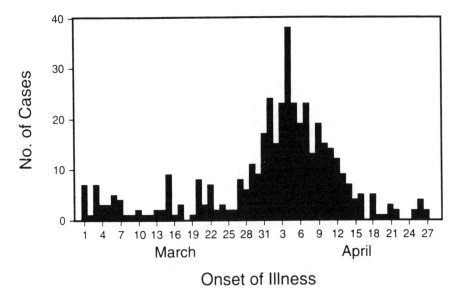

Figure 11–3. Reported date of onset of watery diarrhea during the period March 1–April 28, 1993, in 436 cases of cryptosporidium infection identified by a telephone survey of the Greater Milwaukee area (from MacKenzie et al., 1994). Reprinted by permission of N Engl J Med 331:165, 1994, Massachusetts Medical Society.

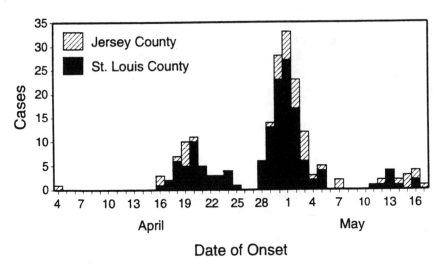

Figure 11–4. Number of measles cases, by date of onset of rash and by location, St. Louis County, Missouri, and Jersey County, Illinois, April 4–May 17, 1994 (from Centers for Disease Control, 1994).

al., 1994). Similar curves might be seen if the exposure is constant but the contamination is intermittent.

Propagative, or *progressive, epidemic curves* result from epidemics involving the spread of a pathogen from one susceptible individual to another. Such epidemics may be propagated by human-to-human spread with or without an intermediate host such as an animal, bird, or arthropod vector. For infectious agents, multiplication in the susceptible host usually occurs. The generation time influences the epidemic curve. A propagative epidemic is illustrated in Figure 11–4 for an outbreak of measles that occurred April 4–May 17, 1994, among students who were Christian Scientists and did not accept routine vaccinations. The outbreak involved two communities 30 miles apart with 180 cases reported to the St. Louis County, Missouri, Health Department and 49 to the Jersey County, Illinois, Health Department. The infection was carried by a high school student infected in Colorado who commuted between the two locations (Centers for Disease Control, 1994).

Figure 11–5 shows a curve of person-to-person spread of an influenza-

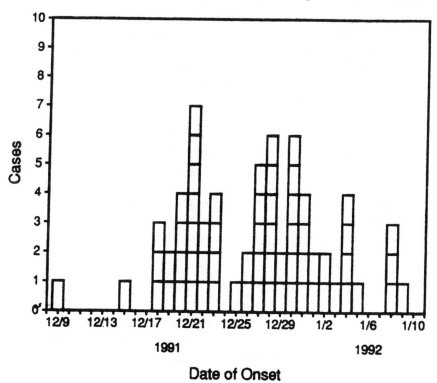

Date of Onset

Figure 11–5. Influenza-like illness (characterized by fever ≥100°F (≥38°C) with cough or sore throat) among nursing home residents by date of onset, New York, December 9, 1991–January 10, 1992 (from Centers for Disease Control, 1992).

like illness in a nursing home in which 65 residents (19%) developed the illness, and 34 developed pneumonia (Centers for Disease Control, 1992). Two large peaks and a small one are observed. Irregular peaks frequently occur in propagative epidemics, reflecting the number of infected sources and the numbers of susceptible and exposed persons. The magnitude of the peaks may vary according to the age of those exposed, because the proportion of those infected who develop *clinical* illness depends in part upon the age at the time of infection for many infectious agents. Prior immunity, nutrition, physical activity, and other factors also vary according to age. Noninfectious agents may simulate person-to-person spread because of the spread of behavioral or cultural characteristics that affect either the distribution of the pathogen or the number of persons exposed to it.

In addition to "copy cat," "cultural," and "peer-pressure" spread are the occurrence of outbreaks of phenomena having the marks of hysteria or religious fervor. The "dancing manias" of the Middle Ages fall into this category. An occurrence of this type is described under the term *koro syndrome* (Sachdev and Shukla, 1982), which took place in four Indian villages with a total population of 600 persons. It involved 60 males and females aged 20–40 years who were from lower socioeconomic groups. The symptoms usually began between 7 and 11 p.m. with tingling in the legs that spread to the rest of the body, sensations of intense heat, anxiety, and the feeling that the genitalia were going inward. This was accompanied by a fear of impending death.

Mixed types of curves, such as a single large peak followed by successive smaller peaks, may be seen when (a) a common-source outbreak of an infectious agent occurs with secondary person-to-person spread, or (b) the main group of susceptibles is initially exposed and is followed either by later exposure of the same groups to the common source or by later recontamination of the source involving the same exposed population. In the latter instance, a decrease of susceptibles usually occurs because of the acquisition of immunity by some members of the group.

STUDY DESIGNS

Because an epidemic is by definition an increase in the number of cases for a given period and place over that of past experience, the potential outbreak must meet this criterion before being called an epidemic. Thus, virtually all epidemic investigations are retrospective, at least in part. If no new cases occur after the epidemic starts, then the analysis will be fully retrospective. If all persons are infected from a common source and all exposed and susceptible persons have not developed the disease at the time of its identification as an epidemic, then the follow-up of additional people known to have been exposed but who are not yet ill would constitute a prospective cohort study. Persons known to be exposed to a source that continues to exist could similarly be followed prospectively. Rarely, a contamination source can be identified early and the persons exposed to it identified and followed before illness develops, such as when exposure to known contaminated water or food or to a known or suspected hazard in the occupational environment occurs. In these instances, truly prospective cohort studies can be undertaken.

In general, the urgency of solving an epidemic precludes long-term planning of a study and procedures that take a long time to implement. For instance, identification of cohort members for a retrospective cohort study may be incomplete. Controls in a case-control study may of necessity be chosen partly for convenience rather than because they are the ideal control group. Furthermore, people may have a vested interest in whether to cooperate with the investigation, thus creating an additional potential source of bias (Dwyer et al., 1994).

Case-control methods are being employed in epidemic investigations with increasing frequency. The reader is referred to a recent article by Dwyer et al. (1994) for a more thorough discussion of case-control studies of outbreaks. In a food-borne outbreak, the usual approach is to list all of the relevant items on the menu, determine by questionnaire the proportions of ill and of non-ill persons who ate each of the items, and identify the food item with the biggest difference in proportion between cases and controls. Usually one food item stands out as showing the greatest difference in proportions, and it is taken as the probable source of illness. One can also determine the odds ratio of illness among those eating a specific food item relative to those not eating the food item among all persons known to have eaten the meal, although the odds ratio will not be a good approximation to the risk ratio if the occurrence of disease is common in the cohort under study (Dwyer et al., 1994). It should be kept in mind that recall may in some instances be inaccurate, depending mostly on the time elapsing between the suspect meal and the interval until illness develops (incubation period).

The case-control approach can also be applied to epidemics not related to food. In a *Giardia lamblia* outbreak that had been identified by the Colorado State Laboratory (Wright et al., 1977), the differences in the extent of exposure to a variety of activities were compared between cases and controls, the latter having been drawn from the same home towns as the cases by use of a telephone directory. A questionnaire was administered to cases and controls, and camping and mountain climbing were found to be risk factors. The contamination of mountain water by infected humans and/or beavers was identified as the source of infection.

If the source of the pathogen is known or strongly suspected, often a retrospective cohort study can be constructed and the "attack rate" (risk for a specified group over a limited time period) or mortality rate among those exposed and among those not exposed determined. For example, John Snow suspected that sewage-contaminated water might be the means of transmission of cholera. In his classical studies, he compared death rates from cholera in households in neighborhoods that were supplied by one of two water companies in London (Snow, 1855). The mortality rate from cholera in households provided with water by the Lambeth Company, which drew its water from the Thames River far above the sewage of the city, was only 5 per 10,000 houses, whereas the death rate in those provided with water by the Southwark and Vauxhall Companies from a polluted area of the Thames River was 71 per 10,000 houses. The death rate in London as a whole was 9 per 10,000 houses, indicating a specific risk associated with the Southwark and Vauxhall water. A similar recent investigation of the attack rates for cryptosporidium infection in two water sources supplying the city of Milwaukee illustrates the sophistication of epidemiologic and laboratory techniques that have emerged in the 150 years since John Snow's investigation (MacKenzie et al., 1994).

In a retrospective cohort approach to a food-borne outbreak, the attack rate is determined among those who ate or did not eat each food or beverage. The food item showing the biggest difference in the attack rate between those who ate the item and those who did not eat it usually identifies the vehicle of infection. An example of this is shown in Table 11–3 from an outbreak of diarrhea in a college dormitory that involved 366 students among 3000 eating in the dining halls; the peak incubation period was 14 hours (Helstad et al., 1967). The table indicates that the 65% difference in the attack rate between those who ate gravy (69.9%) and those who did not eat gravy (4.9%) clearly exceeded any other difference. *Clostridium perfringens* was isolated from 19 of 20 ill students who had eaten the gravy and from none of 13 non-ill students who had not. In this instance, leftover gravy in which to search for the organism was not available.

GENERAL CONSIDERATIONS IN EPIDEMIC INVESTIGATION

The establishment of the source, method of transmission, and infectious or noninfectious agent causing an outbreak or epidemic is of the utmost importance and urgency as a basis for preventive action to protect the public against further spread. The epidemiologist, clinician, and laboratory specialist must join forces in this investigation. The clinician can assist in establishing a simple working definition of the condition as a basis for reporting and surveillance, and later for defining the spectrum of the dis-

Table 11-3. Analysis of Attack Rate for Different Foods Eaten in a College Outbreak of Diarrhea

Food Item	Ate Food			Did Not Eat Food			Difference in Percentage
	Number	Number Ill	Percentage Ill	Number	Number Ill	Percentage Ill	
Fish	391	16	4.1	715	340	47.6	−43.5
Hamburger	188	15	8.0	918	351	38.2	−30.2
Beef							
With gravy	479	335	69.9	627	31	4.9	+65.0
Without gravy	48	0	0	1,058	366	34.6	−34.6

Source: Helstad et al. (1967).

ease produced. The laboratory worker can identify the appropriate specimens to collect and the proper tests to diagnose the disease.

The initial task of the epidemiologist is essentially one of descriptive epidemiology: to define the circumstances under which the epidemic occurred by identifying the who, what, where, and when of ill persons and those who escaped illness. Establishing the incidence of the disease in various age, gender, racial, socioeconomic, or religious groups, or in different geographic areas or time periods may yield important clues as to the persons at highest risk and the nature of the exposure. A map indicating where cases have occurred geographically (often referred to as a spot map) and an epidemic curve showing when cases have occurred over time are essential elements of defining some of these parameters. The search for a common exposure is important, as are the apparent exceptions to the common exposure. Case-control studies are useful in seeking differences in exposure to the source of infection, the vehicle of transmission, or special host characteristics that result in susceptibility (Dwyer et al., 1994).

The responsibility for investigation usually falls to the local health department, augmented when needed by state and federal help depending on the size, seriousness, or complexity of the outbreak. Because of the need for an epidemiologist and a sophisticated laboratory, most important outbreaks involve the health department of a large metropolitan area, or more commonly of the state health department. The work of the Minnesota State Health Department provides an example of the diversity of problems investigated and of the methods of epidemic investigation. Recent examples of outbreaks of infectious diseases that they have investigated include psittacosis in turkey workers (Hedberg et al., 1989a), *Salmonella enteritides* in a fast food restaurant (Hedberg et al., 1991), *E. coli* colitis from contaminated meat patties (Belongia et al., 1991a), *Herpes gladitorium* in high school wrestlers (Belongia et al., 1991b), and giardiasis in a nursing home (White et al., 1989). Examples of outbreaks of a noninfectious nature are nitrogen-induced respiratory illness among ice hockey players (Hedberg et al., 1989b), eosinophilia-myalgia syndrome associated with the use of tryptophan (Belongia et al., 1990), and a population-based study of drownings (Hedberg et al., 1990). A recent review of their experience with food-borne outbreaks discusses the effects of changing dietary habits, new methods used in food production, new agents, and the particular problems presented by imported foods and large commercial distribution systems (Hedberg et al., 1994). The Minnesota State Health Department has also addressed other epidemiologic problems that involve not only the investigation of epidemics, but also means of preventing them (e.g., vaccination efficacy) and improving or evaluating laboratory methods to establish causation. As examples of these, the Department has studied the efficacy of Hemophilus B polysaccharide vaccine (Holmes et al., 1991), has carried out performance tests for the serologic diagnosis of *Borrelia burgdorferi*, the cause of Lyme disease (Hedberg and Osterholm, 1990), and an evaluation of serologic tests for the human immunodeficiency virus type 1 (HIV-1) in blood banks (MacDonald et al., 1989). These examples are presented because they illustrate the varied and sophisticated techniques employed by a modern state health department in epidemic investigation, vaccine evaluation, and assessment of the reliability of diagnostic tests for diseases of public health significance.

Finally, it must be recognized that some epidemics have defied intensive epidemiologic and laboratory investigation. Kawasaki syndrome is a good example. Despite (a) a well-characterized clinical picture recognized since 1967, with rash, mucocutaneous involvement, fever, leukocytosis, and late involvement of the coronary arteries in some 15%–20% of cases, (b) a well-defined age distribution in which most cases occur in children under 5 years of age, and (c) periodic large outbreaks in Japan and smaller ones in other parts of the world, the mode of transmission, occurrence of subclinical infections, and etiology remain unknown (Evans, 1988a,b).

STEPS IN EPIDEMIC INVESTIGATION

The steps taken in investigating an outbreak of a disease are outlined in Table 11–4. The discussion that follows is derived from two books (Evans, 1989, 1990) and a pamphlet prepared by the Center for Training and Development at the U.S. Centers for Disease Control and Prevention (Centers for Disease Control, 1979), from which many of the figures are derived. The steps outlined vary with different outbreaks, but all encompass the same general principles.

Defining the Problem

The most important immediate issue is to determine whether an epidemic exists. In other words, is there an increase in the number of observed cases in a given time and place over the number expected on the basis of past experience with that condition? In many outbreaks, a working definition of the disease syndrome must be drawn up that will permit the identification and reporting of cases. As the investigation proceeds and the source, method of transmission, or etiologic agent becomes better known, then the working definition can be modified. For example, the initial case definition of Legionnaires' disease during the Philadelphia outbreak was as follows: "A case was considered Legionnaires' disease if it met with clinical and

Table 11–4. Steps in Epidemic Investigation

1. Define the problem.
Is it an epidemic? What is the etiologic agent?
2. Appraise existing data.
Determine the date and hour of onset for acute conditions; make an epidemic curve.
Prepare a spot map of cases; consider home, work, and recreational places and special meetings.
Where did exposure occur?
Calculate attack rates if possible.
Evaluate possible means of transmission.
Seek common sources of exposure and apparent exceptions to the common exposure.
3. Formulate a hypothesis.
Determine the most likely source of infection, method of spread, and possible control.
4. Test the hypothesis.
Search for added cases; evaluate all the data; perform laboratory investigations.
5. Draw conclusions and devise practical applications.
Write a report.
Undertake the long-term surveillance and prevention.

Source: Evans (1989, 1991).

epidemiologic criteria. The clinical criteria required that a person have onset between July 1 and August 18, 1976, of an illness characterized by cough and fever (temperature of 38.9°C or higher) or any fever and chest X-ray evidence of pneumonia. To meet the epidemiologic criteria, a patient either had to have attended the American Legion Convention held July 21–24, 1978, in Philadelphia or had to have entered hotel A between July 1 and the onset of illness" (Fraser et al., 1977). When illness was recognized in persons watching a parade outside the hotel and in other passers-by on Broad Street, the definition was expanded to include persons who met the clinical but not the epidemiologic criteria for Legionnaires' disease and who had been within one block of hotel A between July 1 and the onset of illness.

For outbreaks involving a large number of cases of a disease, in which cases are concentrated in a particular subgroup of the population or in a particular place or time period, or in which mortality is high, public concern and publicity from the news media will usually necessitate an investigation by public health officials regardless of whether the outbreak can be defined as an epidemic. However, when the situation is not clear-cut, the official records of past experience with the disease can be sought in local or national morbidity and mortality reports, such as *Morbidity and Mortality Weekly Report (MMWR)* in the United States or in the *WHO Weekly Epidemiological Record.* State, county, city, or other health records can also be consulted and hospital or clinic records reviewed. In the absence of such data or if a condition is not reportable, then the past experience of local physicians can be ascertained by individual solicitation or through the local medical society. Group practices, health maintenance organizations, and other prepaid medical plans that have computerized records of the diagnosis and duration of various illnesses are an increasingly important resource for both reportable and nonreportable conditions.

Appraising Existing Data and Other Preliminary Steps

The classical features of the descriptive epidemiology of a disease involving time, place, person, incidence data, clinical features, and environment should be identified as early as possible. For short-term epidemics, steps that might be taken in approximately the first 24 hours of the investigation are listed in Table 11–5. This preliminary assessment is usually based on existing clinical records of the cases and on available public health data on past experience with that disease in the community. The completion of the steps outlined in Table 11–5 may sometimes take much longer than the first 24 hours, depending upon when the investigation was started, the nature of the epidemic (common source, propagated), the incubation period of the disease, and the availability of data and staff.

Epidemic Curve Construction and Other Temporal Aspects. An epidemic curve should be constructed to indicate the number of cases on one axis and time (hour, day, or week) on the other. Although sophisticated methods of estimating parameters of epidemic curves using mathematical models are available (Anderson and May, 1991), generally simpler methods are used with the usual time constraints and urgency of epidemic investigation. The nature of the outbreak itself can often be deduced by the appearance of

---

Table 11–5. Preliminary Assessment of Data and Usual Steps Taken in First 24 Hours of Acute Epidemic, If Possible

1. Determine extent of outbreak: contact hospitals, clinics, physicians.
2. Establish the etiologic diagnosis, if possible, by appropriate laboratory tests.
3. Try to identify all persons at risk.
4. Identify the key clinical and epidemiologic features, including age, sex, race, environmental and blood exposures, and date of onset.
5. Obtain basic data on samples from the environment that may be related to the source or transmission of the agent: water, food, air.
6. Arrange for public relations.
7. Obtain any lists of persons at risk of exposure, menus of banquets, home or hotel locations, and other relevant data.
8. Organize the investigative team: epidemiologist, clinician, laboratory worker, sanitarian.
9. Call for added help if needed, such as from local and state health departments and the Centers for Disease Control and Prevention (CDC).

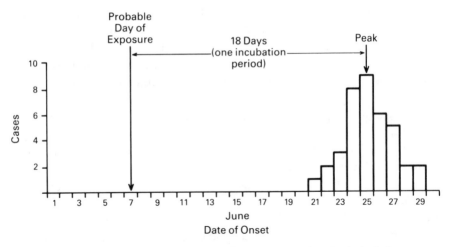

Figure 11–6. Estimation of probable period of exposure in outbreak of rubella by count-ing back the known mean incubation of the disease (18 days) from the first case (from Centers for Disease Control, 1979).

the epidemic curve, as discussed previously. If the etiologic agent has been identified, then the probable time of exposure in a common source out-break can be estimated by knowledge of the incubation period. Two meth-ods are commonly employed. One is to determine from previous studies the mean incubation period and the count back this amount of time from the peak of the epidemic curve. This method is illustrated for an epidemic of rubella in Figure 11–6 (Centers for Disease Control, 1979). A second way is to obtain the minimum incubation period by counting back from the time of occurrence of the first case and then to obtain the maximum incubation period by counting back from the last case. The period in between repre-sents the probable period of exposure.

These methods are often satisfactory to pinpoint a single common source of exposure, but if secondary spread is involved and the incubation period is short enough that the incubation period in the secondary cases overlaps the maximum incubation period from exposure to the first epi-demic cases, then the point of common exposure will be obscured. Other problems are illustrated in Figure 11–7, which represents an outbreak of hepatitis A subsequent to brief exposure to a fruit punch over one day (Centers for Disease Control, 1979). Given an incubation period of 15–50 days, the duration of the subsequent outbreak would be expected to be approximately the difference between these points, or 35 days. The actual duration was shorter (24 days), suggesting a more limited exposure, vari-ability in host response, cases missed toward the end of the epidemic, or

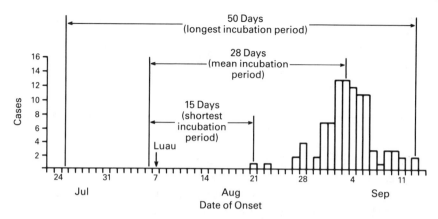

Figure 11–7. Cases of hepatitis A in individuals drinking a fruit punch at a luau, by day of onset of illness, Orange County, California, 1971 (from Centers for Disease Control, 1979).

simply random variation. It must be remembered that these estimated incubation periods represent averages from past experience and depend upon many variables such as the duration of exposure, the dosage and generation time of the organism, the susceptibility of the host, and the portal of entry. The variation in the incubation period resulting from variability in the host response when all other features are held constant was illustrated in Figure 11–2.

Another issue in determining the time of exposure is illustrated in Figure 11–7. Counting back 15 days from the first case points to August 6 as the day of exposure, which is one day *before* the actual exposure took place. Possibly the first apparent case with onset on August 21 was not really hepatitis or resulted from exposure elsewhere; the reported date of onset could be incorrect or vague. The shorter incubation period could also have represented variability in host response. Yet another limitation becomes apparent if one counts back 50 days from the last case; the resulting data of presumed exposure, July 25, is actually 12 days *before* the exposure occurred. In this outbreak, the mean incubation period of 28 days most accurately reflects the probable time of exposure. This variability in calculating the exposure time again emphasizes that the mean, minimum, and maximum incubation periods given in reference texts reflect cumulative experiences and may not always fit well with the individual outbreak being investigated.

The secondary spread of an infectious disease may obscure the temporal aspects of exposure in a common-source outbreak, but it may also provide a useful marker of the means of spread within a family. This is depicted for three different families in Table 11–6 for an illness with an

Table 11–6. Cases of a Disease ("x") that Occurred in Each of Three Families by Day of Onset

Family No.	Cases, by Date of Onset (August)									
	1	2	3	4	5	6	7	8	9	10
1		x		x				x		
2					x			x	x	
3			x							x

incubation period of 2–5 days and period of infectiousness limited to one day (Centers for Disease Control, 1979). In family 1, the temporal relation is compatible with spread from the index case to the second case to the third case because these fall within the 2- to 5-day incubation period of the disease. In family 2, two family members were infected at about the same time by the index case. Data from family 3 suggest that the second case did not represent spread from the first case because the time difference exceeds the incubation period. However, the possibility also exists that another family member may have had an inapparent infection about August 6th and passed the infection on to case 2.

The secondary attack rate in family or institutional settings is the number of cases per number of persons exposed, excluding the index case(s) from both the numerator and denominator. A more meaningful expression, when information on initial susceptibility is available, is the number of infected persons per number of susceptible and exposed persons, again excluding the index case(s). In the latter formula, the number of infected persons (with or without clinical disease) is taken as the numerator and the number of susceptible (i.e., lacking antibody) and exposed persons is taken as the denominator.

Construction of Spot Maps and Other Aspects of Place. A map indicating the place of occurrence of cases may provide leads to the nature and source of the outbreak. The location of cases on the map can reflect their home addresses in a community; their location in a school room, workplace, or hospital setting; or the location of some restaurant, bar, swimming hole, or other place of social activity that they visited. If the persons and places at risk of exposure are not clear-cut on preliminary assessment, several spot maps pertinent to different potential epidemic sources may be needed to illuminate their possible significance. The distributions of cases possibly resulting from spread by water, air, or food, from person to person, or via insect or animal vectors or other routes indicate the number of cases and are not rates; the latter must be based on enumeration of persons at risk. Age- and sex-specific rates may also be needed. When differences in attack rates are found between one place and another, then a case-control study

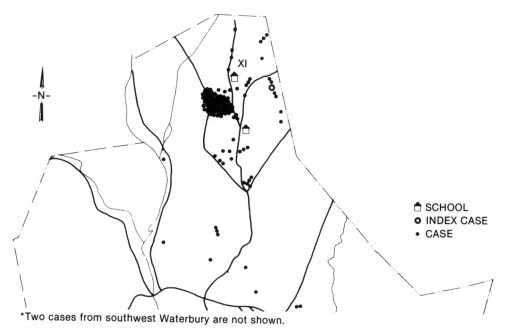

-N-

🏠 SCHOOL
⊙ INDEX CASE
• CASE

*Two cases from southwest Waterbury are not shown.

Figure 11–8. Geographic distribution of measles cases by place of residence, Waterbury, Connecticut, January 31–April 4, 1971 (from Centers for Disease Control, 1979).

can be undertaken in the areas with elevated rates to try to identify the specific exposures responsible for the elevated rates.

Figure 11–8 displays the distribution of cases of measles in an outbreak in Waterbury, Connecticut (Centers for Disease Control, 1979). This map suggests the school as a possible source of spread. If a food-borne outbreak occurred in the summer when schools were not in session, then the location of church picnics, county fairs, and other such gatherings that were held within the probable incubation period should be considered. If water were the suspected source, then attention should be paid to the location of supplies. For outbreaks of noninfectious diseases, consideration needs to be given to occupational exposures to chemicals, gases, skin-sensitizers, metals, aerosols, and other factors in the workplace as well as to home exposures to lead paint, dietary factors, home remedies and medications, and common household substances (e.g., ammonia, chlorine, lime, cleaning fluids). Hunting, fishing, camping, mountain climbing, spelunking, and other recreational activities may also result in potential disease-causing exposures.

Consideration of Characteristics of Persons Affected. The host plays a key role in behavioral, sexual, and cultural patterns affecting exposure, in the

Table 11–7. Attack Rate Per 100 Persons, by Age Group, of Cases of Diarrhea in a Day-Care Center

Years of Age	Number of Children in Regular Attendance	Number of Children With Diarrhea	Attack Rate
1	20	17	85
2	19	15	79
3	39	13	33
4	39	4	10
5	38	5	13
≥6	18	1	6
Total	173	55	32

Source: Centers for Disease Control (1979).

frequency and severity of clinical illness following exposure, and in further transmission of the pathogens to others. These host factors are important in cases of disease that occur both as epidemics and sporadically (haphazardly from time to time and not as epidemics). Some of these host determinants of exposure and disease may yield important clues to the causes and methods of transmission of epidemic diseases.

The *age* distribution of persons with infection and/or disease during an outbreak may lead to hypotheses about the source of infection or to the nature of transmission. The pattern seen in Table 11–7 of an epidemic of diarrhea suggests a highly contagious infectious agent that induces an immunity that most older children have already acquired as a result of prior infection (Centers for Disease Control, 1979). This pattern might be seen in viral gastroenteritis due to rotaviruses. Similar age patterns could occur with Epstein-Barr virus, cytomegalovirus, or hepatitis A virus. The age distribution seen in Table 11–8 of a St. Louis encephalitis outbreak in Chicago shows increasing rates of clinical illness with increasing age (Centers for Disease Control, 1979). This age distribution could indicate (a) more frequent or longer duration of exposure of the older population to the mosquito vector, (b) loss of immunity in older age groups, or (c) a higher rate of *clinical* disease in the aged even though the attack rate for the infection might be similar in all age groups. In considering age distributions, one must assess the roles of exposure and prior immunity as well as the rates of infection and of clinical illness among those infected. A similar pattern to that of the St. Louis encephalitis outbreak occurred with Legionnaires' disease, in which age, smoking, and prior cardiopulmonary disease enhanced the severity of the host response to infection in older persons (Fraser et al., 1977).

In analyzing attack rates by age, 5-year intervals are commonly chosen, but knowledge of the age groups at risk or the nature of the outbreak may

Table 11–8. Attack Rate Per 100,000 Population, by Age Group, of Confirmed and Probable Cases of St. Louis Encephalitis (Encephalitis or Aseptic Meningitis) in the Chicago Standard Metropolitan Statistical Area, 1975

Age Group	No. of Cases	Population	Attack Rate
0–9	8	1,299,952	0.6
10–19	15	1,333,796	1.1
20–29	21	1,014,357	2.1
30–39	20	808,917	2.5
40–49	23	858,176	2.7
50–59	35	757,321	4.6
60–69	49	512,255	9.6
70–79	32	286,632	11.2
≥80	17	107,811	15.8
Total	220	6,978,947	3.2

Source: Centers for Disease Control (1979).

suggest more appropriate intervals. The type of exposure most likely for a given agent, the proportion of persons who are already immune, and the frequency of clinical disease among those infected will also bear on this analysis. When numbers are large enough, smaller divisions by age may be tried at least initially in order to uncover leads that would be obscured by larger groups. Proper investigation and analysis of age-specific attack rates are one of the most useful keys to understanding the source and spread of an epidemic.

Gender may affect the likelihood of the presence and nature of an exposure, but in most situations has little effect on the risk of disease, given equal exposure. Gender, like age, may yield clues to the source of an epidemic. The gender-specific attack rate by age should be calculated in each epidemic if the population at risk can be properly identified. The segregation of persons by gender in school systems, occupations, social organizations, sports, the military, and various avocations is now disappearing in our society so that an a priori assumption of a higher exposure level in one gender in a given situation may be unwarranted. However, custom and behavioral characteristics may occasionally create outbreaks primarily involving one gender or the other. For example, AIDS predominantly involves male but not female homosexuals. Among those exposed and infected, clinical disease may be more common in one gender than the other. Smoking, chronic lung disease, and rigorous physical exercise are generally more common in men than women and may lead to a higher incidence of clinical diseases such as *Legionella* pneumonias or poliomyelitis among those infected.

The attack rate of a disease according to *occupation* may provide clues as to the source of the infection. Within a given setting, such as an industry or hospital, the specific jobs of members of each group at risk should be ascertained. If differences in attack rates within occupational groups or particular subsets of the occupational groups are found, then further analysis of these higher risk groups can be made. For example, nurses working in a nursery may experience an outbreak of hepatitis A because infection in infants is inapparent and unrecognized.

Other characteristics of persons that should be considered in an unexplained outbreak include ethnic group, behavioral features (e.g., sexual behavior, drug use, smoking habits, alcohol consumption), cultural and dietary habits, and other factors. The calculation of attack rates according to subgroup, and the presence or absence of differences in attack rates among the various subgroups, are key factors in the formulation of hypotheses. In some epidemics, special attention should be directed to the first or index case to find out if a travel history might suggest the nature of the causative agent.

Possible Means of Transmission. The means of transmission may be identified either when there is a much higher attack rate in persons exposed to one common source (e.g., air, water, milk, specific food, infected persons, animals, insects) than another or when one pathogen responsible for the outbreak can be identified in one source and not in another. Thus, both epidemiologic and laboratory expertise are required.

Common Exposures and Apparent Exceptions. The major focus of epidemic investigation is to seek the exposure associated with the highest incidence rates for the epidemic disease. At the same time the investigator should be alert as to why certain persons so exposed did not become ill and why some unexposed persons did develop the illness. These exceptions may involve some special characteristics of time, place, or person that could provide a clue to the source of the outbreak or its means of transmission. For example, in John Snow's classic investigation of the Broad Street pump outbreak of cholera (Snow, 1855), one woman who carried water from the pump to an area outside the Broad Street area developed cholera whereas a group of brewery workers in the Broad Street area who had their own water supply used for making beer did not develop cholera. These observations provided still stronger evidence that the well water was the source of the disease.

Formulating Hypotheses about the Cause(s) of the Epidemic

The formulation of hypotheses about the source and means of spread of an epidemic after the available data are gathered and analyzed provides the basis for the first steps in controlling the outbreak. The original hypotheses may change if further data do not support them.

Testing the Hypotheses about the Presumed Cause(s) of the Epidemic

Evaluating whether a given hypothesis about the source of an epidemic is correct may consist of further analysis, analytic studies, laboratory investigations, or demonstration of the efficacy of a control measure directed to the putative source or its putative method of transmission. Often, a hypothesis is not tested in one discrete study but rather hypotheses are formulated, tested, and possibly modified as the investigation progresses (Dwyer et al., 1994). Generally, after a hypothesis is formulated, one should be able to show that (a) all additional cases, laboratory data, and epidemiologic evidence are consistent with the initial hypothesis, and (b) no other hypothesis fits the data as well. In addition, the observation that the greater the degree of exposure (or the higher the dosage of the putative pathogen) the higher the incidence rate of disease adds quantitative support to the hypothesis. The statistical demonstration of a significant difference between those exposed to one source or one method of transmission compared to another, or of having a much higher incidence in the presence of one risk factor than another, lends added weight to the validity of the hypothesis.

The current outbreak of AIDS provides an example of an epidemic in which knowledge about causation developed over a period of several years as hypotheses were formulated, tested, and refined. The first focus was the surveillance of cases, the identification of the persons at highest risk (male homosexuals, hemophiliacs, and intravenous drug users), the possible mechanism of transmission (via blood and blood products and semen), and the environmental settings in which infection occurred (bathhouses, gay bars, urban parties with intravenous drug use). These descriptive epidemiologic studies were followed by case-control analyses comparing characteristics of AIDS patients with characteristics of (a) urban age-matched homosexuals from a clinic, and (b) urban age-matched homosexuals from a private practice (Jaffe et al., 1983). These comparisons led to the identification of multiple sexual partners, exposure to feces during sex, a history of syphilis or non-A, non-B hepatitis, and having been treated for illnesses resulting from various illicit drugs as important risk factors. The third phase was the identification of the human immunodeficiency virus type 1 (HIV-1) as the possible causative agent (Vilmer et al., 1984; Gallo et al., 1984). The fourth phase was the initiation of large retrospective and prospective cohort studies to identify the rates of AIDS in high-risk populations in relation to HIV-1 and various characteristics of the host. As a result of these studies, HIV-1 has been definitively established as the causative agent. The development of the ELISA test for antibody and its confirmation by the Western blot test has permitted identification of HIV-1 infected individuals who are also infectious to others, because both virus and antibody can coexist. Such tests are widely used to exclude HIV-1–positive persons from giving blood. The isolation of the virus in lymphocyte cultures and its detection in blood and other tissues by the polymerase chain reaction (PCR) have enabled identification of which babies are infected from the mother, have facilitated measurement of the magnitude of viral load as a predictor of AIDS, and have allowed demonstration of HIV-1 even in frozen or paraffin-embedded tissues.

With such techniques now available to detect the infectious agent, and simplified tests to measure CD4+ (as a marker of helper lymphocytes) and CD8+ (as a marker of suppressor lymphocytes), much information has been gained from cohort studies about the pathogenesis of AIDS and of the factors that predict the development of clinical disease in HIV-1 infection. New sensitive tests to detect the HIV-1 virus have shown the almost universal presence of the virus antigen prior to the development of antibody, its persistence, and its presence in various body secretions. The absolute number of helper lymphocytes (as indicated by CD4+) cells has been a reliable predictor of the risk of clinical illness and has served as a guide to the use of AZT or other drugs even prior to symptoms.

Epidemiologic findings from prospective cohort studies have identified a high risk of HIV-1 infection among recipients of anal intercourse and a low risk associated with oral-genital contact. Kaposi's sarcoma has been found to be generally limited to homosexual males, suggesting the presence of a yet unidentified infectious agent that may be spread by oral-anal means.

Another example of the methods used in formulating and testing hypotheses is that of the eosinophilia-myalgia syndrome. First identified by the State Health Department of New Mexico in three patients with an unexplained acute illness characterized by intense myalgia, rash, edema, dyspnea, and eosinophilia, a nationwide outbreak was recognized within weeks of this report. By August 1990, 1536 cases had been reported to CDC (Varga et al., 1992). Case-control studies by several state health departments unequivocally demonstrated an association of the syndrome with products containing L-tryptophan (Centers for Disease Control, 1989). Clinical studies revealed both an acute and chronic form of the syndrome, and the occurrence in about half of the cases of a late sequela consisting of diffuse scleroderma-like lesions (Varga et al., 1992). Intensive studies were made by a team organized by the Minnesota State Health Department (Centers for Disease Control, 1989). A case-control analysis of 52 cases and controls revealed that cases were older than controls (median age 45 vs. 43), were mostly female, and had consumed more tryptophan-containing products per month over a shorter time than controls. A single manufacturer was identified in 29 of the 30 cases who had consumed the product in the month before they became ill. Analysis of the manufacturing process indicated that lots used by patients were prepared using a different strain of *B. amyloliquefaciens* and a lower amount of powdered carbon as an adsorbent, producing a product that showed a peak, called E, by high performance liquid chromatography. Some toxin contained in this peak, or reflecting its presence, was the cause of the syndrome (Belongia et al., 1990). The tryptophan-containing products were subsequently removed from the retail market by the Food and Drug Administration.

In the absence of a randomized controlled trial, the demonstration that the removal of a given agent decreases or eliminates the disease is generally considered to be one of the strongest pieces of evidence for the validity of a causal association. If the source of the pathogen or toxin or its means of transmission is controlled and the epidemic ceases, this helps to validate the hypothesis. Cessation of the outbreak does not, of course, offer absolute proof because other reasons for the cessation of the epidemic, such as the exhaustion of the susceptibles, may also explain the termination of the outbreak. In most settings, ethical considerations do not permit a randomized controlled trial.

Conclusions and Practical Application

The practical objectives of epidemic investigation are to stop the current epidemic and to establish measures that would prevent similar outbreaks in the future. The methods described form the basis for initiating measures that would (a) eliminate the source of the pathogen or the exposure of susceptibles to it, (b) interrupt the spread from the source to the susceptibles, and (c) protect the susceptibles from the consequences of exposure even when the source or method of transmission cannot be controlled. Table 11–9 outlines these steps and gives examples of their application. If the outbreak is a serious one in terms of mortality or widespread morbidity, public concern and pressure may force the epidemiologist to initiate one or more control measures before the true nature, source, and means of spread are fully established, much like the physician who gives antibiotic therapy before the etiologic agent is definitely identified.

Reporting epidemics to health authorities is important at two points in time. First, at the time of its recognition, the epidemic should be reported to local and state health departments and to the CDC in order to alert others to the possibility of a similar epidemic in other areas and to mobilize

Table 11–9. Elements of Epidemic Control

Action	Example
1. Control the source of the pathogen.	Remove the source of contamination. Remove persons from exposure. Inactivate or neutralize the pathogen. Isolate and/or treat the infected person.
2. Interrupt the transmission.	Sterilize or interrupt environmental sources of spread (water, milk, air). Control mosquito or insect transmission. Improve personal sanitation (wash hands, etc.).
3. Control or modify the host response to exposure	Immunize the susceptibles. Use prophylactic chemotherapy.

an investigative team, including personnel from the CDC, if warranted. Second, at the end of the investigation it is important to provide information on the nature, spread, and control measures employed as a point of reference for similar outbreaks in the future. Even if the nature of an outbreak has not been completely elucidated, it is nevertheless important not only to prepare a final report, but also to freeze infectious secretions, sera from cases, and sample materials from potentially contaminated environmental sources because these materials may later yield the causative agent when new techniques for their identification are developed or new pathogens are discovered. For example, sera from cases of an undiagnosed outbreak of pneumonia in 1957 permitted the serologic diagnosis of Legionnaires' disease some 25 years later (Osterholm et al., 1983). Another example is that of Lyme disease, which was presumed to have occurred first in Lyme, Connecticut, in 1975. However, recent studies of the DNA of its spirochetal pathogen, *Borrelia burgdorferi,* have identified the presence of this organism in ticks in 1940, and even in museum ear specimens from white-footed mice collected in 1894 (Marshall et al., 1994).

REFERENCES

Agocs MM, Markowitz LE, Straub I, Domok I. 1992. The 1988–1989 measles epidemic in Hungary: assessment of vaccine failure. *Int J Epidemiol* 21:1007–1013.

Anderson RM, May RM. 1991. Infectious Diseases of Humans: Dynamics and Control. New York, Oxford University Press.

Belongia EA, Hedberg CW, Gleich GJ, White KE, Mayeno AN, Loegering DA, Dunnette SL, Pirie PL, MacDonald KL, Osterholm MT. 1990. An investigation of the cause of the eosinophilia-myalgia syndrome associated with tryptophan use. *N Engl J Med* 323:357–365.

Belongia EA, MacDonald KL, Parham GI, White KE, Korlath JA, Lobato MN,

Strand SM, Casale KA, Osterholm MT. 1991a. An outbreak of *Escherichia coli* 0157:H7 colitis associated with consumption of precooked meat patties. *J Infect Dis* 164:338–343.

Belongia EA, Goodman JL, Holland EJ, Andres CW, Homann SR, Mahanti RL, Mizener MW, Erice A, Osterholm MD. 1991b. An outbreak of herpes gladitorium at a high-school wrestling camp. *N Engl J Med* 325:906–910.

Biggar RJ. 1990. Cancer in acquired immunodeficiency syndrome: an epidemiological assessment. *Semin Oncol* 17:251–260.

Centers for Disease Control. 1979. Investigation of disease outbreaks, principles of epidemiology. *Homestudy Course 3030-G, Manual 6*, pp 1–79. Atlanta, GA.

Centers for Disease Control. 1989. Eosinophilia-myalgia syndrome and L-tryptophan–containing products—New Mexico, Minnesota, Oregon, and New York, 1989. *MMWR* 38:785–788.

Centers for Disease Control. 1990a. Update: Ebola-related filovirus infection in nonhuman primates and interim guidelines for handling nonhuman primates during transit and quarantine. *MMWR* 39:22–24.

Centers for Disease Control. 1990b. Update: Filovirus infection in animal handlers. *MMWR* 39:266–267.

Centers for Disease Control. 1991. Tuberculosis among residents of shelters for the homeless—Ohio, 1990. *MMWR* 40:869–871, 877.

Centers for Disease Control. 1992. Outbreak of influenza A in a nursing home—New York, December 1991–January 1992. *MMWR* 41:129–131.

Centers for Disease Control. 1993a. Multistate outbreak of viral gastroenteritis related to consumption of oysters—Louisiana, Maryland, Mississippi, and North Carolina, 1993. *MMWR* 42:945–948.

Centers for Disease Control. 1993b. Update: Hanta virus pulmonary syndrome—southwestern United States. Interim recommendations for risk reduction. *MMWR* 42 (No. RR-11):1–13.

Centers for Disease Control. 1993c. Update: Multistate outbreak of *Escherichia coli* infections from hamburgers—western United States. *MMWR* 42:258–263.

Centers for Disease Control. 1994. Outbreak of measles among Christian Science students—Missouri and Illinois, 1994. *MMWR* 43:463–465.

Dwyer DM, Strickler H, Goodman RA, Armenian HK. 1994. Use of case-control studies in outbreak investigations. *Epidemiol Rev* 16:109–123.

Evans AS. 1988a. Epidemiological considerations from the epidemiological picture. In Proceedings of the Third International Kawasaki Disease Symposium. Tokyo, Keidandren Kihan, pp 52–53.

Evans AS. 1988b. Etiology. In Proceedings of the Third International Kawasaki Disease Symposium. Tokyo, Keidandren Kihan, pp 105–108.

Evans AS. 1989. Epidemiological concepts and methods. In: AS Evans, Ed. Viral Infections of Humans. Epidemiology and Control. New York, Plenum, pp 1–57.

Evans AS. 1991. Epidemiological concepts. In: AS Evans, PS Brachman, Eds. Bacterial Infections of Humans. Epidemiology and Control. New York, Plenum, pp 3–57.

Fraser DW, Tsai TR, Orenstein W, Parkin WE, Beecham HJ, Sharrar RG, Harris J, Mallison GF, Martin SM, McDade JE, Shepard CC, Brachman PS, the Field Investigation Team. 1977. Legionnaires' disease: description of an epidemic of pneumonia. *N Engl J Med* 297:1189–1197.

Gallo RC, Shearer GM, Kaplan M, Haynes BF, Palker TJ, Redfield R, Oleske J,

Safai B, Foster P, Markham PD. 1984. Frequent detection and isolation of cytopathic retroviruses (HTLV-III) from patients with AIDS and at risk for AIDS. *Science* 224:500–503.

Hedberg CW, MacDonald KL, Osterholm MT. 1994. Changing epidemiology of food-borne disease: a Minnesota perspective. *Clin Infect Dis* 18:671–682.

Hedberg CW, Osterholm MT. 1990. Serologic tests for antibody to *Borrelia burgdorferi*. Another Pandora's Box for medicine? *Arch Intern Med* 150:732–733.

Hedberg K, White KE, Forfang JC, Korlath JS, Friendshuh KA, Hedberg CW, MacDonald KL, Osterholm MT. 1989a. An outbreak of psittacosis in Minnesota turkey industry workers: implications for modes of transmission and control. *Am J Epidemiol* 130:569–577.

Hedberg K, Hedberg CW, Iber C, White KE, Osterholm MT, Jones DB, Flink JR, MacDonald KL. 1989b. An outbreak of nitrogen dioxide–induced respiratory illness among ice hockey players. *JAMA* 262:3014–3017.

Hedberg K, Gunderson PD, Vargas C, Osterholm MT, MacDonald KL. 1990. Drownings in Minnesota, 1980–85: a population-based study. *Am J Public Health* 80:1071–1074.

Hedberg K, White KE, Johnson JA, Edmonson LM, Solar JT, Korlath JA, Theurer LS, MacDonald KL, Osterholm MT. 1991. An outbreak of *Salmonella enteritidis* infection at a fast-food restaurant: implications for foodhandler-associated transmission. *J Infect Dis* 164:1135–1140.

Helstad AG, Mandel AD, Evans AS. 1967. Thermostable *Clostridium perfringens* as a cause of food poisoning outbreak. *Public Health Reports* 82:157–161.

Holmes SJ, Lucas AH, Osterholm MT, Froeschle JE, Granoff DM. 1991. Immunoglobulin deficiency and idiotype expression in children developing Haemophilis influenzae type b disease after vaccination with conjugate vaccine. The Collaborative Study Group. *JAMA* 266:1960–1965.

Jaffe HW, Choi K, Thomas PA, Haverkos HW, Auerbach DM, Guinan ME, Rogers MF, Spira TJ, Darrow WW, Kramer MA, Friedman SM, Monroe JM, Friedman-Kien AE, Laubenstein LJ, Marmor M, Safai B, Dritz SK, Crispi SJ, Fannin SL, Orkwis JP, Kelter A, Rushing WR, Thacker SB, Curran JW. 1983. National case control of study of Kaposi's sarcoma and *Pneumocystis carinii* pneumonia in homosexual men: Part 1. Epidemiologic results. *Ann Intern Med* 99:145–151.

Klitzman RL, Alpers MP, Gajdusek DC. 1984. The natural incubation period of kuru and the episodes of transmission in three clusters of patients. *J Neuroepidemiology* 3:3–20.

Last JM, Ed. 1995. A Dictionary of Epidemiology. Third Ed. New York, Oxford University Press.

MacDonald KL, Jackson JB, Bowman RJ, Poleskly HF, Rhame FS, Balfour HD, Osterholm MT. 1989. Performance characteristics of serologic tests for human immunodeficiency virus type 1 (HIV-1) antibody among Minnesota blood donors. Public health and clinical implications. *Ann Intern Med* 110:617–621.

MacKenzie WR, Hoxie NJ, Proctor ME, Gradus MS, Blair KA, Peterson DE, Kazmierczak JJ, Addiss DG, Fox KR, Rose JB, Davis JP. 1994. A massive outbreak in Milwaukee of cryptosporidium infection transmitted through the public water supply. *N Engl J Med* 331:161–167.

Marshall WF, Telford SR III, Rys PN, Rutledge BJ, Mathieson D, Malawista SE,

Spielman A, Persing DH. 1994. Detection of *Borrelia burgdorferi* DNA in museum specimens of *Peromyscus leucopus*. *J Infect Dis* 170:1027–1032.

Osterholm MT, Chin TDY, Osborne DO, Dull HB, Dean AG, Fraser DW, Hayes PS, Hall WN. 1983. A 1957 outbreak of Legionnaires' disease associated with a meat packing plant. *Am J Epidemiol* 117:60–67.

Parr LW. 1945. Host variation in the manifestations of disease with particular reference to homologous serum jaundice in the Army of the United States. *Dist of Columbia Med Assoc* 14:443–449.

Sachdev PS, Shukla A. 1982. Epidemic koro syndrome in India. *Lancet* 2:1161.

Snow J. 1855. On the mode of communication of cholera. London; reprinted in Snow on Cholera. WH Frost, Ed. New York, Commonwealth Fund, 1936.

Varga J, Uitto J, Kimenez SA. 1992. The cause and pathogenesis of the eosinophilia-myalgia syndrome. *Ann Intern Med* 116:140–147.

Vilmer E, Barre-Sinoussi F, Rouzioux C, Gazengel C, Brun FV, Dauguet C, Fischer A, Manigne P, Chermann JC, Griscelli C, Montagneir L. 1984. Isolation of new lymphotrophic retrovirus from two siblings with hemophilia B, one with AIDS. *Lancet* 1:753–757.

White KE, Hedberg CW, Edmonson LM, Jones DB, Osterholm MT. 1989. An outbreak of giardiasis in a nursing home with evidence of multiple modes of transmission. *J Infect Dis* 160:298–304.

Wright RA, Spencer HC, Brodsky RE, Vernon TM. 1977. Giardiasis in Colorado: an epidemiologic study. *Am J Epidemiol* 105:330–336.

EXERCISES

Answer each section before proceeding to the next.

Introduction

As health officer of the city of Philadelphia, you receive a telephone call that cases of severe and often fatal pneumonia are occurring among the delegates attending the 58th annual meeting of the American Legion, Department of Pennsylvania, July 21–24, 1976, most of whom are housed in hotel A. The illness is characterized by dry cough, pains in various muscles, occasional gastrointestinal symptoms, and ultimately, in the most severe cases, cardiovascular collapse and evidence of dysfunction of other major organs. It is midsummer, and the nation has been warned to expect an outbreak of swine influenza.

1. How would you decide that this was an "epidemic"?

2. List three or more possible infectious causes of this clinical syndrome and the specific diagnostic steps you would take to establish or eliminate these as the causative agent.

3. Outline the immediate steps you would take in the first 24 hours to investigate the situation.

Background

The 58th annual convention of the American Legion, Department of Pennsylvania, was held in Philadelphia, July 21–24, 1976. The headquarters of the convention was in hotel A. During the same period, the 58th annual convention of the American Legion Auxiliary, Department of Pennsylvania was also held in Philadelphia, with headquarters in hotel B. Persons who attended the conventions included American Legion delegates, delegates of the Ladies Auxiliary, members of the families of Legion and Auxiliary delegates, and other Legionnaires with no formal role at the conventions.

Official activities of the American Legion Convention included meetings for all delegates, a parade, a testimonial dinner, a dance, committee meetings, regional caucuses, and a breakfast. Unofficial activity centered about the hotel A lobby, a sidewalk in front of the hotel, and several hospitality rooms. Each of the 13 candidates for major office reserved a room or a suite of rooms in hotel A to serve as a hospitality room for entertaining delegates. Each district and many of the local posts had their own hospitality rooms, which were scattered throughout several hotels. Liquor—most commonly beer and whiskey with or without mixers and ice—was served along with simple snacks.

Hotel A was constructed in 1904 and had been extensively modified and renovated since. Hotel guests were housed in approximately 700 rooms on the 2nd through 16th floors. The lobby floor, which is slightly above street level, included a registration desk, a counter for the sale of newspapers and sundries, several shops and airline offices, ladies' and men's rooms, and two restaurants and lounges. Meeting rooms were on the 1st and 18th floors. The air-conditioning system consisted of two water chillers in the subbasement from which chilled water was circulated to approximately 60 air-handling units in the building.

"A case was considered Legionnaires' disease if it met clinical and epidemiological criteria. The clinical criteria required that a person have onset between July 1 and August 18, 1976, of an illness characterized by cough and fever (temperature of 38.9 degrees or higher) or any fever and chest x-ray evidence of pneumonia. To meet the epidemiologic criteria, a patient either had to have attended the American Legion Convention held July 21–24, 1976, in Philadelphia, or had to have entered hotel A between July 1 and the onset of illness."

4. What are the advantages and disadvantages of this definition of Legionnaires' disease?

It was soon found that cases were occurring not only in persons in hotel A, but also in persons walking on Broad Street outside. *Broad Street pneumonia* was defined as occurring in a person who met the clinical but not the epidemiologic criteria for Legionnaires' disease and had been within a block of hotel A between July 1, 1976, and the onset of illness.

5. How do you define the numerator and denominator (those at risk)? How does Broad Street pneumonia affect the numerator? How accurate is it? How does one define the denominator?

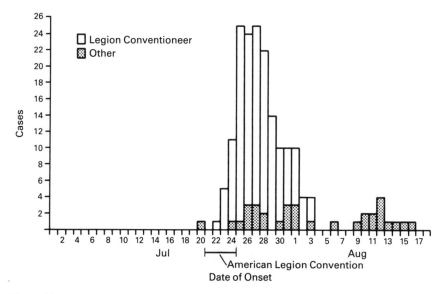

Figure 11–9. Legionnaires' disease (total 180 cases; date of onset unknown for 2), by date of onset, Philadelphia, July 1–August 18, 1976 (from Fraser et al., 1977a). Reprinted by permission of N Engl J Med 297:1193, 1977, Massachusetts Medical Society.

Analysis of the Outbreak

Figure 11–9 (Fraser et al., 1977a)* gives the data on 180 cases of Legionnaires' disease by date of onset.

6. What type of outbreak does this resemble?

7. What is the estimated incubation period?

8. Explain the incidence in nonconventioneers during July 20–August 3.

9. Why are cases occurring exclusively in non-Legionnaires from August 6 to 16?

Clinical data on the first 94 cases are shown in Table 11–10 (Fraser et al., 1977b).

The chest x-ray was abnormal in 90%. The risk of death was greater in older patients. No antibiotic was clearly effective; tetracycline (3/30 died) and erythromycin (2/18 died) were best.

In 182 patients finally identified, 81% were hospitalized and 16% died; 58/94 had a record of preexisting illness, 10 pulmonary in nature. The white blood count (WBC) was over 10,000 per cm³ in 59% and over 14,000 in 20%.

*References cited in this section are listed at the end of the Exercises.

Table 11–10. Symptoms and Signs of Legionnaires' Disease from Review of Hospital Charts of 94 Cases

	Initial	Total Present	Absent
Symptoms			
Feverishness	66	90	1
Cough	38	68	18
Malaise	36	59	11
Chills	39	53	19
Dyspnea	20	39	24
Headache	26	35	34
Myalgia	26	34	27
Sputum	9	31	40
Chest pain	11	31	32
Diarrhea	14	31	44
Vomiting	8	18	62
Hemoptysis	2	13	48
Purulent sputum	5	11	44
Abdominal pain	4	11	48
Conjunctivitis	1	3	53
Hematemesis	0	2	56
Epididymitis	1	1	55
Signs			
Rales	39	72	17
Rhonchi	24	38	43
Consolidation	5	20	58
Obtundation	6	18	67
Abdominal tenderness	7	18	68
Hepatomegaly	4	9	70
Stool heme	—	9	30
Splenomegaly	1	3	80
Focal signs	1	1	82

Source: Fraser et al. (1977b).

10. Are these data compatible with an epidemic of influenza? If not, which features do not fit?

11. What other laboratory or epidemiologic evidence would you wish in order to include or exclude the diagnosis of influenza?

Further epidemiologic analysis on 149 cases had now been obtained as a result of hotel guest, hotel employee, roommate, and hospital surveys and by a two-page questionnaire sent to the commanders of each of 1,002 local American Legion posts in Pennsylvania; 3,683 of these questionnaires were returned by persons who attended the convention, of whom 51.6% were delegates. The results are given in Table 11–11.

12. Which groups were at highest risk of Legionnaires' disease by age, gender, convention status, and hotel?

13. Can you postulate why these rates varied in the different groups?

A separate analysis was made of delegates alone, which gave very similar results but a slightly higher attack rate (6% versus 4%).

Table 11–11. Number of Cases of Legionnaires' Disease by Age, Gender, Convention Status, and Hotel for Persons Attending the American Legion Convention, Philadelphia, July 21–24, 1976

Age (Years)	No. of Respondents	No. of Cases
<40	610	11
40–49	805	25
50–59	1428	58
60–69	538	36
≥70	254	19
Total	3635	149

Gender	No. of Respondents	No. of Cases
Male	2292	123
Female	1380	26
Total	3672	149

Convention Status	No. of Respondents	No. of Cases
Delegate	1849	125
Auxiliary	701	4
Family member	268	17
Nondelegate	762	3
Total	3580	149

Hotel	No. of Respondents	No. of Cases
A	1161	75
D	1046	21
E	403	19
F	312	12
G	104	4
Other	210	7
Home	294	8
Unknown	153	3
Total	3683	149

Source: Fraser et al. (1977b).

Investigation now made clear that cases of severe pneumonia were not limited to persons in hotel A but included persons exposed on Broad Street outside the hotel. An analysis of the occurrence of disease in this group as compared with Legionnaires' disease is portrayed in Figure 11–10 (Fraser et al., 1977b).

14. Comment on the temporal occurrence of cases not in hotel A.

The possibility of exposure outside the hotel was also explored by analysis of persons in other hotels. The results are given in Table 11–1? (Fraser et al., 1977b).

15. Comment on the geographic and temporal aspect of the findings.

16. Given a common source in hotel A, how do you explain the other cases?

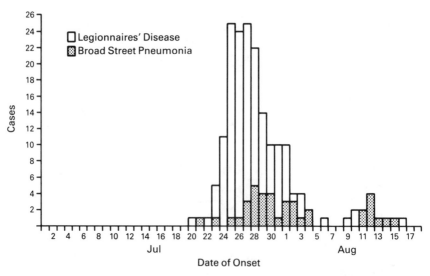

Figure 11–10. Broad Street pneumonia compared with Legionnaires' disease, by date of onset, Philadelphia, July 1– August 18, 1976 (from Fraser et al., 1977b).

Further Analysis of Epidemic

Additional epidemiologic analyses were made, including case-control studies. More cases than controls attended hospitality room A on the 14th floor ($p < 0.05$), but all other rooms surveyed showed no difference between cases and controls. No illness associations were found for specific foods or restaurants or alcohol consumption patterns, for roommate exposure, for water supply, or for contact with birds, mammals, or souvenirs.

Data on cigarette smoking are given in Table 11–13 (Fraser et al., 1977a).

17. Was smoking a factor? If so, why? What was the odds ratio?

Analysis of the cumulative time spent in the lobby of hotel A by Legionnaire

Table 11–12. Illness Resembling Legionnaires' Disease in Random Samples of Guests in Four Philadelphia Hotels by Week of Registration July 6–August 7, 1976

| Hotel | Week of Registration | | | | |
	7/6–7/10	7/11–7/17	7/18–7/24	7/25–7/31	8/1–8/7
A	1/142[a]	0/130	15/180	0/106	0/88
B	—	1/70	2/100	0/95	0/78
C	—	1/90	1/84	0/92	0/58
D	—	—	5/144	—	—

[a]No. ill/no. surveyed.

Table 11–13. History of Cigarette Smoking among Cases and Controls at the American Legion Convention, Philadelphia, July 1976

	Cases	Controls	Total
Smoker	31	19	50
Nonsmoker	21	33	54
Total	52	52	104

Source: Fraser et al. (1977a).

delegates resident at hotel A was significantly greater for the delegate cases than for delegates who were not ill ($p < 0.01$) as shown in the table:

	Mean No. of Minutes in Lobby A	
	Cases	Controls
Residents of A	249	142
Other Legionnaires	133	86

It was found that 62/125 of ill delegates resided in hotel A versus 356/1006 who resided elsewhere.

18. What hypotheses of spread are compatible with the evidence thus far?

Laboratory Studies

Vigorous initial attempts to isolate or identify a common cause of Legionnaires' disease and/or Broad Street pneumonia were unsuccessful. The microbiologic and serologic methods included attempts by fluorescent antibody and eight other methods to visualize the agent, isolation attempts on 14 bacteriologic and mycologic media and 13 virologic host systems, and tests of patients' serum against 77 infectious agents (McDade et al., 1977). Tissue samples were analyzed for abnormal concentrations of more than 30 metallic elements. Tissue and urine were also tested for a broad spectrum of organic toxic substances. Comparison of case and control data failed to show the consistent presence of any unusual component or elevated levels of toxins that might be related to the epidemic (McDade et al., 1977).

There were some early leads. "The histologic findings in the lungs in fatal cases were those of an acute bacterial pneumonia, whether primary or secondary, accompanied by alveolar damage, but with no evidence of bacteria by the conventional Gram stains" (Kass, 1977). Thin-section electron microscopy of lung tissue of 10 fatal cases revealed thin-walled bacteria in seven. Guinea pigs inoculated as part of the rickettsial investigation yielded an agent from four of six lung specimens from fatal cases—three from cases of Legionnaires' disease and one from a case of Broad Street pneumonia (McDade et al., 1977). The disease in guinea pigs was characterized by fever, watery eyes, and eventual prostration. An exudate containing numerous bacilli was seen in the peritoneum, especially on the liver and spleen of animals killed when moribund. The bacterial agent could then be passed into embryonated eggs, producing death in 4–7 days. It has now been grown on

Mueller-Hinton medium with 1% hemoglobin and 1% Isovitalex under 5% CO_2 (Centers for Disease Control, 1977a). When stained by the Gimenez method, the bacilli were 0.3–0.4 μm in width and usually 2–3 μm long, although longer forms up to 50 μm were occasionally seen. The bacterial agent was gram-negative but not acid fast. It also grew in primary chick-embryo cell cultures but was not pathogenic for mice. The agent was as yet unclassified and was of unknown environmental source. In histologic section, the Dieterle silver-impregnation stain had been the most sensitive method for identification and had successfully detected the bacterium in the lung tissue of 18 of 26 cases, 15 of whom had Legionnaires' disease and three Broad Street pneumonia (Chandler et al., 1977). A technique based on indirect immunofluorescence with the agent was developed for serologic diagnosis.

Seroepidemiologic Studies

The results of indirect immunofluorescent tests for IgG antibody on 136 patients with Legionnaires' disease are shown in the table:

Category	No. of Patients	Highest Titer Observed for Each Patient						
		<32	32	64	128	256	512	≥1024
Seroconversion	62	0	0	4	11	14	16	17
Positive only	39	0	0	0	10	14	13	2
Negative	10	4	2	4	0	0	0	0
Questionable	25	9	7	9	0	0	0	0
Total	136							

19. Given the diagnostic criteria of "seroconversion" as a twofold increase in titer with the highest titer of ≥1:64, and "positive only" as a single titer of ≥1:128, what percentage of the cases were serologically confirmed?

20. What reasons can you suggest for failure to confirm the others?

21. What other class of antibodies might yield better data in a *single* serum?

Nine of 14 cases of Broad Street pneumonia were also serologically positive.

Some Legionnaires had mild respiratory illness that did not meet the clinical criteria for a case, but no properly timed serum specimens were available from 98 such delegates identified by questionnaire. Such mild illness was more common in registrants in hotels A and B (delegates and Legion auxiliary) than in hotels C and D (few or no Legionnaires) (Fraser et al., 1977a). Serum specimens drawn in August and September, 1976, from 21 Legionnaires who had attended the convention and remained well did not show serologic evidence of infection.

22. What do these data suggest about mild and inapparent illness?

Pennsylvania Health Department employees who handled specimens associated with the epidemic were tested close to the start of this exposure and several months later. No clinical illness occurred in this group and no serologic evidence of inapparent infection was observed. None had a titer of ≥1:64. The IFA titers of hotel A employees were tested according to the year in which they started work. The distribution of titers is shown below (here ≥1:64 is taken as positive):

IFA Titer	No. Positive by Year			
	Before 1970	1970–74	1975–76	Total
<64	10	4	19	33
≥64	7	13	6	26
Total	17	17	25	59

23. Assuming a titer of ≥1:64 as significant, can you determine if the employees were involved in the current outbreak? Is the risk of high titers greater in persons employed before 1975 than after this date?

24. Are the data compatible with a long-term, continuing exposure to the agent in hotel A? Contrast with Pennsylvania Health Department employees.

25. What added information do you want?

26. Postulate why employees working in the lobby escaped illness.

An analysis was also made of delegates watching a parade from the sidewalk in front of hotel A because of the occurrence of cases from Broad Street who had not been in hotel A. The data are given in the table:

Watched Parade from	Seropositive and Ill	Well or Seronegative	Total
Sidewalk in front of hotel A	15	155	170
Elsewhere	12	432	444
Total	27	587	614

27. Is there an increased risk from watching the parade from in front of hotel A? What is the relative risk? Any explanation?

We have already mentioned that case delegates spent more time in the lobby of hotel A than did controls, and this was true both in residents of hotel A and delegates who lived elsewhere. With the serologic test now available, it was shown that 82% of seropositive case delegates had spent more than 6 hours in hotel A on July 23, as compared with 54% of the controls ($p < 0.0001$ by chi-square). Among the serologically proven cases, a linear trend for more time spent on the sidewalk in front of hotel A was seen as compared with controls ($p < 0.05$). Independent of hotel residence, 55% of the confirmed cases versus 26% of the controls had watched the parade from the sidewalk in front of hotel A (Fraser et al., 1977a).

The relation of apparent exposure, date of onset, and date of death could also be determined on 72 proven cases, 67 of whom attended the convention or were near the hotel from July 1 to July 24. Figure 11–11 (Fraser et al., 1977a) portrays this information. This is a complicated figure: each dot represents the date of onset of each case, and the stippled bar and hatched bar at the same level as the dot indicate the duration of exposure in hotel A or at the American Legion Convention (stippled area) or within a block of hotel A during the time period shown (hatched area). The longest horizontal bar with hatched area thus represents one person exposed within a block of the hotel from July 1 to August 18 who became ill on July 28. The circled crosses indicate deaths.

28. Was a single day of exposure sufficient to lead to illness? If so, when?

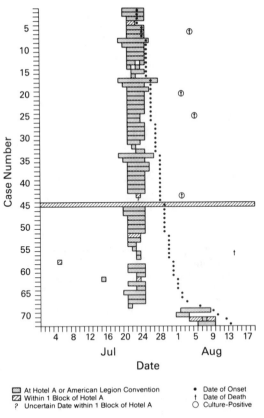

Figure 11–11. Days of apparent exposure, date of onset, and date of death among culture-positive or seroconverting cases of Legionnaires' disease or Broad Street pneumonia (from Fraser et al., 1977a). Reprinted by permission of N Engl J Med 297:1194, 1977, Massachusetts Medical Society.

29. Why were Broad Street pneumonia cases spread over such a range as compared with delegates?

The availability of diagnostic tools also permitted the serologic investigation of those prior outbreaks of severe respiratory disease studied by CDC in which sera had been collected and stored. One such outbreak had occurred in patients in a large psychiatric hospital in Washington, D.C., in July 1965, with 81 cases and 12 deaths (Fraser et al., 1977a; Centers for Disease Control, 1965). Appropriately timed specimens were available from 23 patients. Another outbreak of an acute febrile illness *without pneumonia* that involved personnel and visitors in an office of the county health department of Pontiac, Michigan, in July 1968 was also studied (Fraser et al., 1977a; Centers for Disease Control, 1968). There were 144 cases and no deaths. The clinical illness included fever, chills, myalgia, and minor respiratory symptoms. There were paired sera available from 37 cases and from 10 nonexposed controls. The results are given in the table:

	Washington, DC	Pontiac, MI
Seroconversion	17	31
Positive only	4	1
Negative	2	5
Total	23	37

All sera from the 10 controls in Pontiac lacked antibody.

30. What percent of the cases in each outbreak were serologically confirmed on the basis of the criteria given before (see Question 22)?

31. Based on all evidence presented thus far, what is the biologic spectrum of infection associated with the agent of Legionnaires' disease?

32. How would you set up a study to determine what other clinical syndromes, if any, are associated with *Legionella pneumophilia?*

33. Do you have any evidence that a vaccine might work?

Serologic tests of other cases of *sporadic* severe pneumonia on whom sera had been stored at CDC revealed 9 of 170 positive for Legionnaires' disease agent as well as 49 positives on whom a clinical diagnosis of Q fever had been made (Fraser et al., 1977a). The cases were widely scattered geographically. Cases in at least 29 states, as well as in visitors to Spain in 1973, have now been identified (Kass, 1977). By October 31, 1977, 64 sporadic cases in the United States had been confirmed in addition to confirmed outbreaks in Ohio, Vermont, and Tennessee (Centers for Disease Control, 1977b). In the sporadic cases, there were 49 men and 15 women (3.3:1) with a mean age of 51.6 years (range, 25–72) and a case-fatality rate of 25%. The clinical picture has been predominantly that of pneumonia. No other cases in household members or in work or community contacts were identified. The source of infection in these sporadic cases remains unknown (Centers for Disease Control, 1977b).

The occurrence of such cases is shown in Figure 11–12 for 1976–1977 (Centers for Disease Control, 1977b).

"Epidemiologic investigations to date of these 64 cases have not revealed other cases in household members or in work or community contacts. Investigation of many of these sporadic cases is ongoing by state health departments. The source of infection in these cases remains unknown" (as reported by State Epidemiologists from 24 states and the District of Columbia, Viral Diseases Division, Bureau of Laboratories, and Bacterial Diseases Division, Bureau of Epidemiology, CDC).

34. How do you account for the increased number of cases?

35. How would you determine the worldwide distribution of infection? Of disease? Assume that you are in charge of Communicable Diseases for the WHO.

References to Exercises

Centers for Disease Control. 1965. Institutional outbreak of pneumonia. *MMWR* 14:265–266.

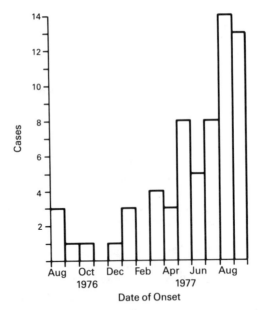

Figure 11–12. Confirmed sporadic cases of Legionnaires' disease by month of onset, 1976–1977 (from Centers for Disease Control, 1977b).

Centers for Disease Control. 1968. Epidemic of obscure illness—Pontiac, Michigan. *MMWR* 17:315, 320.

Centers for Disease Control. 1977a. Follow-up on respiratory disease—Pennsylvania. *MMWR* 26:93. See also Glick TH, Gregg MB, Berman B, Mallison G, Rhoades WR Jr, Kassanoff I. 1978. Pontiac fever. An epidemic of unknown etiology in a health department. *Am J Epidemiol* 107:149–160.

Centers for Disease Control. 1977b. Sporadic cases of Legionnaires' disease—United States. *MMWR* 26:369.

Chandler RW, Hicklin MD, Blackmon JA. 1977. Demonstration of the agent of Legionnaires' disease in tissue. *N Engl J Med* 297:1218–1220.

Fraser DW, Tsai TR, Orenstein W, Parkin WE, Beecham HJ, Sharrar RG, Harris J, Mallison GF, Martin SM, McDade JE, Shepard CC, Brachman PS, the Field Investigative Team. 1977a. Legionnaires' disease—description of an epidemic of pneumonia. *N Engl J Med* 297:1189–1197.

Fraser DW, et al. 1977b. Legionnaires' disease. Presented at American Epidemiologic Society, April 1–2.

Kass EH. 1977. Legionnaires' disease. *N Engl J Med* 297:1229–1230.

McDade JE, Shepard CC, Fraser DW, Tsai TR, Redus MA, Dowdle WR, the Laboratory Investigative Team. 1977. Legionnaires disease—isolation of a bacterium and demonstration of its role in other respiratory disease. *N Engl J Med* 297:1197–1203.

12

Methods of Sampling and Estimation of Sample Size

The preceding chapters have described study designs and methods of statistical analysis commonly used in epidemiology. The remaining chapters cover certain other methodologic issues that need to be considered when planning epidemiologic studies. Specifically, Chapter 12 first discusses common methods of sampling used by epidemiologists and then methods of estimating sample size. Chapters 12 through 15 are concerned with issues related to measurement in epidemiologic studies.

IMPORTANCE OF SAMPLING

Most epidemiologic studies require sampling. For instance, in the Framingham prospective cohort study of heart disease a sample of the population of Framingham between the ages of 30 and 59 years was selected for study, not the entire population in that age range. In case-control studies, it is common for all patients meeting the study criteria in a defined population or seen at certain medical facilities to be included as cases, but usually people free of the disease of interest are sampled in order to obtain a control group. Prevalence studies often involve sampling the general population in order to determine the prevalence of disease in the population as a whole and in those exposed and those not exposed to a putative risk factor. If the validity and reliability (discussed in Chapter 13) of a measurement are to be estimated, they are usually assessed on only a subsample of the participants.

There are two major reasons to use sampling instead of making measurements on an entire population. One is to save time and money, because it is obviously less expensive and less time-consuming to make a few hundred measurements, for instance, than many thousands of measurements. A second reason is that measurements are often more accurate if they are made on a sample of the population rather than on an entire population, because more effort can be spent on ensuring high-quality measurements if they are made on a smaller number of individuals. Training and monitoring five interviewers is easier than training and monitoring 25.

These basic purposes of sampling should be kept in mind when deciding which sampling method to use, as the choice is usually the method that gives the highest degree of accuracy and precision for a given amount of money. Before defining and discussing formal sampling procedures, however, consideration will be given to why formal sampling is usually necessary even though other options exist that are considerably less expensive.

One option is to ask for volunteers to participate in a study. The hazards of doing this are well illustrated in a study by Cochrane and colleagues (Cochrane et al., 1956) of the prevalence of pulmonary diseases in miners. An especially high prevalence of pneumoconiosis, for which workers' compensation is given, was found among the first group of miners to volunteer for this study, whereas in the last enrolled group, who agreed to participate only after some urging, the prevalence of tuberculosis, for which the workers could lose their jobs, was particularly high. More recently, Paganini-Hill et al. (1993) found that early respondents to a health questionnaire sent through the mail tended to be "worried well," whereas people reporting problems with their mental and emotional status were overrepresented among the late responders. Time and again, people who volunteer are observed to be different from those who do not. Another way of accruing a sample is to let the interviewers do the selection. However, interviewers are likely to select individuals who are easiest to find or who are most likely to be cooperative or who they feel might benefit most from the study. These individuals may well differ from the rest of the population in the characteristics studied. Similar lack of representativeness almost invariably occurs in a readily accessible population, such as one in close geographic proximity to the investigator, or patients seen by a particular physician. It used to be believed, for instance, that thromboangiitis obliterans (Buerger's disease) was restricted to Jewish individuals, but it was later realized that the study reporting this association was carried out in a Jewish hospital. In the medical literature, one frequently sees descriptions of particularly interesting or severe cases; similarly, cases in which there is a positive association with a putative risk factor tend to be reported.

The question sometimes arises as to whether these informal procedures will result in less biased estimates if larger numbers of participants are recruited, biased meaning that on the average the results deviate from the truth. The answer is definitely not, because the same sources of bias still will be present. In fact, false confidence may be placed in the resulting estimates because of the larger sample size. Although these informal methods of obtaining participants may be relatively inexpensive and easy to carry out, studies based on them should be regarded as very preliminary and need to be followed by more rigorous sampling procedures before any conclusions are reached. In addition, if probability sampling procedures such as those described later in this chapter are used, then the sampling error can be measured and described; this cannot be done unless probability sampling is used.

Once a scientifically sound sampling procedure is decided upon, the investigator should ensure that as many of those selected for the sample participate as possible; otherwise, despite the intention to use good sampling procedures, the sample may still give biased results. Methods of obtaining favorable response rates are discussed in Chapter 14, but typically, studies employing in-person interviewing obtain participation rates of 75% or less, whereas studies requiring clinical examination tend to obtain response rates of 55%–65%, and studies collecting data by postal questionnaire obtain response rates of less than 60% even after three mailings. When possible, sampling the nonrespondents and applying intensive efforts to obtain at least some information from them are useful, so that characteristics of respondents and nonrespondents can be compared and adjustments made in estimates. Respondents and nonrespondents almost always differ in important ways. If one is trying to learn about the prevalence of disease in a population, for instance, those with serious disease may not be well enough to participate, whereas those who feel completely healthy may have little interest in participating. Thus, the respondents may include a disproportionate number of people who are not completely healthy but who have no life-threatening disease. Such conditions as arthritis and back pain are commonly overrepresented among respondents, not only because these people are not too ill to participate, but also because many people with these conditions have not found any effective treatment and hope that the study will in some way help them, even though it is explained to them that the study is being undertaken for research purposes. In any event, obtaining as high a response rate as possible is of critical importance.

DEFINITIONS

The *sampling unit* is the basic unit (e.g., person, household) around which a sampling procedure is planned. For instance, if one wanted to estimate the prevalence of chronic bronchitis in a population, the sampling unit would be a person. If one wanted to know the number of households with one or more persons affected by an infectious disease, the household would be the sampling unit. The *sampling frame* is the list of all the sampling units in the population. This might be an alphabetic listing of residents of a community, or a list of households arranged by street address. The *sample*, then, consists of the sampling units chosen (usually by one of the methods described below) from the population eligible to be included. Finally, *probability sampling* is sampling in which each sampling unit has a known, nonzero probability of being included in the sample.[1]

The methods of probability sampling to be described below include simple random sampling, systematic sampling, stratified sampling, cluster sampling, multistage sampling, and ratio estimation. Textbooks of sampling (Cochran, 1977; Levy and Lemeshow, 1991) provide a more detailed description and theoretical justification of these sampling methods. Although means and standard errors obtained in examples of certain sampling procedures are given, formulas used in their estimation are not emphasized, but are given in Table 12–8 for interested readers; their derivations may be found in sampling textbooks. In this textbook, the reader should focus on the nature of the sampling methods and on their advantages and limitations.

SIMPLE RANDOM SAMPLING

Simple random sampling is a form of probability sampling in which each sampling unit in the population has an equal chance of being included in the sample. Table 12–1 gives the heights of 32 students in an epidemiology class listed by the order in which they were sitting around a table. These 32 students constitute the population from which the sample is to be taken. The mean height in this population is 66.34 inches. If an investigator were to take a simple random sample of 10 heights, he or she could take 10 numbers between 1 and 32 either from a table of random numbers or from a list of random numbers generated by a computer. Suppose that the numbers selected were 6, 30, 16, 10, 6, 21, 25, 30, 27, and 4. The corresponding values of heights are shown in Table 12–2, with a mean of 65.6 inches and a standard error of 1.18 inches. It may be noted that the sixth and thirtieth students were each selected twice. When, as in this example, selected individuals are placed back in the pool from which the sample is being taken, the sampling is said to be *with replacement*. If selected individuals are not placed back in the population being sampled and therefore can be selected only once, the sampling is said to be *without replacement*. A

Table 12–1. Heights, in Inches, of 32 Students in an Epidemiology Class

66, 67, 71, 68, 67, 64, 63, 68, 65, 65, 67, 64, 66, 61, 73, 74, 62, 65, 64, 70, 60, 66, 67, 71, 65, 64, 68, 66, 72, 64, 68, 62

Population mean = 66.34

Table 12–2. Heights, in Inches, of Simple
Random Sample with Replacement of 10 Individuals in Table 12–1

64, 64, 74, 65, 64, 60, 65, 64, 68, 68

Mean = 65.6
Standard error (mean) = 1.18

simple random sample without replacement from this same population is shown in Table 12–3. Here the mean is 65.8, and the standard error is 0.81. Because sampling without replacement permits coverage of a wider range of sampling units, on average it yields an estimate with a smaller standard error and therefore should be used in epidemiologic studies. Sampling with replacement is generally employed only for certain theoretical calculations.

Simple random sampling has the advantages of being simple to carry out and understand and of permitting easy calculation of means and variances. However, it is usually not the most efficient method of sampling in that it often does not provide the most precise estimates for a given amount of money. Also, it requires knowledge of the complete sampling frame in advance, a requirement not necessary in some of the other methods of probability sampling to be described.

In addition, one has to be careful that each unit really does have an equal chance of being included in the sample. In the first armed forces draft lottery in the United States, slips of paper with birthdates were selected at random from a bowl. Because the slips of paper had not been adequately mixed, men with birthdates at the end of the year had a greater probability of inclusion than those at the beginning of the year. If one wanted to estimate average family size of children in a school, one could list all the children in the school and find out the number of family members. However, this method would be biased because families with large numbers of children would be more likely to be included than families with small numbers of children. The sampling unit should be families rather than children. Some biased ways of obtaining samples from the general population include sampling from city directories or sampling from telephone directories; not all people are listed in these directories, so the sampling

Table 12–3. Heights, in Inches, of Simple
Random Sample without Replacement of 10
Individuals in Table 12–1

68, 64, 66, 64, 65, 61, 67, 65, 68, 70

Mean = 65.8
Standard error (mean) = 0.81

frame is incomplete. In summary, if one decides to take a simple random sample of a population, one has to be certain that all members actually do have equal chances of being included.

SYSTEMATIC SAMPLING

In systematic sampling, the selected sampling units are spaced regularly throughout the sampling frame; that is, every kth (e.g., third, tenth) unit is selected. If the investigator were to sample every third height from those listed in Table 12–1, the sampled heights, in inches, would be 67, 67, 68, 67, 61, 62, 70, 67, 64, 72, and 62, with a mean of 66.1, if the randomly selected starting point were the second height listed. Systematic sampling has three major advantages. First, the investigator does not need to know the sampling frame in advance; the frame can be constructed as the study progresses, so that the ordering is by time of accrual. If it were desired to perform a screening test on a sample of newborn infants in a hospital during the course of a year, constructing a sampling frame in advance would be impossible because it would not be known exactly how many deliveries would take place. However, a rough estimate could be made of the expected annual number of births, and on the basis of this a decision made as to whether to take a one-in-two sample, a one-in-ten sample, or some other fraction.

A second advantage to a systematic sample is that it is often simpler to implement under field conditions than other sampling methods. It is easier, for instance, for an interviewer to visit every fifth house on a block than to determine which houses are to be visited by means of a table of random numbers or by rolling dice. If one is to select a sample of cards in a drawer, it is likewise easier to sample systematically every nth card than to take a random sample of cards.

A third advantage is that if a trend is present in the sampling frame, such as from units with small values of a variable of interest to units with large values of the variable of interest, a systematic sample will ensure coverage of the spectrum of units. If one were to order the people whose heights are listed in Table 12–1 from shortest to tallest, as in Table 12–4, and a large enough systematic sample were taken, then it would be certain that short, medium, and tall people would all be included. For instance, if one were to take the third, sixth, ninth, . . . persons listed in Table 12–4, then the

Table 12–4. Heights, in Inches, From Table 12–1, Ordered from Shortest to Tallest

60, 61, 62, 62, 63, 64, 64, 64, 64, 64, 65, 65, 65, 65, 66, 66, 66, 66, 67, 67, 67, 67, 68, 68, 68, 68, 70, 71, 71, 72, 73, 74

Table 12–5. Heights, in Inches, from Table
12–1, Ordered by Row

74, 73, 72, 71, 71, 70, 68, 68
68, 68, 67, 67, 67, 67, 66, 66
66, 66, 65, 65, 65, 65, 64, 64
64, 64, 64, 63, 62, 62, 61, 60

sampled heights would consist of, in inches, 62, 64, 64, 65, 66, 66, 67, 68, 70, and 72, with a mean of 66.4.

Two important disadvantages of systematic sampling are that, first, if cyclical trends exist in the data, then it is possible that a poor estimate of the mean will be obtained; this could occur if the systematic sample consistently included peaks or troughs. If the individuals in Table 12–1 were arranged as in Table 12–5 (as if they were having their pictures taken, with short people in the front and tall people in the back), and a one-in-four systematic sample were taken by proceeding in turn down each column, it would be possible to obtain a mean as low as 62.9 inches if the sample includes persons 4 (64″), 8 (64″), 12 (64″), 16 (63″), 20 (62″), 24 (62″), 28 (61″), and 32 (60″), or as high as 70.9 by taking persons 1 (74″), 5 (73″), 9 (72″), 13 (71″), 17 (71″), 21 (70″), 25 (68″), and 29 (68″). Cyclical trends could occur when selecting houses on a block, household members for interview, or time of the year during which an interview was to take place. The prevalence of bronchitis would be considerably higher if one sampled every twelfth month starting in January than every twelfth month starting in July.

Systematic sampling has a second disadvantage in that the variance associated with a single systematic sample cannot be estimated (unless one assumes that a systematic sample from a randomly ordered population is the same as a simple random sample). If one takes two smaller systematic samples instead of one large one, as, for instance, two one-in-ten samples instead of a single one-in-five sample, then the variance can in fact be estimated.

STRATIFIED SAMPLING

In stratified sampling, the population is divided into strata, or groups of units having certain characteristics in common, and a sample of units is drawn from each stratum. The population represented in Table 12–1 could be divided into males and females, as in Table 12–6, and a simple random sample taken from each of these two strata, as in Table 12–7.

Stratified sampling is widely used and has several advantages over simple random sampling. First, the investigator can make certain that each

Table 12-6. Heights, in Inches, of Population in Table 12–1, Stratified by Gender

Females: 66, 67, 68, 67, 64, 63, 65, 65, 67, 64, 66, 61, 62, 65, 64, 60, 66, 67, 65, 64, 68, 66, 64, 68, 62

Mean = 64.96

Males: 71, 68, 73, 74, 70, 71, 72

Mean = 71.29

subgroup of the population is represented. This guarantees that the mean heights of males and females can be estimated separately in addition to the overall mean. Second, when the population can be subdivided into subgroups that are more homogeneous than the population as a whole, on the average more precise estimates of population parameters are obtained than when a simple random sample is taken, because the variance computed from the entire sample is based on each within-stratum variance. In Table 12–7, it may be noted that the standard error is 0.64 inches, which is in fact less than the standard error of 0.81 for the simple random sample in Table 12–3.

Strata can be constructed such that those that are least expensive to study or have the largest variances or largest number of individuals of interest can be sampled most heavily. For instance, determination of whether a person has osteoarthritis requires x-ray. One might, by means of a questionnaire, determine which members of a large sample have symptoms suggestive of osteoarthritis and then divide the group into one stratum of people without symptoms and another stratum of people with symptoms. The stratum of people with symptoms then could be sampled more heavily when individuals are invited for x-ray. An additional advantage of stratified sampling is that sometimes it is administratively easier to deal with strata. A geographic area or a period of time can be divided into smaller areas or periods of time and the strata handled as separate administrative units with similar procedures applied.

The main potential disadvantage of stratified sampling is that loss of

Table 12-7. Heights, in Inches, of Sample from Population Stratified by Gender in Table 12–6

Females: 66, 64, 65, 61, 67, 67, 62

Mean = 64.6

Males: 71, 68, 73

Mean = 70.7

Stratified sample mean = 65.9
Standard error (mean) = 0.64

precision can occur if very small numbers of units are sampled within individual strata. Nevertheless, under most other circumstances, any time the population can be subdivided into subgroups more homogeneous with respect to the variable of interest than the population as a whole, precision can be increased by using these subgroups for stratification. Stratification should thus be considered whenever sampling is being planned.

Many examples of stratified sampling can be found in the literature. In a study to determine the extent to which a questionnaire on bronchial symptoms could predict bronchial response to histamine (Burney et al., 1989), all adults aged 18–64 years in two areas of southern England were asked to fill out the questionnaire; all persons who stated on the questionnaire that they had had wheezing or whistling in the chest at any time and about 20% of those without symptoms were invited to visit a local clinic for a bronchial challenge test. In a study of dietary intake in three English towns (Cade and Margetts, 1988), it was desired to have approximately equal numbers of people in each 5-year age group from 35–54 years of age, and to have equal numbers of men and women within each 5-year age group. Stratified sampling from General Practitioner lists, with 5-year age groups within each gender as strata, was used to achieve this.

CLUSTER SAMPLING

Cluster sampling is a procedure in which clusters (e.g., classrooms) rather than individual units (e.g., children) are first sampled from all of the clusters in a defined area and then observations are made on all individual units (e.g., all children) in each sampled cluster. If one wanted to know the prevalence of dental caries in elementary school children in a large city, one could compile a list of all children enrolled in these schools (by all accounts a difficult task), draw a random sample, and then examine each selected child. It would be much easier, however, to select certain classes (clusters) at random, visit these classes, and examine all the children in the selected classes. This example illustrates the two major advantages of cluster sampling. First, one need not enumerate the entire population in advance; rather, just the members of the selected clusters are enumerated. Second, cluster sampling may enable the investigator to make more economical use of available resources than does simple random sampling. Although for the same sample size the variance is greater for cluster sampling, in cluster sampling larger numbers can be taken to reduce the variance. When population parameters are estimated from cluster sampling, these factors are taken into account.

An example of cluster sampling comes from a study to determine the relationship of various gastrointestinal signs and symptoms to *Schistosoma mansoni* infection in a small city in Brazil (Proietti and Antunes, 1989). All blocks (clusters) were assigned numbers, a random sample of blocks selected, and all inhabitants of all households on the selected blocks asked to supply stool samples.

MULTISTAGE SAMPLING

Multistage sampling is a procedure in which primary (larger) sampling units (e.g., municipalities) are first selected from a population, and then secondary (smaller) units (e.g., city blocks) are sampled from within each chosen primary unit. This may be extended so that tertiary units (e.g., households) or further units (e.g., individuals) are selected within these secondary units. Multistage sampling differs from cluster sampling in that the secondary units are sampled, whereas in cluster sampling all secondary units are included.

Multistage sampling may include, at different stages, several sampling procedures. For instance, the Baltimore Eye Survey (Tielsch et al., 1990) was undertaken to determine the prevalence of blindness and visual impairments in blacks and whites in the eastern and southeastern health districts of Baltimore, Maryland. Since a major aim of the survey was to compare prevalence rates of ocular disease in blacks and whites, a sampling plan was devised such that approximately equal numbers of blacks and whites would be identified, with a total sample size of about 5000 people. Census tracts (geographically defined areas into which a city such as Baltimore is divided by the U.S. Bureau of the Census) were first divided into three strata based on their racial characteristics: (a) predominantly black, (b) predominantly white, and (c) mixed race. Within each of the three strata, census tracts were ordered geographically from east to west, and systematic samples were taken within each stratum. Six predominantly black census tracts, eight predominantly white census tracts, and two mixed race census tracts were thereby selected. Within each census tract, all residential dwelling units were identified and screened to identify those eligible for the survey (nontransient residents 40 years of age or older). Cluster sampling, with census tracts as clusters, enabled the investigators to minimize the distance between sampled homes and each neighborhood screening center, to use neighborhood leaders efficiently, and to use the media to encourage participation. In summary, three sampling methods were used at different stages of this multistage scheme: stratification was undertaken to ensure that blacks and whites were included in approximately equal numbers; systematic sampling was employed to ensure representation from different geographic areas; and cluster sampling was used for efficiency and economy of resources.

In a study relating air pollution to chronic bronchitis in Britain (Lambert and Reid, 1970), all local administrative districts were first stratified by region and degree of urbanization to ensure representation from different regions and various presumed levels of air pollution. A total of 298 administrative districts were randomly selected from within these strata, with all strata represented. Households were then sampled systematically from electoral registers supplemented by rating lists. Because the investigators desired to compare the prevalence of chronic bronchitis in British migrants in the United States to the prevalence of chronic bronchitis in persons of similar origin who remained in England, and because 30% of British migrants to the United States were of Scottish birth, the sampling fraction for Scottish districts was increased fourfold. Here, stratification was used first to ensure representation from all subpopulations of interest and then to allow the inclusion of a disproportionate number of individuals from a subgroup of particular interest (the Scottish).

In a study to determine the frequency and health implications of consanguinal marriages in Jordan (Abbas and Walker, 1986) a three-stage sampling procedure was used. First, localities (defined as aggregates of blocks forming a settlement, village, town, or city) were classified into nine strata according to the size of the locality. Localities were randomly selected from within each stratum, with sampling proportional to the number of households in the strata. Seventy-three out of 1008 localities were selected at this first stage. Second, blocks (defined as aggregates of buildings demarcated by street intersections) were randomly sampled from the selected localities. Interviewers then visited all households on the sampled blocks to determine the year of marriage of married household members. About 2.1% of all households were included at this second stage. Third, reported marriages over the 10 years prior to 1979 were stratified by year and sampled proportionate to the size of the stratum to give 20% of marriages. The wife in each of these marriages was then interviewed.

RATIO ESTIMATION

This is a method of estimation in which sample observations are used to estimate the ratio of the unknown population mean (or total or proportion) for one variable to a known population mean (or total or proportion) for some other variable. For instance, suppose one wants to estimate the incidence of hip fracture in the state of New Mexico over a period of one year. Because hip fracture is almost always treated in a hospital, one should be able to identify hip fractures through hospital discharge lists, which are often computerized. However, it is likely that the hospital discharge lists will miss some cases, so that it will be worth examining operating room log books or x-ray log books as well; the operating-room and x-ray log books are likely to be quite complete and should permit estimation of the extent of underascertainment by hospital discharge lists alone. Because looking through lists of diagnoses and operations in log books is extremely tedious and time-consuming, it is much more practical to check a sample of log books than to review them all. Suppose that through computerized discharge lists one finds 300 cases, and that by taking a sample of log books, one finds that for the 100 cases found in the sampled log books, only 75 were identified by the discharge lists and that none of the cases identified by the discharge lists were missed by log books. The ratio of total number of cases to cases identified by the discharge list is accordingly estimated to be 100 to 75 or 4 to 3, and the total number of cases occurring in the state during that year can be estimated to be $4/3 \times 300 = 400$. In general, $rX = Y$, where r is the estimated ratio of the number of cases from the complete source to the number of cases from the incomplete source, X is the total number of cases found through the incomplete source, and Y is the estimated total number of cases when the proportion estimated to have been missed by the incomplete source is taken into account. Ratio estimation is useful when (a) either Y/X is easier to obtain than Y itself or Y/X is less variable than Y itself, and (b) the total X for the population is known. In the instance of hip fracture, X and the estimate of Y/X were much easier to obtain than Y itself.

The ratio estimate is appropriate when if $X = 0$, $Y = 0$, and when the ratio Y/X is constant over all values of X. For instance, the line in Figure 12–1 can be represented by the formula $Y = X/2$, so that $Y/X = 2$ regardless of the value of X. However, for a situation such as that shown in Figure

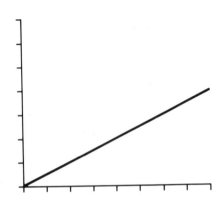

Figure 12–1. Ratio estimation.

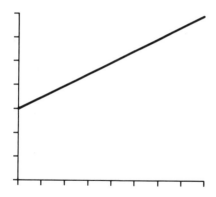

Figure 12–2. Regression estimation.

12–2 (when $X = 0$, $Y = 3$), a ratio estimate would not be appropriate, and a regression equation, which in this instance would be $Y = 3 + X/2$, should be used to represent the relationship.

FORMULAS FOR CALCULATIONS OF MEANS, PROPORTIONS, AND STANDARD ERRORS FOR COMMON METHODS OF SAMPLING

Table 12–8 gives formulas for the calculation of means, proportions, and standard errors for the common methods of sampling. Table 12–9 defines the symbols used in Table 12–8, and Table 12–10 illustrates the use of Table 12–8 with an example.

OTHER METHODS OF SAMPLING

A few other less commonly used methods of sampling should also be mentioned briefly. *Area sampling* is a type of multistage or cluster sampling in which a geographic area is divided into smaller areas, and a sample of these smaller areas is randomly selected. Within these areas, secondary sampling units are enumerated and either all are included (cluster sampling) or a random sample is taken (multistage sampling). *Multiphase sampling* involves obtaining some information from the entire sample and other information from subsamples of the full sample. *Sequential sampling* is any procedure in which units are drawn and observed singly or in small groups, and the results of each observation or group of observations are used to determine the subsequent sampling procedure. Sequential sampling is most commonly used in clinical trials, when ethical considerations may dictate that the trial be stopped if it appears that one treatment is clearly better than anoth-

Table 12–8. Formulas for Estimates of Means, Proportions, and Standard Errors Selected Methods of Sampling

Method	Mean $\bar{x}$		Proportion p_y	
	Estimate	Standard Error	Estimate	Standard Error
Simple random sampling	$\displaystyle\sum_{i=1}^{n}\frac{x_i}{n}$	$\left(\dfrac{s_x}{\sqrt{n}}\right)\left(\dfrac{N-n}{N}\right)^{1/2}$	$\displaystyle\sum_{i=1}^{n}\frac{y_i}{n}$	$\left(\dfrac{p_y(1-p_y)}{n-1}\right)^{1/2}\left(\dfrac{N-n}{N}\right)^{1/2}$
Systematic sampling, repeated	$\bar{\bar{x}}=\displaystyle\sum_{i=1}^{m}\frac{\bar{x}}{m}$	$\left[\left(\dfrac{1}{m}\right)\dfrac{\displaystyle\sum_{i=1}^{m}(\bar{x}_i-\bar{\bar{x}})^2}{m-1}\left(\dfrac{M-m}{M}\right)\right]^{1/2}$		
Stratified sampling	$\displaystyle\sum_{h=1}^{L}\frac{N_h\bar{x}_h}{N}$	$\left[\displaystyle\sum_{h=1}^{L}(N_h^2)\left(\dfrac{s_{hx}^2}{n_h}\right)\left(\dfrac{N_h-n_h}{N_h}\right)\dfrac{1}{N^2}\right]^{1/2}$	$\displaystyle\sum_{h=1}^{L}\frac{N_h p_{hy}}{N}$	$\left\{\dfrac{\displaystyle\sum_{h=1}^{L}(N_h^2)\left[\dfrac{p_{hy}(1-p_{hy})}{n_h-1}\right]\left(\dfrac{N_h-n_h}{N_h}\right)}{N^2}\right\}^{1/2}$
Cluster sampling, one stage	$\bar{\bar{x}}=\displaystyle\sum_{i=1}^{k}\frac{x_i}{k\bar{N}}$	$\left(\dfrac{1}{\sqrt{kN}}\right)(\hat{\sigma}_{1x})\left(\dfrac{K-k}{K-1}\right)^{1/2}$		
Ratio estimation, simple random sampling	$r=\dfrac{\bar{x}}{\bar{y}}$	$\left(\dfrac{r}{\sqrt{n}}\right)(V_x^2+V_y^2-2\hat{\rho}_{xy}V_x V_y)^{1/2}\left(\dfrac{N-n}{N-1}\right)^{1/2}$		

Source: Levy and Lemeshow (1980).

Table 12-9. Definitions

Simple Random Sampling

x_i = value of unit i in the sample
n = number of units in the sample
N = number of units in the population
y_i = value of unit i in the sample
　　($y_i = 1$ if attribute is present, $y_i = 0$ if attribute is absent)

$$s_x = \left\{ \frac{\sum\limits_{i=1}^{n} (x_i - \bar{x})^2}{n - 1} \right\}^{1/2} = \text{estimate of standard deviation of } x$$

Systematic Sampling

m = number of systematic samples taken
M = total number of possible systematic samples

Stratified Sampling

L = number of strata
N_h = population size of stratum h
n_h = sample size of stratum h
$x_{h,i}$ = value of unit i in stratum h
$\bar{x}_h$ = estimate of mean value in stratum h
p_{hy} = estimate of the proportion of units in stratum h having a given dichotomous attribute

$$s_{hx}^2 = \frac{\sum\limits_{i=1}^{n_h} (x_{h,i} - \bar{x}_h)^2}{n_h - 1}$$

Cluster Sampling

k = number of clusters in sample
K = number of clusters in population
$\bar{N} = N/K$ = average number of units per cluster in the population
x_i = total of values for all units in cluster i

$$\bar{x}_{\text{clu}} = \frac{\sum\limits_{i=1}^{k} x_i}{k} = \text{estimate of mean of total within clusters}$$

$$\hat{\sigma}_{1x} = \left[\frac{\sum\limits_{i=1}^{k} (x_i - \bar{x}_{\text{clu}})^2}{k - 1} \right]^{1/2} \left(\frac{K - 1}{K} \right)^{1/2} = \text{standard deviation over all clusters}$$

Ratio Estimation

$$s_x^2 = \frac{\sum\limits_{i=1}^{n} (x_i - \bar{x})^2}{n - 1} \qquad s_y^2 = \frac{\sum\limits_{i=1}^{n} (y_i - \bar{y})^2}{n - 1}$$

$$\hat{V}_x^2 = \left(\frac{N - 1}{N} \right) \left(\frac{s_x^2}{\bar{x}^2} \right)$$

$$\hat{V}_y^2 = \left(\frac{N - 1}{N} \right) \left(\frac{s_y^2}{\bar{y}^2} \right)$$

$$\hat{\rho}_{xy} = \frac{\sum\limits_{i=1}^{n} (x_i - \bar{x})(y_i - \bar{y})}{(n - 1)s_x s_y}$$

Table 12-10. Example of Use of Table 12-8. (Data from Stratified Sample in Table 12-7)

$$\text{Mean} = \frac{\sum_{h=1}^{L} N_h \bar{x}_h}{N} = \frac{(25)(64.6) + (7)(70.7)}{32} = 65.9$$

$$\text{SE (mean)} = \left[\frac{(25)^2 \left(\frac{5.619}{7}\right)\left(\frac{25-7}{25}\right) + (7)^2 \left(\frac{6.335}{3}\right)\left(\frac{7-3}{7}\right)}{(32)^2} \right]^{1/2} = 0.64$$

er. Finally, *quota sampling* is a nonprobability method of sampling in which the interviewer is told how many individuals in various subgroups are needed, such as specific age and gender groups, and the interviewer chooses the sample. Quota sampling is in some ways similar to stratified sampling, but the units within the strata are not randomly selected and the results therefore cannot be reliably generalized to any known population.

METHODS OF IMPUTATION

In the course of almost any study, missing values will occur for some participants. The most frequent way of handling missing data is to exclude all incomplete information from the analysis. However, this procedure may lead to biased estimates of the parameters of interest because it assumes that the observations that are complete are representative of all observations that would have been made if there had been no missing data. *Imputation* refers to the process of converting incomplete data into a data set in which values for all people included in the study are present. Sophisticated but computationally complex methods of imputation have been described in the recent statistics literature (Rubin, 1987; Little and Rubin, 1989), and the interested reader is referred there for further information on this topic. Also, Greenland and Finkle (submitted for publication) have reviewed and summarized these methods. Briefly, the major methods of imputation include (a) multiple imputation methods, in which multiple copies of the original data set are generated, each with missing values randomly generated according to some set of assumptions; the results from the different data sets are then combined in a way that takes into account their variability; (b) maximum-likelihood and maximum pseudo-likelihood methods that take into account the joint disease and covariate distribution; and (c) weighted estimating equation methods, in which weights for regression analysis are provided by a model for the missing data process. More detailed descriptions of these methods are beyond the scope of this book.

DETERMINATION OF SAMPLE SIZE: INTRODUCTION

In the second part of this chapter, we turn to another important aspect of planning an epidemiologic study, that is, deciding how large a sample to include. Before starting a study, it is important for the investigator to determine that the size of the sample is large enough that estimates will be sufficiently precise and that any differences of importance are likely to be detected. An odds ratio of 2.8, for instance, could have confidence limits as wide as 0.8 and 10.0, in which case the investigator could not rule out with a reasonable degree of certainty a wide range of values for the odds ratio, even if the value of 2.8 were biologically plausible. If one had known prior to undertaking the study that the estimate obtained would turn out to be so imprecise and therefore uninformative, then one would probably not have embarked on the research or would have included a larger sample size.

Fortunately, methods are available for assessing at the planning stage whether the proposed study will achieve sufficient precision to be informative. Given information on certain characteristics of the population under study and given a specified sample size, it is possible to calculate the power of the study, that is, the probability of detecting as statistically significant an association of a particular magnitude. Alternatively, it is possible to specify the desired power and to calculate the sample size that is required to achieve that power. The following sections describe how these two types of calculations are performed.

POWER CALCULATIONS

Power calculations usually are based on the sampling distribution of the difference between means or proportions for the groups being compared. Figure 12–3 illustrates the basic principle underlying power calculations for a normally distributed variable. The symbol d denotes the mean value of the difference when the null hypothesis is true (typically $d = 0$), and d_c denotes the value for the difference that is just significantly different from d at the significance level α, say $\alpha = 0.05$, leading to rejection of the null hypothesis. When the null hypothesis is false and the actual value of the difference in means or proportions between the populations is not zero, then the portion of the sampling distribution of the estimator d^* that is to the left of d_c represents the probability of inappropriately failing to reject the null hypothesis. The portion of the distribution to the right of d_c represents the power of detecting the association, that is, the probability of appropriately rejecting the null hypothesis when the mean value of the measure of association in the population is d^*.

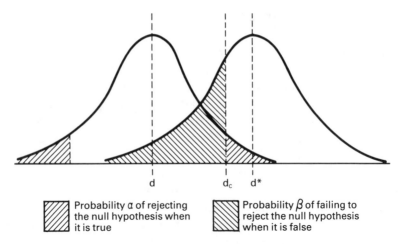

Figure 12–3. Sampling distribution of a measure of association when the null hypothesis is true and when it is false. The symbol d denotes the null mean value of the measure of association, $d*$ denotes the non-null mean value of the measure, and d_c denotes the value of the measure that is just significant at the significance level α.

By reference to the standard normal distribution, d_c may be expressed equivalently as $d + Z_{\alpha/2}\text{s.e.}(d)$ or as $d* - Z_{\beta}\text{s.e.}(d*)$, where $Z_{\alpha/2}$ denotes the standard normal deviate corresponding to the position of d_c on the distribution around d, Z_{β} denotes the standard normal deviate corresponding to the position of d_c on the distribution around $d*$, and s.e. denotes the standard error. Therefore we have the following equality:

$$d + Z_{\alpha/2}\text{s.e.}(d) = d* - Z_{\beta}\text{s.e.}(d*)$$

The symbol $Z_{\alpha/2}$ is used in what is called a two-tailed test of the difference. Use of a two-tailed test makes provision for the possibility that the difference between groups might be either positive or negative. One-tailed tests are sometimes used but are not illustrated here because they require the investigator to ignore a statistically significant difference in the direction opposite to that which has been hypothesized. When use of a one-tailed test is planned, Z_{α} rather than $Z_{\alpha/2}$ is used.

Solving the above equation for Z_{β} yields the following expression:

$$Z_{\beta} = \frac{d* - d - Z_{\alpha/2}\text{s.e.}(d)}{\text{s.e.}(d*)}$$

Consequently, based on the values of d and $d*$ and their respective standard errors, it is possible to obtain a standard normal deviate corresponding to the power of the proposed study to detect a difference when its value in the population is $d*$. Because the standard errors of d and $d*$ are generally very

Table 12–11. Definitions of Symbols Used in Equations for Calculating Power and Required Sample Size

Symbol	Definition
$d*$	Non-null value of the difference in proportions or means (i.e., the magnitude of difference one wishes to detect)
n	In a cohort or cross-sectional study, the number of exposed individuals studied; in a case-control study, the number of cases
r	In a cohort or cross-sectional study, the ratio of the number of unexposed individuals studied to the number of exposed individuals studied; in a case-control study, the ratio of the number of controls studied to the number of cases studied
σ	Standard deviation in the population for a continuously distributed variable
p_1	In a cohort study (or a cross-sectional study), the proportion of exposed individuals who develop (or have) the disease; in a case-control study, the proportion of cases who are exposed
p_0	In a cohort study (or a cross-sectional study), the proportion of unexposed individuals who develop (or have) the disease; in a case-control study, the proportion of controls who are exposed
p	$\dfrac{p_1 + rp_0}{1 + r}$ = weighted average of p_1 and p_0

close in value, a good approximation that simplifies many of the calculations is given by:

$$Z_\beta = \frac{d* - d}{\text{s.e.}(d*)} - Z_{\alpha/2}$$

Table 12–11 gives definitions of the symbols used here in the formulas for power and sample size. In order to calculate power, one must specify the significance level (α), the magnitude of the difference that one is interested in detecting ($d*$), the sample size for the exposed group in a cohort or cross-sectional study or for the case group in a case-control study (n), and the ratio (r) of the sample size for the comparison group (unexposed group in a cohort or cross-sectional study, or the control group in a case-control study) to the sample size for the exposed group or case group. If the difference between two proportions is of interest, then an estimate of the value of the proportion of the unexposed with the disease in a cohort or cross-sectional study or of the proportion of the controls with the exposure in a case-control study is required (p_0). If the difference between two means for a continuously distributed variable is of interest, then an estimate of the standard deviation of that variable (σ) is needed.

Formulas for the calculations of power are given in Table 12–12 for differences in means and proportions. Also given are conversion formulas that permit the use of the formula for the risk difference when one wishes to

Table 12–12. Formulas for Use in Calculating the Power of a Study to Detect an Association

Z_β for difference in means: $\dfrac{d^*}{\sigma} \sqrt{\dfrac{nr}{r+1}} - Z_{\alpha/2}$

Z_β for difference in proportions: $\left[\dfrac{n(d^*)^2 r}{(r+1)\bar{p}(1-\bar{p})} \right]^{1/2} - Z_{\alpha/2}$

Value of p_1 in terms of p_0 and a specified odds ratio (OR): $p_1 = \dfrac{p_0 OR}{1 + p_0(OR-1)}$

Value of p_1 in terms of p_0 and a specified risk ratio (RR) (for use in cohort or cross-sectional studies only): $p_1 = p_0 RR$

calculate the power for detecting risk ratios or odds ratios of a given magnitude.

As an illustration of how power calculations are performed, consider a cohort study designed to assess whether smoking during pregnancy is associated with an increased frequency of low birthweight (that is, weight of 2500 grams or less) in offspring. Based on earlier studies, it is known that for every pregnant woman who smokes during her pregnancy, there are about three who do not (Streissguth et al., 1983). Therefore, in a study in which subjects are selected without respect to their smoking habits, the value of r is 3. Previous studies also indicate that the overall proportion of birthweights of 2500 grams or below is 0.07 (Chase, 1977). Suppose it is feasible to study a total of 1200 pregnant women, of whom an n of $1/4 \times 1200 = 300$ would be expected to smoke during pregnancy. Suppose also that a difference of $d^* = 0.04$ between exposure groups in the proportion of low-birthweight offspring is of interest. In this situation, the overall proportion (0.07) of low-birthweight infants is related to the proportion p_0 of low-birthweight offspring among women who do not smoke by the equation $0.07 = (0.25)(p_0 + 0.04) + (0.75)(p_0)$. Solving for p_0 then yields a value of 0.06. The value of p_1 is $0.06 + 0.04 = 0.10$, and the value of $\bar{p}$ is of course $[0.10 + (3)(0.06)]/[1 + 3] = 0.07$, as above. If the significance level (α) is set at 0.05, then from Table 12–13 the corresponding value of $Z_{\alpha/2}$ is

Table 12–13. Value of $Z_{\alpha/2}$ for Frequently Used Significance Levels

Significance Level (α)	$Z_{\alpha/2}$
.001	3.291
.005	2.807
.01	2.576
.02	2.326
.05	1.960
.10	1.645

1.960. Based on the appropriate formula from Table 12–12, the value of Z_β for this example is calculated as follows:

$$Z_\beta = \left[\frac{300(0.04)^2(3)}{(3 + 1)(0.07)(0.93)} \right]^{1/2} - 1.96 = 0.39$$

Table 12–14 gives the data required for converting a value of Z_β to the actual value for the power of the study. In this example, the power for

Table 12–14. Conversion of Z_β to the Percentage Corresponding to the Power for Detecting an Association

Z_β	0.00	0.01	0.02	0.03	0.04	0.05	0.06	0.07	0.08	0.09
−1.3	9.7	9.5	9.3	9.2	9.0	8.9	8.7	8.5	8.4	8.2
−1.2	11.5	11.3	11.1	10.9	10.7	10.6	10.4	10.2	10.0	9.9
−1.1	13.6	13.3	13.1	12.9	12.7	12.5	12.3	12.1	11.9	11.7
−1.0	15.9	15.6	15.4	15.2	14.9	14.7	14.5	14.2	14.0	13.8
−0.9	18.4	18.1	17.9	17.6	17.4	17.1	16.9	16.6	16.4	16.1
−0.8	21.2	20.9	20.6	20.3	20.0	19.8	19.5	19.2	18.9	18.7
−0.7	24.2	23.9	23.6	23.3	23.0	22.7	22.4	22.1	21.8	21.5
−0.6	27.4	27.1	26.8	26.4	26.1	25.8	25.5	25.1	24.8	24.5
−0.5	30.9	30.5	30.2	29.8	29.5	29.1	28.8	28.4	28.1	27.8
−0.4	34.5	34.1	33.7	33.4	33.0	32.6	32.3	31.9	31.6	31.2
−0.3	38.2	37.8	37.4	37.1	36.7	36.3	35.9	35.6	35.2	34.8
−0.2	42.1	41.7	41.3	40.9	40.5	40.1	39.7	39.4	39.0	38.6
−0.1	46.0	45.6	45.2	44.8	44.4	44.0	43.6	43.3	42.9	42.5
−0.0	50.0	49.6	49.2	48.8	48.4	48.0	47.6	47.2	46.8	46.4
0.0	50.0	50.4	50.8	51.2	51.6	52.0	52.4	52.8	53.2	53.6
0.1	54.0	54.4	54.8	55.2	55.6	56.0	56.4	56.7	57.1	57.5
0.2	57.9	58.3	58.7	59.1	59.5	59.9	60.3	60.6	61.0	61.4
0.3	61.8	62.2	62.6	62.9	63.3	63.7	64.1	64.4	64.8	65.2
0.4	65.5	65.9	66.3	66.6	67.0	67.4	67.7	68.1	68.4	68.8
0.5	69.1	69.5	69.8	70.2	70.5	70.9	71.2	71.6	71.9	72.2
0.6	72.6	72.9	73.2	73.6	73.9	74.2	74.5	74.9	75.2	75.5
0.7	75.8	76.1	76.4	76.7	77.0	77.3	77.6	77.9	78.2	78.5
0.8	78.8	79.1	79.4	79.7	80.0	80.2	80.5	80.8	81.1	81.3
0.9	81.6	81.9	82.1	82.4	82.6	82.9	83.1	83.4	83.6	83.9
1.0	84.1	84.4	84.6	84.8	85.1	85.3	85.5	85.8	86.0	86.2
1.1	86.4	86.7	86.9	87.1	87.3	87.5	87.7	87.9	88.1	88.3
1.2	88.5	88.7	88.9	89.1	89.3	89.4	89.6	89.8	90.0	90.1
1.3	90.3	90.5	90.7	90.8	91.0	91.1	91.3	91.5	91.6	91.8
1.4	91.9	92.1	92.2	92.4	92.5	92.6	92.8	92.9	93.1	93.2
1.5	93.3	93.4	93.6	93.7	93.8	93.9	94.1	94.2	94.3	94.4
1.6	94.5	94.6	94.7	94.8	94.9	95.1	95.2	95.3	95.4	95.4
1.7	95.5	95.6	95.7	95.8	95.9	96.0	96.1	96.2	96.2	96.3
1.8	96.4	96.5	96.6	96.6	96.7	96.8	96.9	96.9	97.0	97.1
1.9	97.1	97.2	97.3	97.3	97.4	97.4	97.5	97.6	97.6	97.7
2.0	97.7	97.8	97.8	97.9	97.9	98.0	98.0	98.1	98.1	98.2
2.1	98.2	98.3	98.3	98.3	98.4	98.4	98.5	98.5	98.5	98.6
2.2	98.6	98.6	98.7	98.7	98.7	98.8	98.8	98.8	98.9	98.9
2.3	98.9	99.0	99.0	99.0	99.0	99.1	99.1	99.1	99.1	99.2
2.4	99.2	99.2	99.2	99.2	99.3	99.3	99.3	99.3	99.3	99.4

Note: For values of Z_β less than −1.39, the power is less than 8.2%; for values of Z_β greater than 2.49, the power is greater than 99.4%.

detecting a difference of 0.04 in the proportion of low-birthweight deliveries is found to be approximately 65%.

As another example of the calculation of power, suppose that a case-control study is planned for assessing the relationship between smoking during pregnancy and low birthweight in offspring. Cases would be women giving birth to babies weighing 2500 grams or below, and controls would be women giving birth to babies weighing over 2500 grams. Because only a small minority of the population falls into the case group, the overall prevalence of smoking in the general population of pregnant women serves quite well as an estimate of p_0, which in a case-control study denotes the proportion of controls who have the exposure. Suppose that an odds ratio of 1.8 is regarded as important to detect, that 175 cases are available for study, and that a control-to-case ratio (r) of 2 is planned. Based on the formula given in Table 12–12, the value of p_1 corresponding to an odds ratio of 1.8 is calculated as $(0.25)(1.8)/[1 + (0.25)(1.8 - 1)] = 0.375$, and the difference $d* = 0.375 - 0.250 = 0.125$. The value of $\bar{p}$ is therefore $[0.375 + (2)(0.25)]/[1 + 2] = 0.29166$. Based on the appropriate formula from Table 12–12, the value of Z_β for this example is calculated as follows:

$$Z_\beta = \left[\frac{(175)(0.125)^2(2)}{(2 + 1)(0.29166)(0.70834)} \right]^{1/2} - 1.96 = 1.01$$

Reference to Table 12–13 yields a power of 84.4% for detecting an odds ratio of 1.8.

CALCULATIONS OF REQUIRED SAMPLE SIZE

The formulas given in Table 12–12 can be solved for n in order to obtain expressions for the sample size required to achieve a specified power for detecting an association. The resulting expressions for n are given in Table 12–15. The expression $(Z_{\alpha/2} + Z_\beta)^2$ occurs in the numerators of both equations in the table. Therefore, in order to simplify the calculations, the

Table 12–15. Formulas for Use in Calculations of Required Sample Size

Difference in means:

$$n = \frac{(Z_{\alpha/2} + Z_\beta)^2 \sigma^2 (r + 1)}{(d*)^2 r}$$

Difference in proportions:

$$n = \frac{(Z_{\alpha/2} + Z_\beta)^2 \bar{p}(1 - \bar{p})(r + 1)}{(d*)^2 r}$$

where $d*$, r, σ, and $\bar{p}$ are as defined in Table 12–11

Table 12–16. Values of $(Z_{\alpha/2} + Z_{\beta})^2$ for Frequently Used Combinations of Significance Level and Power

Significance Level (α)	Power $(1 - \beta)$	$(Z_{\alpha/2} + Z_{\beta})^2$
0.01	0.80	11.679
	0.90	14.879
	0.95	17.814
	0.99	24.031
0.05	0.80	7.849
	0.90	10.507
	0.95	12.995
	0.99	18.372
0.10	0.80	6.183
	0.90	8.564
	0.95	10.822
	0.99	15.770

values of $(Z_{\alpha/2} + Z_{\beta})^2$ for several frequently used combinations of significance level and power are given in Table 12–16.

As an illustration of the calculation of required sample size, consider the example involving smoking and low birthweight. The earlier calculations indicated that for a case-control study with an n of 175 (total sample size of $3 \times 175 = 525$), the power of the study to detect an odds ratio of 1.8 was 84%. Using the appropriate expression from Table 12–15, it is possible to calculate the sample size that would be required to increase the power of the study to any desired value. In order to achieve a power of 90%, the required sample size for this example is calculated as follows:

$$n = \frac{(10.507)(0.29166)(0.70834)(3)}{(0.125)^2(2)} = 208.4$$

Rounding to the next higher integer, it is found that approximately 209 cases and $2 \times 209 = 418$ controls would have to be included. As before, the calculations incorporate the assumption that 7% of deliveries are of low-birthweight infants; also, 25% of the control group is assumed to be exposed, and the significance level is $\alpha = 0.05$.

When calculating either power or required sample size, it is important to consider the possible effects of measurement error. As discussed in Chapter 13, the usual effect of such error is to attenuate a measure toward its null value and thereby to reduce the power of a study. Consequently, in order to ensure that adequate power will be achieved, the non-null value of the difference (d^*) incorporated into the calculations should not be the biologically relevant magnitude of association, but instead the value one would actually expect to observe, given the anticipated attenuation due to measurement error. Tabulations presented in Chapter 13 provide some guidance as to the amount of attenuation one would anticipate on the basis of particular magnitudes of measurement error.

SMALLEST DETECTABLE ASSOCIATION

Occasionally one is interested in knowing the smallest value for a measure of association that can be detected with a specified power, given a fixed sample size. Appropriate calculations are discussed elsewhere (Schlesselman, 1982; Walter, 1977). Frequently, it is useful to consider the smallest detectable association for a number of different values for the desired power (e.g., 60%, 80%, 90%, 95%). Alternatively, it may be equally informative to use the methods of calculating power described above and to apply these methods to a series of values of interest for the magnitude of the association (e.g., odds ratio = 1.5, 2.0, 3.0, 5.0).

PROBLEMS OF CENSORING AND OTHER LOSSES

When planning a study, it is important to bear in mind that not all persons selected are likely to be included. For example, in many studies it is difficult to enroll more than 80% of the individuals initially selected for inclusion. The required sample size should therefore be inflated to protect against the anticipated losses. If, for example, an n of 500 is required to achieve the desired power for detecting an association, then the number of people selected should be $500/0.80 = 625$.

Calculations of power and of required sample size are complicated considerably in cohort studies because of the incompleteness of the data for the many cohort members who die or are otherwise lost to follow-up without having experienced the event of interest (e.g., incidence of a particular cancer). Methods appropriate for use when the observations are censored in this way have been proposed (George and Desu, 1974; Lachin, 1981), but these methods require a number of assumptions that may be seriously violated in actual research settings, such as constant incidence over the period of follow-up.

The factor of overriding importance in determining the power and required sample size for detecting associations involving infrequent events is the number of members of the cohort who are expected to experience the event, given the time frame and relevant censoring processes for the planned study. Consequently, careful estimation of the expected number experiencing the event and incorporation of this estimate into the equations given for the calculation of power and sample size yield acceptably accurate results for infrequent events.

Accurate estimation of the number of members of the cohort who will experience a particular event within the study period often requires fairly detailed calculations. Consider, for example, a long-term study of cancer incidence in a large cohort. In order to obtain an accurate estimate of the total number expected to develop a particular cancer within the study period, one must assemble schedules of age- and gender-specific rates for mortality and for cancer incidence. One may then consider a number of subgroups of the cohort based on gender and on age at entry into the study and calculate the expected outcome for each subgroup over each successive year of the proposed study. Thus, the schedule of age-specific mortality rates would be applied to calculate the anticipated loss due to death in each year. The schedule of cancer incidence rates would be applied to those still at risk at a given point in the follow-up. Numbers of expected cancers would then be accumulated over all subgroups and over the entire study period to obtain an estimate of the total number expected to develop the cancer. Provided that the study and referent groups do not differ greatly in terms of the pattern of losses, crude power estimates may then be obtained by dividing the total number of expected events by the initial size of the cohort and by using this proportion as p_0 in the calculations. Estimates of required sample size may also be calculated using this value of p_0.

In performing these calculations, one must also bear in mind the possibility that not all cancers that occur will be ascertained. For example, if cancers are to be identified through linkages with a tumor registry for the geographic region in which the cohort is initially enrolled, then cancers diagnosed in persons subsequent to moving from the local area cannot be included. Consequently, estimates of the annual percentage moving out of the area should be applied to each successive year of follow-up in the same way that one takes account of losses due to mortality. Failure to take adequate account of such losses results in an inflated estimate of the proportion of the cohort that will be found to develop the cancer over the period of the study, and thus the resulting estimates of power will be overly optimistic.

MATCHED STUDIES

When persons in the referent group have been matched to persons in the study group, the methods described above for calculating power and sample size are not strictly appropriate. Furthermore, the power of a matched study is not necessarily as great as the power of an unmatched study (Greenland and Morgenstern, 1990). Although formulas for matched designs have been derived, the information required for their application in practice is often lacking (Schlesselman, 1982). An important determinant of the efficiency of a matched study is the degree to which the matching process induces concordance among the members within matched sets. Particularly when participants have been matched on a number of variables, it is difficult to estimate the degree of that concordance prior to actually executing the study. As in any situation where sample size calculations are based on the incorporation of questionable estimates, it is wise to err on the side of a somewhat larger sample size. If frequency matching has been employed, the methods of estimating sample size are similar to those used when control for confounding is anticipated. This situation is described next.

CONTROL FOR CONFOUNDING AND DETECTION OF EFFECT MODIFICATION

When it is necessary to control in the analysis for confounding variables, the sample size and power calculations presented above are also not entirely accurate. However, unless the confounding variable is strongly associated with both the disease and exposure of interest (odds ratios of 5 or more), power is reduced only slightly (Smith and Day, 1984). Methods for taking account of confounding in the calculation of power and sample size when the data are arranged as a series of 2×2 tables are discussed by Gail (1973) and by Schlesselman (1982). These methods are appropriate only when frequency matching has been performed and when the outcome of interest is fairly frequent in the sample. Methods for calculation of power and sample size for data arranged in tables with more than two variables have been provided by Greenland (1985).

If detection of effect modification is an important objective of the study, then a much larger sample size will be needed. This issue is discussed for dichotomously distributed variables by Smith and Day (1984). These authors show that even under optimal conditions, that is, when about 50% of the study population is classified as exposed to the risk factor and about 50% is exposed to the potential effect modifier, about four times as many participants will be needed as for the detection of a main effect. If the prevalence of the risk factor or effect modifier is lower or higher than 50%, then still larger sample sizes will be needed. If the potential effect modification involves a matching variable, then under most circumstances an even larger sample size will be required (Thomas and Greenland, 1985). Thus, when planning a study, an investigator must be cautious in claiming the ability to detect effect modification unless the sample size really is sufficiently large. Greenland (1985) has presented methods that can be used to calculate power and sample size for detecting effect modification.

OPTIMAL ALLOCATION

Throughout the discussion of power and required sample size, it has been assumed that the relative size of the referent group versus the study group (r) is fixed. When the investigator has some degree of flexibility in choosing a value for this ratio, he or she generally hopes to select a value that is optimal in terms of the precision of estimation of a particular measure of association. Assuming that power to detect an association is of primary importance, it can be shown (Gail et al., 1976; Miettinen, 1969) that if C denotes the ratio of the cost of studying a member of the study group to the corresponding cost for a member of the referent group, then the optimal value of r for fixed total costs is approximately the square root of C. Thus, if the costs for studying the two types of individuals are equal, then the optimal strategy is to select equal numbers. In contrast, if the cost of studying a person in the study group is twice as great as the cost of studying a person in the referent group, then the optimal value for r is approximately $\sqrt{2} = 1.41$.

Practical constraints on the availability of participants often preclude the use of an optimal value of r. For example, case-control studies often include all available cases. Because it is not possible to augment further the precision for estimating the exposure history of cases, one often attempts to maximize the precision of the study as a whole by including a large group of controls. In so doing, one employs a value of r that is often considerably larger than its optimal value for a fixed sample size. Nevertheless, increasing the value of r beyond 4 or 5 when $C = 1$ generally results in very little further improvement in precision when estimating odds ratios. Increasing r may, however, considerably enhance precision for detecting effect modification (Breslow et al., 1983).

PRECISION OF ESTIMATING A SINGLE MEAN OR PROPORTION

Occasionally it is of interest to estimate a single mean or proportion rather than a measure of association (Snedecor and Cochran, 1967). If L denotes the margin of error within which the investigator wishes to estimate these quantities, then the required sample size is given by $n = Z^2\sigma^2/L^2$ for the estimation of a mean and $n = Z^2p(1 - p)/L^2$ for a proportion, p, where Z is the normal deviate corresponding to the desired proportion of the time that the estimate is to be within the desired margin of error. For instance, suppose that it is desired to estimate the proportion of the population having a particular exposure within 0.04. If the proportion exposed is thought to be around 0.40, then the sample size needed to estimate it within 0.04 is $(1.96)^2(0.40)(0.60)/(0.04)^2 = 576$. Provided that a sample size of this magnitude is used, there is a 95% probability that the estimate obtained will be within 0.04 of the population value.

REFERENCES

Abbas AA, Walker GJA. 1986. Determinants of the utilization of maternal and child health services in Jordan. *Int J Epidemiol* 15:404–407.

Breslow NE, Lubin JH, Marek P, Langholz B. 1983. Multiplicative models and cohort analysis. *J Am Stat Assoc* 78:1–12.

Burney PGJ, Chinn S, Britton JR, Tattersfield AE, Papacosta AO. 1989. What symptoms predict the bronchial response to histamine? Evaluation in a community survey of the Bronchial Symptoms Questionnaire (1984) of the International Union Against Tuberculosis and Lung Disease. *Int J Epidemiol* 18:165–173.

Cade JE, Margetts BM. 1988. Nutrient sources in the English diet: Quantitative data from three English towns. *Int J Epidemiol* 17:844–848.

Chase HC. 1977. Time trends in low birth weight in the United States, 1950–1974. In: DM Reed, FJ Stanley, Ed. The Epidemiology of Prematurity. Baltimore, MD, Urban and Schwarzenberg.

Cochran WG. 1977. Sampling Techniques. New York, Wiley.

Cochrane AL, Davies I, Chapman PJ, Rae S. 1956. The prevalence of coalworkers' pneumoconiosis: its measurement and significance. *Br J Ind Med* 13:231–250.

Gail M. 1973. The determination of sample sizes for trials involving several independent 2 × 2 tables. *J Chron Dis* 26:669–673.

Gail M, Williams R, Byar DP, Brown C. 1976. How many controls? *J Chron Dis* 29:723–731.

George SL, Desu MM. 1974. Planning the size and duration of a clinical trial studying the time to some critical event. *J Chron Dis* 27:15–24.

Greenland S. 1985. Power, sample size, and smallest detectable effect determination for multivariate studies. *Stat Med* 4:117–127.

Greenland S, Finkle WD. 1995. A critical look at methods for handling missing covariates in epidemiologic regression analyses. *Am J Epidemiol,* 142:1255–1264.

Greenland S, Morgenstern. 1990. Matching and efficiency in cohort studies. *Am J Epidemiol* 131:151–159.

Lachin JM. 1981. Introduction to sample size determination and power analysis for clinical trials. *Controlled Clin Trials* 2:93–113.

Lambert PM, Reid DC. 1970. Smoking, air pollution, and bronchitis in Britain. *Lancet* 1:853–857.

Levy PS, Lemeshow S. 1980. Sampling for Health Professionals. Belmont, CA, Lifetime Learning Publications.

Levy PS, Lemeshow S. 1991. Sampling of Populations: Methods and Applications. New York, Wiley.

Little RJA, Rubin DB. 1989. Statistical Analysis with Missing Data. New York, Wiley.

Miettinen OS. 1969. Individual matching with multiple controls in the case of all-or-none responses. *Biometrics* 25:339–355.

Paganini-Hill A, Hsu G, Chao A, Ross RK. 1993. Comparison of early and late respondents to a postal health survey questionnaire. *Epidemiology* 4:375–379.

Proietti FA, Antunes CMF. 1989. Sensitivity, specificity and positive predictive value of clinical signs and symptoms associated with *Schistosomiasis mansoni*. *Int J Epidemiol* 18:680–683.

Rubin DB. 1987. Multiple Imputation for Nonresponse in Surveys. New York, Wiley.

Schlesselman JJ. 1982. Case-Control Studies: Design, Conduct, Analysis. New York, Oxford University Press.

Smith PG, Day NE. 1984. The design of case-control studies: the influence of confounding and interaction effects. *Int J Epidemiol* 13:356–365.

Snedecor GW, Cochran WG. 1967. Statistical Methods. Ames, IA, Iowa State University Press.

Streissguth AP, Darby BL, Barr HM, Smith JR, Martin DC. 1983. Comparison of drinking and smoking patterns during pregnancy over a six-year interval. *Am J Obstet Gynecol* 145:716–724.

Thomas DC, Greenland S. 1985. The efficiency of matching in case-control studies of risk-factor interactions. *J Chron Dis* 38:569–574.

Tielsch JM, Sommer A, Witt K, Katz J, Royall RM. 1990. Blindness and visual impairment in an American urban population. *Arch Ophthalmol* 108:286–290.

Walter SD. 1977. Determination of significant relative risks and optimal sampling procedures in prospective and retrospective comparative studies of various sizes. *Am J Epidemiol* 105:387–397.

EXERCISES

1. What method(s) of sampling would you use to determine the following? Give brief reasons for your choice.

a. Prevalence rates of dental caries in 4-year-old residents in _____ (nearest large city).

b. Prevalence rates of osteoarthritis of the hands in residents of _____ (nearest large city) by social class. (Symptoms give some indication of the presence of osteoarthritis and lack of symptoms provides some indication of the absence of osteoarthritis, but definitive diagnosis requires x-ray.)

c. Incidence rates by age and sex of bladder cancer among Iowa residents.

d. Prevalence at birth of congenital dislocation of the hip among births in _____ (nearest large city). (Definitive and consistent diagnosis would require someone trained by the investigator to administer a test to infants within a few days of birth.)

e. Whether mortality statistics for hip fractures published in the *Vital Statistics* are a good indication of death from hip fractures in _____ (your state).

f. Whether there are differences in prevalence rates of chronic bronchitis in residents in _____ (one nearby city with relatively high levels of air pollution) and _____ (another nearby city with relatively low levels of air pollution).

g. Total number of hospitalizations for hysterectomy in _____ (nearest large hospital) from 1980 to 1984.

2. Assume that the annual incidence rate for breast cancer among those exposed to oral contraceptives is 4.4 per 10,000, and among those not exposed is 2.2 per 10,000.

a. How large a sample must be studied in order to detect this difference in risk in one year? (Assume that equal numbers of exposed and unexposed individuals are studied.)

b. How large must the sample be if the study is to last for 10 years?

c. If 1000 exposed people and 1000 unexposed people are available for study, then how many years must they be followed for the investigator to detect the difference in risk?

d. A case-control study of the same problem is planned using cases and an equal number of unmatched controls. Again, the risk for breast cancer is assumed to be twice as great among those exposed to oral contraceptives as among those not exposed. If 25% of women in the general population are exposed to oral contraceptives then how many cases and controls will be needed?

e. What would the corresponding number be if only 10% of women in the general population were exposed?

f. Using the 25% exposure figure, what is the power of a study with 200 cases and 200 controls?

g. Using the 25% exposure figure, what is the power of a study of 200 cases if a control-to-case ratio of 3 rather than 1 is used?

NOTE

1. Sometimes what is called "probability sampling" here is referred to as "random sampling," but the former term will be used in this book so as to minimize confusion between the terms "random sampling" and "simple random sampling." Simple random sampling, described in the next section, is one specific type of probability sampling.

13

Measurement Error

A certain amount of error is intrinsic to any measurement process. In the conduct of epidemiologic research, measurement error is potentially a major problem that may invalidate the results of otherwise well-designed studies. For instance, if a case-control study is undertaken to address the issue of whether past dietary fat consumption affects the risk of breast cancer, assessment of food items consumed many years ago may be so inaccurate that it is not worth undertaking the study. Although measurement error can seldom if ever be eliminated, an appreciation of the sources of measurement error, of the nature of its impact on study results, and of methods for minimizing that impact can contribute greatly to the quality of epidemiologic studies and to the appropriateness of the conclusions drawn from them.

In the two chapters following this one, several of the measurement techniques used most frequently in epidemiology will be discussed in detail. Particular emphasis will be given to methods for ensuring that the data obtained are as accurate and as free from systematic bias as possible, given practical constraints. The purpose of the present chapter is to address a number of more general quantitative issues that arise in assessing the magnitude of measurement error and in judging and controlling its likely impact on study results. The reader is also referred to a book by Armstrong et al. (1992) on exposure measurement in epidemiology.

Errors occur in the measurement of exposure variables, disease occurrence, and confounding variables. Because much information on exposure to risk factors is obtained from questionnaires, the quality of the data obtained is often no better than the imperfect memory of individuals about such factors as their dietary habits, their exposure to chemicals in the workplace, or their use of medications. Data obtained from questionnaires present special problems of measurement in case-control studies because information on exposure must often be obtained only after the disease has manifested itself, sometimes decades after the relevant exposure has taken place. Even when exposure information is available from sources other than the reports of the respondents themselves, such as from medical records, employer's records, and direct biologic assays, there are often no assurances that the data are any more accurate, particularly if they have been collected for purposes other than those of the study.

Errors of classification in terms of disease status are also frequent in epidemiologic studies. Even when clear-cut diagnostic criteria are available for use in a clinical setting, the necessary diagnostic tests may be impractical or unethical for use in large-scale epidemiologic studies. Additionally, there may be a spectrum of disease, so that it is virtually impossible to classify all individuals either as clearly having a particular disease or as clearly not having it.

Errors in the measurement of confounding variables are another important concern in the execution and interpretation of observational studies. Often the critical confounding variables are just as difficult to measure as the exposure of primary interest. Some potentially confounding variables, such as socioeconomic status and general level of medical care utilization, pose their own formidable problems of conceptualization and measurement. When planning an epidemiologic study, one's attention is often concentrated on measurement issues relating to the exposure and disease under study, sometimes at the expense of concern for measuring confounding variables. However, as will be discussed in detail below, inadequate measurement of important confounding variables can lead to biases just as serious as those biases arising from errors in the measurement of exposure or disease.

Here we consider measurement error in the context of studies of individual persons. Discussion of measurement error in ecological studies is available in Chapter 10 and elsewhere (Brenner et al., 1992; Greenland, 1992).

INDICES OF THE ACCURACY OF MEASUREMENT

The *accuracy*, or *validity*, of a measurement refers to the extent to which the measurement represents the true value of the attribute being assessed. In order to obtain something more than an impressionistic idea of the quality of one's measurement of a given variable, it is useful to calculate quantitative indices of the accuracy of measurement. Several such indices have been proposed. The choice of a particular index depends on whether the variable is discrete (e.g., smoker versus nonsmoker) or continuously distributed (e.g., diastolic blood pressure in millimeters of mercury).

For a discrete variable that is binary, there are two separate aspects of the accuracy of measurement. One is *sensitivity*, which is defined as the proportion of those who truly have the characteristic that are correctly classified as having it by the measurement technique. The other is *specificity*,

Table 13-1. Definitions of Sensitivity and Specificity

		True classification	
		Present	Absent
Imperfect classification	Present	a	b
	Absent	c	d
		$a + c$	$b + d$

$$\text{Sensitivity} = \frac{a}{a + c}$$

$$\text{Specificity} = \frac{d}{b + d}$$

$$\text{False negative rate} = \frac{c}{a + c}$$

$$\text{False positive rate} = \frac{b}{b + d}$$

which is defined as the proportion of those who truly do not have the characteristic that are correctly classified as not having it by the measurement technique. Table 13-1 gives the definitions of sensitivity and specificity in terms of the cells of a 2 × 2 table, where a denotes the number of true positives; b, the number of false positives; c, the number of false negatives; and d, the number of true negatives. The complements of sensitivity and specificity are often referred to as the false negative rate and the false positive rate, respectively, although these quantities are not actually rates in the formal sense discussed in Chapter 2.

Measurement of a binary characteristic is perfect only when both sensitivity and specificity are 100%. When sensitivity is equal to 100% minus specificity, then the measurement method is no better than an entirely random means for classifying individuals. That is, the probability of being classified as having the characteristic is the same for those who do not have the characteristic as for those who do. In order for a measurement technique to be useful in epidemiologic research, it must be substantially better than a random method of classification. Unfortunately, the ideal of near-perfect sensitivity and specificity is seldom achieved in practice.

Figure 13-1 illustrates a variety of patterns of measurement error for a continuously distributed variable such as blood pressure. Two important aspects of the correspondence, or lack of correspondence, between the variable of interest and the variable as measured are bias and correlation. Bias refers here to the difference between the mean value as measured and the mean of the true values. In the figure, and throughout this discussion,

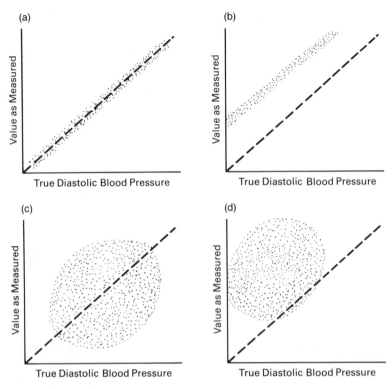

Figure 13–1. Illustration of four possible patterns of measurement error for diastolic blood pressure. (a) High correlation and no bias, (b) high correlation and some bias, (c) low correlation and no bias, (d) low correlation and some bias.

we consider only the special instance where the bias does not vary in magnitude according to the value of the variable of interest; thus, in part b of the figure, the points cluster around a straight line that is parallel to the dotted line. Because the importance of a bias of a given magnitude can often be assessed only in relation to the total variability, it is useful to calculate the *standardized bias* as follows:

$$\frac{\text{Mean of measurements} - \text{True mean}}{\text{Standard deviation of true values}}$$

For example, if a given technique for measuring diastolic blood pressure systematically overestimates the true value by 4 mm Hg and the standard deviation for "true" pressures in the population is 15 mm Hg, then the measurement technique has a standardized bias of $4/15 = 0.27$. That is, the imperfect measurement technique tends to yield values that are 0.27 of a standard deviation higher than the true values.

Correlation is denoted here by $corr_{xX}$, where x denotes the imperfectly measured value and X denotes the true value. The measure $corr_{xX}$ indexes the extent to which the imperfectly measured values tend to fall in the same position relative to their mean as do the corresponding true values relative to the true mean. The square of $corr_{xX}$ denotes the proportion of the total variation in true values that is captured by the imperfect measurement technique.

INDICES OF RELIABILITY

The indices of the accuracy of measurement discussed in the preceding section (sensitivity, specificity, $corr_{xX}$, and the standardized bias) are readily interpretable quantitative measures of the adequacy of one's measurement techniques. Unfortunately, a major obstacle to their use is the frequent lack of information regarding true values in order that the imperfect measurement technique can be evaluated against a criterion.

In the absence of a criterion measure, some sense of the quality of one's measurement can be obtained by comparing multiple imperfect measurements to each other rather than by comparing them to true values. Thus, rather than assessing the accuracy or validity of the measurement, one of necessity settles for assessing its reliability. *Reliability,* or *reproducibility,* refers to the extent to which results of a measurement can be replicated. One might, for example, assess the reliability of an imperfect set of operational criteria for diagnosing rheumatoid arthritis by having two observers independently classify the same patients as each meeting or not meeting the criteria for rheumatoid arthritis. The extent of their agreement in classifying the individuals would then reflect the reliability, or what is often termed the *inter-rater reliability,* of the diagnostic process. Similarly, in order to assess the reliability of blood pressure measurements, a single technician might take two blood pressure readings on each of several individuals, and the two sets of readings would then be compared. This latter type of reliability is often called *test-retest reliability.* Additional types of reliability, such as *split-half* and *alternative-forms reliability,* are employed primarily in the psychometric area (Nunnally, 1978). In many epidemiologic studies, it is important to assess the degree of correspondence of two qualitatively different methods of measurement, such as information on use of medications obtained through interviews compared with similar information obtained through review of records. Although somewhat distinct from inter-rater reliability and test-retest reliability, assessment of the agreement between different measures entails many of the same conceptual issues.

Several indices have been proposed for the quantification of reliability (Bishop et al., 1975; Fleiss, 1975; Nunnally, 1978). Here just two are presented, namely, the kappa coefficient and the correlation coefficient of reproducibility.

The *kappa coefficient* is appropriate for discrete variables. Only binary variables are considered in this chapter. Extensions to discrete variables with more than two values are straightforward (Fleiss, 1981), but are not discussed here. The kappa coefficient, which was first proposed by Cohen (1960), has the important characteristic of correcting for the chance agreement that would be expected to occur if the two classifications were completely unrelated. Failure to take into account chance agreement can lead to erroneous conclusions about the quality of measurement. Chance-expected agreement for a binary variable is given by $p_1 p_2 + (1 - p_1)(1 - p_2)$, where p_1 is the observed proportion classified as having the characteristic by the first imperfect classification, and where p_2 is the observed proportion classified as having the characteristic by the second imperfect classification. The kappa coefficient is defined as follows:

$$\frac{\text{Observed agreement} - \text{Expected agreement}}{1 - \text{Expected agreement}}$$

When the two measurements agree only at the chance level, the value of kappa is zero. When the two measurements agree perfectly, the value of kappa is one. Methods are available for calculating confidence intervals for computed values of kappa (Fleiss, 1981).

Table 13–2 illustrates the calculation of the kappa coefficient for a study of the agreement between information on reserpine use obtained from interview and from medical records. The value of 0.39 for kappa indicates that the observed agreement between the two imperfect classifications concerning a history of use of reserpine is 39% of the way between chance agreement and perfect agreement. Note that failure to take proper account of chance agreement would have resulted in a serious overestimate of agreement between the measures. The observed agreement (0.85) is much larger than the chance-corrected value of kappa.

Whereas kappa is appropriate for discrete variables, the *correlation coefficient of reproducibility* is appropriate for continuously distributed variables, with the caveat that the magnitude of the measurement error does not vary systematically according to the value of the variable of interest. When two measurements, x and x', have been made for each individual, this coefficient $(corr_{xx'})$ is simply the product-moment correlation between the first and second sets of imperfect measurements. The coefficient indexes the extent to which measurements of one type tend to fall in the same position relative to their mean as do measurements of a second type relative to their mean. This coefficient does not reflect possible differences between the mean values for the two sets of measurements and therefore indexes only

Table 13-2. Example of the Calculation of Kappa: Agreement between Personal Interview and Medical Chart Concerning Use of Reserpine among Controls from a Case-Control Study of Breast Cancer in Two Retirement Communities

		History of use of reserpine according to medical chart		
		Yes	No	
History of use of reserpine according to patient's report	Yes	14	7	21
	No	25	171	196
		39	178	217

$$\text{Chance-expected agreement} = \frac{(21)(39) + (196)(178)}{(217)^2} = 0.7583$$

Observed agreement = $(14 + 171)/217 = 0.8525$

$$\text{Kappa} = \frac{0.8525 - 0.7583}{1 - 0.7583} = 0.39$$

Source: Paganini-Hill and Ross (1982).

one aspect of agreement between the two sets of measurements. The square of the correlation coefficient of reproducibility is interpretable as the proportion of the variation in one set of measurements that is captured by the other set of measurements.

The value of kappa or the correlation coefficient of reproducibility is of greatest interest to epidemiologists when it reflects something about accuracy of measurement rather than simply reliability. Provided that the errors made in the two measurements are independent (i.e., the same errors do not tend to be repeated), then the algebraic relationship between measures of accuracy and measures of reliability can be specified. For continuous variables, this relationship is simply $corr_{xx'} = (corr_{xX})(corr_{x'X})$. If the two imperfect measurements are equally accurate, then $corr_{xX} = corr_{x'X} = \sqrt{corr_{xx'}}$ (Nunnally, 1978). The relationship of kappa to sensitivity and specificity under the assumption of independent errors is more complex and is a function not only of these two indices of accuracy, but also of the true proportion of the population that in fact has the characteristic of interest (Kraemer, 1979; Thompson and Walter, 1988). Consequently, even for fixed values of sensitivity and specificity, the value of kappa can vary widely, so that inferences about accuracy based on the value of kappa are difficult to draw.

Relating either kappa or the correlation coefficient of reproducibility to the accuracy of measurement is frequently made difficult by the lack of independence of the errors for two imperfect sets of measurements. Misclassification involving two measurements is considered *independent* if the degree of misclassification for one measurement does not depend on the degree of misclassification for the other. Misclassification is considered *dependent* if the degree of misclassification of one measurement depends on the degree of misclassification of the other. For example, it is often possible to achieve excellent reliability when classifying individuals as diseased or not diseased according to a very specific set of diagnostic criteria. However, much of the reliability could represent consistently erroneous misclassification of diseased individuals as nondiseased and of nondiseased individuals as diseased. Similarly, if information on a man's drinking habits is obtained both from the man himself and from his wife, then errors in reporting are likely to be correlated (i.e., dependent), because a man who is motivated to conceal or exaggerate his drinking when interviewed might also have misled his wife in a similar manner. Even if the wife is fully aware of her husband's drinking habits, similarities between husband and wife concerning the social acceptability of reporting various patterns of alcohol use might still induce a correlation of errors.

Because of these problems of interpretation, indices of reliability are primarily useful for providing negative information about the accuracy of measurement. If reliability is low, then accuracy must be low as well. However, if reliability is high, then accuracy may or may not be acceptably high.

EFFECTS OF MEASUREMENT ERROR ON MEASURES OF ASSOCIATION

In light of the very common occurrence of measurement error, it is important to understand its effects on observed associations between exposure and disease. In this section, the distinction between differential and nondifferential measurement error is discussed and the quantitative impact of nondifferential measurement error on measures of association is illustrated.

Measurement error in one variable is *differential* with respect to a second variable if the magnitude of error in the first variable differs according to the true value of the second variable. For example, consider a case-control study of the possible relationship between intrauterine exposure to ionizing radiation and the occurrence of congenital malformations. If information on exposure to pelvic radiation during pregnancy is obtained retrospectively from reports of the mothers and if the mothers of infants with congenital malformations recall radiation to which they were exposed to a greater extent than do the control mothers, then the measurement error is said to be differential with respect to disease status.

Measurement error in one variable is *nondifferential* with respect to a second variable if the magnitude of error in the first variable does not vary according to the value of the other variable of interest. For instance, in a case-control study assessing the relationship between age at menarche and ovarian cancer, many ovarian cancer cases and their controls may not remember their age at menarche, but it is unlikely that the magnitude of error will depend on whether a person is a case or control. For a binary variable, measurement error is nondifferential if both sensitivity and specificity remain constant irrespective of the value of the other variables. For a continuous variable, measurement error is generally regarded as nondifferential if the bias (i.e., the magnitude of any difference between the true mean and the mean for the imperfect measurement) and precision remain constant irrespective of the values of the other variable of interest.

When measurement error is differential, the effects on measures of association can be in any direction. That is, the apparent magnitude of the measure may be increased or reduced, or the direction of the association may even be reversed. Spurious associations may be found between an exposure and a disease when in fact no association exists.

The effect of nondifferential and independent misclassification on a measure of association in a single 2×2 table is always to bias or attenuate the measure toward the null value (Newell, 1962; Gullen et al., 1968; Copeland et al., 1977). For two continuously distributed variables, nondifferential and independent misclassification also biases the correlation coefficient towards the null, except in the unusual situation that a perfect linear relationship exists between the variable as measured and the true values (i.e., $corr_{xX} = 1.0$).

The magnitude of the attenuation induced by nondifferential and independent measurement error is illustrated in Table 13–3 for the situation in which exposure and disease are both binary. The measure of the association between exposure and disease is the odds ratio. For simplicity, it is assumed that only the exposure variable is subject to measurement error. Results are given for a number of combinations of sensitivity, specificity, and prevalence of exposure. The results indicate that even for fairly high values of sensitivity and specificity, the degree of attenuation of the odds ratio can be substantial. Specificity is particularly critical when only a small minority of the study population has the exposure, as is sensitivity when the great majority have the exposure. Note also that for fixed values of sensitivity and specificity, the degree of attenuation can vary considerably, depending on the prevalence of exposure. For a given sensitivity and specificity, the degree of attenuation tends to be greatest when the prevalence of exposure differs substantially from 50%.

As an illustration of the type of calculations on which Table 13–3 is based, consider a case-control study in which 40% of cases and 25% of controls have the exposure of interest. The true odds ratio is therefore $(0.40/0.60)/(0.25/0.75) = 2.0$. If the sensitivity and specificity for classify-

Table 13-3. Effect on the Odds Ratio of Nondifferential Error in the Measurement of a Binary Exposure Variable[a]

Sensitivity	Specificity	Prevalence of Exposure	True Odds Ratio 1.5	2.0	5.0	10.0
0.60	0.60	0.01	1.00	1.01	1.03	1.07
		0.50	1.08	1.14	1.31	1.39
		0.99	1.00	1.00	1.01	1.01
0.60	0.90	0.01	1.03	1.05	1.21	1.46
		0.50	1.24	1.42	1.99	2.31
		0.99	1.01	1.01	1.02	1.02
0.60	0.99	0.01	1.19	1.37	2.47	4.24
		0.50	1.30	1.54	2.29	2.74
		0.99	1.01	1.01	1.02	1.02
0.90	0.60	0.01	1.01	1.02	1.08	1.18
		0.50	1.26	1.48	2.40	3.16
		0.99	1.02	1.03	1.04	1.05
0.90	0.90	0.01	1.04	1.08	1.33	1.73
		0.50	1.38	1.72	3.29	4.79
		0.99	1.03	1.04	1.07	1.08
0.90	0.99	0.01	1.24	1.47	2.89	5.24
		0.50	1.43	1.82	3.63	5.42
		0.99	1.03	1.05	1.08	1.09
0.99	0.60	0.01	1.01	1.02	1.10	1.22
		0.50	1.35	1.68	3.61	6.46
		0.99	1.14	1.23	1.43	1.51
0.99	0.90	0.01	1.05	1.09	1.36	1.82
		0.50	1.45	1.89	4.44	8.35
		0.99	1.19	1.31	1.61	1.75
0.99	0.99	0.01	1.25	1.50	3.00	5.50
		0.50	1.49	1.97	4.77	9.09
		0.99	1.20	1.33	1.67	1.82

[a]The entries in the body of the table are the attenuated values of the odds ratio resulting from the effects of the nondifferential error in measuring exposure. Classification in terms of disease status is assumed to be error free.

ing cases into exposure groups are 80% and 95%, respectively, then the expected proportion of cases classified as exposed would be $(0.40)(0.80) + (1 - 0.40)(1 - 0.95) = 0.35$. If the misclassification is nondifferential with respect to disease status, then the sensitivity and specificity will also be 80% and 95%, respectively, for controls. The expected proportion of controls classified as exposed would then be $(0.25)(0.80) + (1 - 0.25)(1 - 0.95) = 0.2375$. Given this level of measurement error, the expected value of the odds ratio would be $(0.3500/0.6500)/(0.2375/0.7625) = 1.73$.

Under certain circumstances the kappa coefficient bears a fairly close relationship to the degree of attenuation of the odds ratio (Thompson, 1990). Specifically, the magnitude of kappa is a rough indicator of the proportion of the true elevation in the odds ratio that will be captured when two groups are compared in terms of the frequency of the imperfectly classified variable. For example, if the true odds ratio is 3.0 and the kappa for the reliability of the imperfect classification of exposure is 0.60, then the attenuated odds ratio will be approximately $(0.60)(3.0 - 1.0) + 1.0 = 2.2$. Thus, even in the absence of estimates of sensitivity and specificity, some quantitative statements may sometimes be made regarding the degree of attenuation from nondifferential and independent misclassification.

It is generally believed that when discrete variables assume more than two values, nondifferential and independent misclassification again usually results in attenuation of measures of association, but this is not always the case. A hypothetical counter-example has been presented by Dosemeci et al. (1990) in which the direction of a trend is reversed because of non-differential misclassification of the exposure. However, such a reversal of direction of trend cannot occur if the mean value of the measured exposure always increases as the true exposure increases (Weinberg et al., 1994).

It has also been pointed out that in both case-control and cohort studies, when exposure categories are formed from continuous variables or when more than two categories are collapsed to two categories, non-differential measurement error in the original metrics does not guarantee nondifferential misclassification in the 2×2 table (Wacholder et al., 1991; Flegal et al., 1991). Thus, combining multiple exposure categories into smaller numbers of categories should be undertaken cautiously.

Table 13-4 illustrates the attenuation induced by error in the measurement of a continuously distributed exposure variable. As is true for a binary variable, imperfect measurement of a continuously distributed variable can be seen to result in a substantial attenuation of the association.

In Tables 13-3 and 13-4, it is assumed that the measurement of the

Table 13-4. Effect on the Odds Ratio of Nondifferential Error in the Measurement of a Continuously Distributed Exposure Variable[a]

Correlation between Imperfect Measure of Exposure and True Exposure	True Value of the Odds Ratio for a Difference in Exposure of One Standard Deviation			
	1.5	2.0	5.0	10.0
0.10	1.04	1.07	1.17	1.26
0.20	1.08	1.15	1.38	1.58
0.50	1.22	1.41	2.24	3.16
0.80	1.38	1.74	3.62	6.31
0.90	1.44	1.87	4.26	7.94
0.95	1.47	1.93	4.61	8.91

[a]The entries in the body of the table are the attenuated values of the odds ratio for a difference of one standard deviation in the imperfectly measured exposure variable. Classification in terms of disease status is assumed to be error free.

exposure is imperfect, but that measurement of a binary disease variable is subject to no error. If instead the measurement of a binary disease variable or some continuously distributed outcome such as blood pressure were imperfect but a binary exposure were subject to no measurement error, then the attenuation would be of the same magnitude as in the tables. When both of the variables involved in the association are continuously distributed and one is subject to error, then the attenuated value of the correlation coefficient is the product of the correlation between the true values for the two variables and the correlation between the imperfect measurement and the true values for the variable subject to measurement error (Nunnally, 1978).

For the more typical situation in which both variables are subject to nondifferential measurement error, the magnitude of attenuation will be greater than when one of the two variables is error-free. Furthermore, in order to be certain that this bias is in the direction of the null value, it must be known that the errors in the two variables are independent (Kristensen, 1992; Chavance et al., 1992). For example, in a cross-sectional study the same individuals who fail to report their disease may also fail to report their exposure, particularly if both the exposure and the disease have a certain amount of social stigma attached to them. This correlation of errors can induce a spurious association where none in fact exists, even if the measurement error for each of the variables is nondifferential with respect to an individual's true value for the other variable.

EFFECTS OF MEASUREMENT ERROR WHEN THE INVESTIGATOR CONTROLS FOR CONFOUNDING VARIABLES

As has been emphasized in previous chapters dealing with the analysis of specific types of studies, it is seldom sufficient in observational research to examine only the magnitude of the "crude" association between exposure and disease. Because the investigator must typically control in the analysis for one or more confounding variables, it is important to consider the effects of measurement error on multivariate analyses.

When the confounding variable is measured without error but the exposure (or disease) is imperfectly measured, then the effect of the measurement error is typically to induce apparent effect modification when none exists (Greenland, 1980). Consider an imperfectly measured binary exposure for which sensitivity is 90% and specificity is also 90% within each of the four combinations of disease status and binary confounding variable. Suppose further that the true odds ratio for the association between exposure and disease is 2.0 within both categories of the confounding variable.

From Table 13–3, it can be seen that if the prevalence of exposure differs considerably across the two categories of the confounding variable, then the degree of attenuation may also differ markedly. This differing attenuation occurs because less than perfect specificity contaminates the exposed group with unexposed individuals proportionately more when the exposure is of low prevalence. For example, Table 13–3 shows that if the prevalence of exposure is 1% in the first category and 50% in the second, then there will appear to be virtually no association in the first category (attenuated odds ratio of 1.08) but a more substantial association in the second category (attenuated odds ratio of 1.72). Consequently, whenever a confounding variable is strongly related to an imperfectly measured binary variable, observed differences in the magnitudes of the stratum-specific odds ratios may be in large part an artifact of measurement error. In such circumstances, the investigator must proceed cautiously in interpreting these differences in the magnitudes of the stratum-specific odds ratios.

When the confounding variable itself is subject to nondifferential measurement error, then the same sort of spurious effect modification may result. Another important consequence of error in measuring a confounding variable is prevention of the complete removal of confounding through stratification or other means of adjustment or even a reversal of the direction of a trend for a variable with several categories (Greenland, 1980; Savitz and Baron, 1989; Brenner, 1993). Table 13–5 illustrates the magnitude of the residual confounding that remains after stratification by an imperfectly measured binary confounding variable. In each instance, the true value of the odds ratio is assumed to be 1.0, after the true value of the confounding variable is controlled for. Table 13–5 shows that after an imperfectly measured confounding variable is controlled for, the residual confounding will often result in an odds ratio greater than 2.0. The magnitude of this residual confounding depends to a great extent on the strength of the relationship of the true value of the confounding variable to both the exposure and the disease. In the table, it is assumed that the association between the confounder and the disease is strong (odds ratio = 10.0); the magnitude of the association between the confounder and the exposure is then varied systematically. Only when both of these associations are rather strong is there substantial residual confounding due to error in measuring the confounding variable.

When both the exposure and the confounder are subject to nondifferential measurement error, the effects are less predictable. In that instance the measurement error, even though nondifferential and independent, may yield an adjusted estimate of the odds ratio that is more seriously biased than is a crude estimate that ignores the confounding variable entirely (Greenland, 1980).

Table 13–5. Effect on the Summary Odds Ratio of Nondifferential Error in the Measurement of a Binary Confounding Variable[a]

Sensitivity for Measure of Confounding Variable	Specificity for Measure of Confounding Variable	True Prevalence of Confounding Factor	Odds Ratio for the Relation between the Confounding Variable and Exposure			
			1.5	2.0	5.0	10.0
0.60	0.60	0.1	1.14	1.25	1.62	1.84
		0.5	1.18	1.33	1.94	2.53
		0.9	1.03	1.06	1.14	1.18
0.60	0.90	0.1	1.12	1.21	1.51	1.70
		0.5	1.14	1.25	1.68	2.10
		0.9	1.03	1.06	1.13	1.16
0.60	0.99	0.1	1.07	1.13	1.32	1.43
		0.5	1.11	1.20	1.54	1.87
		0.9	1.03	1.05	1.12	1.16
0.90	0.60	0.1	1.13	1.24	1.57	1.77
		0.5	1.14	1.25	1.68	2.10
		0.9	1.03	1.05	1.11	1.15
0.90	0.90	0.1	1.09	1.16	1.38	1.52
		0.5	1.06	1.12	1.31	1.51
		0.9	1.02	1.04	1.08	1.11
0.90	0.99	0.1	1.03	1.05	1.12	1.17
		0.5	1.03	1.06	1.17	1.27
		0.9	1.02	1.03	1.07	1.09
0.99	0.60	0.1	1.12	1.23	1.55	1.74
		0.5	1.11	1.20	1.54	1.87
		0.9	1.02	1.03	1.07	1.09
0.99	0.90	0.1	1.08	1.14	1.33	1.45
		0.5	1.03	1.06	1.17	1.27
		0.9	1.00	1.01	1.02	1.03
0.99	0.99	0.1	1.01	1.02	1.06	1.08
		0.5	1.00	1.01	1.03	1.05
		0.9	1.00	1.00	1.01	1.01

[a]It is assumed throughout the table that the true value of the summary odds ratio is 1.0, i.e., there is no association between the exposure and disease within true categories of the confounding variables. The entries in the body of the table are the values of the summary odds ratio for the association between exposure and disease, controlling for the imperfectly measured confounding variable. The odds ratio for the relation between the confounding variable and disease is set at 10.0 throughout. Measure of exposure and disease is assumed to be error free, with 50% of the study group exposed and 10% having the disease.

CORRECTING ESTIMATES FOR ERRORS OF KNOWN MAGNITUDE

Recognition of the likely effects of measurement error on study results helps the investigator to avoid drawing inappropriate conclusions from epidemiologic data. Although appropriately tempered conclusions are certainly preferable to unwarranted ones, if possible one should go beyond general statements about the nature of the impact of measurement error on study results and obtain quantitative estimates of what the study results would have been, were it possible to measure the variables without error. Here we consider only simple situations involving just two variables, one of which is subject to measurement error.

If the accuracy or, under certain circumstances, the reliability of measurement for a particular variable is known from previous studies, then it is theoretically possible to employ that information to correct for the effects of measurement error on the magnitude of the observed association in a given study. As applied to correlations among continuously distributed variables, this approach is generally referred to as "correction for attenuation" in the psychometric literature (Nunnally, 1978). If $corr_{xy}$ denotes the observed correlation between two imperfectly measured continuous variables, and if $corr_{XY}$ denotes the true correlation, then ancillary information on the accuracy of each of the two measures ($corr_{xX}$ and $corr_{yY}$) can be used to estimate the true correlation from the observed correlation as follows:

$$corr_{XY} = \frac{corr_{xy}}{corr_{xX} \, corr_{yY}}$$

Suppose, for example, that the correlations of the mismeasured x and y with the true X and Y are 0.60 and 0.80, respectively, and that the observed correlation between the two variables is 0.24. The true value of the correlation that would have been obtained had it been possible to measure both X and Y perfectly is therefore estimated to be $0.24/[(0.60)(0.80)] = 0.50$. As noted earlier in the chapter, measures of the reliability of a measure sometimes yield information about its accuracy. If x and x' are equally accurate measures of X and if the errors in x and x' are independent, then $\sqrt{corr_{xx'}}$ could be used in place of $\sqrt{corr_{xX}}$, and under similar circumstances $\sqrt{corr_{yy'}}$ could be substituted for $corr_{yY}$.

When the odds ratio or some other measure of association appropriate for binary variables is employed, then estimates of accuracy, if available, can be used to correct for measurement error (Copeland et al., 1977). Consider the proportion of cases who are exposed in a case-control study. If P denotes the true proportion exposed, then the observed proportion exposed, here denoted by p, is given by:

$$p = (P)(\text{Sensitivity}) + (1 - P)(1 - \text{Specificity})$$

Solving for P yields the following expression for P in terms of the observed proportion p and available estimates of sensitivity and specificity:

$$P = \frac{p + \text{Specificity} - 1}{\text{Sensitivity} + \text{Specificity} - 1}$$

As an example of error correction when misclassification is nondifferential and independent with respect to case-control status, assume observed prevalences of 0.65 and 0.55 for cases and controls, respectively. The observed odds ratio would in this instance be $[(0.65)(0.45)]/[(0.55)(0.35)] = 1.52$. If the sensitivity and specificity for the classification of exposure are 0.75 and 0.80, respectively, for both cases and controls, then the corrected prevalences of exposure are $(0.65 + 0.80 - 1)/(0.75 + 0.80 - 1) = 0.82$ and $(0.55 + 0.80 - 1)/(0.75 + 0.80 - 1) = 0.64$. The corrected odds ratio is $[(0.82)(0.36)]/[(0.64)(0.18)] = 2.56$. Because nondifferential misclassification of a binary exposure biases the odds ratio toward 1.0, correction in situations such as this leads to corrected odds ratios that are further away from 1.0 than is the observed odds ratio calculated from the misclassified data.

As an example of correction when misclassification is differential, suppose that the observed proportion of cases exposed is 0.40 and that sensitivity and specificity for classifying cases in terms of their exposure is known from previous research to be 0.70 and 0.90, respectively. Then, the true proportion of cases exposed is estimated to be $(0.40 + 0.90 - 1)/(0.70 + 0.90 - 1) = 0.50$. Suppose further that the sensitivity and specificity for classifying controls as exposed are known to be 0.35 and 0.95, respectively. Then if the observed proportion of controls exposed is 0.30, the true proportion of controls exposed is estimated to be $(0.30 + 0.95 - 1)/(0.35 + 0.95 - 1) = 0.83$. Whereas the observed odds ratio is calculated as $[(0.40)(0.70)]/[(0.30)(0.60)] = 1.56$, the corrected odds ratio that takes appropriate account of the differential misclassification of exposure is estimated to be $[(0.50)(0.17)]/[(0.83)(0.50)] = 0.20$. Here correction actually leads to a reversal in the direction of the association, with the exposure initially appearing to increase the risk of disease, but after correction appearing to be protective. The reason for the reversal is that, relative to cases, controls are less likely to report exposure that actually occurred and also less likely to erroneously report exposure that did not occur. Consequently, although the apparent prevalence of exposure among controls is lower than among cases, with correction for misclassification, the actual prevalence is found to be substantially higher.

When information on sensitivity and specificity is not available from previous studies, the investigator may wish to obtain this information from a sample of study participants. For instance, if a relatively accurate measure is available, but is too expensive or difficult to use in all participants, an investigator may use a less accurate but less expensive measure for all participants and use the more accurate and more expensive measure in a small sample of participants. The results from such a *validation substudy* can be used to obtain improved estimates of measures of association. Greenland (1988) has provided guidance as to when it will be more cost effective to take a smaller sample using the more accurate (but more expensive) measure in all participants and when it will be more cost effective to use the less accurate (but less expensive) measure in the main study combined with a validation substudy to assess the impact of measurement error. In general, when the sensitivity or specificity of the less expensive measure is low, or when there is differential misclassification, using the more accurate and expensive measure is generally advisable, even if the sample size must be smaller. Greenland (1988) also gives guidance about the optimal sample size of a validation substudy. Unfortunately, correcting estimates by these methods may be limited in practice by the absence of existing information on sensitivity and specificity, and the inability to undertake a validation substudy. Green (1983) has considered correction of the risk ratio in cohort studies when the disease rather than the exposure is subject to misclassification, the misclassification of disease is nondifferential with respect to exposure, and the disease affects only a relatively small proportion of the group studied. Under these circumstances, the only ancillary information needed to obtain a corrected value for the risk ratio is an estimate of the proportion of those in the unexposed group classified as having the disease who truly do (i.e., the positive predictive value). Although this method was developed specifically for use in cohort studies when an infrequent disease is imperfectly measured, the method is equally applicable to case-control studies in which an exposure of low prevalence is imperfectly measured. In that instance, the observed value of the odds ratio would be used in place of the risk ratio and the relevant positive predictive value would be the proportion of controls classified as exposed who are truly exposed. An illustration of the application of the method to case-control studies is provided in a study of infertility and breast cancer (Gammon and Thompson, 1990).

In this discussion of correcting measures of association for the effects of measurement error, only point estimates have been considered. Although the calculation of confidence intervals for corrected estimates is complex and beyond the scope of this text, such intervals are often considerably wider than would be the corresponding intervals for estimates based on perfectly measured variables. Measurement error thus has the dual adverse effects of biasing estimates and undermining the precision of estimation. This imprecision results from the inevitable error involved in estimating the measures of accuracy or reliability incorporated into a procedure for correction.

The development of methods for obtaining estimates that correct for the effects of measurement error is an expanding area of epidemiology and biostatistics. Here we have presented only selected simple techniques to familiarize the reader with the general approach. Methods have been developed for more complex situations such as multivariate logistic regression (Rosner et al., 1990). References for more detailed and technical reviews of error correction methods include Armstrong et al. (1992), Thomas et al. (1993), and Willett (1989).

USE OF MULTIPLE MEASUREMENTS TO REDUCE THE EFFECTS OF MEASUREMENT ERROR

When the information required to correct estimates is unavailable, an alternative strategy for the control of measurement error is to obtain multiple imperfect measurements of a given variable rather than to rely on a single one. These multiple measurements are then combined to form a single variable that typically corresponds more closely to the values that would be obtained if the variable could be measured without any error.

When the variable of interest is continuously distributed, the usual method for combining multiple measurements is to calculate the mean value. Thus, because blood pressure measurements are known to be subject to considerable error, the usual practice in epidemiologic studies is to take two or more readings and to average them. Likewise, measurement of a behavioral or psychological characteristic such as depression may be improved by including several relevant items in a questionnaire and summing the responses to obtain a scale that presumably corresponds more closely to the actual state of depression than would the response to any single item. Table 13–6 illustrates how much more strongly the mean of multiple imperfect measurements correlates with the true values than does a single imperfect measurement. The values given incorporate the assumption that the errors are independent, that is, that the same errors do not tend to be repeated. To the extent that the multiple errors are not independent, the actual gains from averaging will be less than in the table. It is evident from the table that the use of multiple measurements can enhance accuracy appreciably, although the gain from each additional measurement falls off

Table 13–6. Magnitude of the Correlation between the Mean of Multiple Imperfect Measurements of a Variable and the True Value for that Variable

Correlation among Measurements of X	Number of Independent Measurements of X					
	1	2	3	4	5	10
0.1	.32	.43	.50	.55	.60	.73
0.2	.45	.58	.65	.71	.75	.85
0.5	.71	.82	.87	.89	.91	.95
0.8	.89	.94	.96	.97	.98	.99

as the number of measurements increases. One note of caution is in order, however. Adding additional measurements of a variable will enhance accuracy only if the measurements are of comparable quality. Adding measurements of inferior quality can actually reduce the magnitude of the correlation between the mean of the multiple measurements and the true values. Thus, for example, it is common practice to eliminate the first of several blood pressure measurements because the first reading is more likely to be influenced by extraneous factors such as anxiety on the part of the participant.

For binary variables, simple averaging of multiple measurements is but one of several approaches. Another approach is to use a "strict" definition and treat as having the characteristic only those individuals who have it according to all measurements, and treating all other individuals as not having the characteristic. An additional approach is to use a "loose" definition and assign all individuals who have the characteristic according to at least one of the multiple measurements to the group defined as having the characteristic. Yet another approach, advocated by Marshall and Graham (1984), is to retain for analysis only those observations that are concordant in the sense that the multiple measurements all agree; measurements for which there is disagreement are eliminated from the analysis.

The latter three approaches are contrasted in Tables 13–7 and 13–8 for various combinations of sensitivity and specificity for the case of two imperfect classifications of equal quality. The true prevalence of the characteristic in the comparison group is set at 10%, the true value of the odds ratio is assumed to be 5.0, and the misclassification is assumed to be nondifferential. The performance of each method is assessed in terms of the attenua-

Table 13–7. Value of the Odds Ratio for Various Methods of Combining Multiple Measurements of a Binary Variable[a]

		Method			
Sensitivity	Specificity	Measurement 1 Only	"Strict" Definition	"Loose" Definition	Concordant Observations Only
0.20	0.90	1.27	1.61	1.28	1.69
	0.99	2.83	3.55	2.89	3.87
	1.00	3.77	3.61	3.95	3.95
0.50	0.90	1.97	3.01	1.96	3.48
	0.99	3.62	3.81	3.81	4.49
	1.00	4.13	3.82	4.51	4.51
0.90	0.90	2.86	4.25	2.45	4.57
	0.99	4.44	4.61	4.37	4.97
	1.00	4.79	4.62	4.98	4.98

[a]The true prevalence of the characteristic is 10% in the comparison group, and the true value of the odds ratio is 5.0.

tion of the odds ratio and in terms of the mean squared error of the sample estimate of the log odds ratio.

The results in Table 13–7 indicate that each of these three methods yields values for the odds ratio that are smaller than the true value of 5.0. The magnitude of this bias is generally less when the two measurements are used than when only one is used. Use of "concordant observations only" yields the least biased value. The "loose" definition can be much worse than the other methods when specificity is low. In that instance, the true positives are swamped by false positives and the odds ratio is greatly attenuated as a result of the nondifferential misclassification.

Table 13–8 gives values of the mean squared error for the same set of parameter values. The examples given in the table indicate that when specificity is high (i.e., there are few false positives), a "loose" definition can lead to a much smaller mean squared error than other methods. However, a "loose" definition can lead to a substantially greater mean squared error than the other methods when specificity is low. The method that employs only concordant observations may have a mean squared error that is substantially greater than other methods even though it is the least biased. The mean squared error for methods that employ two measurements is often greater than for those employing only one measurement. Some prior knowledge of the nature of the errors in measurement is required for judicious choice of a method for handling multiple measures of binary variables. For example, unless one is certain that specificity is extremely high, application of a "loose" definition should be avoided, since it can lead to substantial underestimation of the odds ratio. Also, because a "loose" definition places a relatively large number of individuals into the positive

Table 13–8. Value of the Mean Squared Error of the Logarithm of the Odds Ratio for Various Methods of Combining Multiple Measurements of a Binary Variable[a]

		Method			
Sensitivity	Specificity	Measurement 1 Only	"Strict" Definition	"Loose" Definition	Concordant Observations Only
0.20	0.90	13.3	16.6	12.7	15.9
	0.99	5.3	21.2	3.7	20.9
	1.00	4.8	21.5	2.8	21.2
0.50	0.90	6.5	4.4	6.3	3.6
	0.99	2.3	3.9	1.6	3.5
	1.00	2.0	3.9	1.3	3.5
0.90	0.90	2.7	1.3	3.9	1.2
	0.99	1.1	1.2	1.0	1.2
	1.00	1.1	1.2	1.0	1.2

[a]The magnitude of the mean squared error reflects both bias and variation as: (bias)² + variance. The mean squared error has been divided by the variance of the estimator of the log odds ratio when true status for the characteristic is known. The true prevalence of the characteristic is 10% in the comparison group, and the true value of the odds ratio is 5.0. A sample size of 100 in each of the two groups is assumed.

category, the calculated confidence interval for the odds ratio may be quite narrow. Clearly, a narrow interval for a seriously biased estimate is misleading.

CONCLUSION

The examples presented in this chapter illustrate that measurement error can have a major impact on the results of epidemiologic studies. Although an appreciation of the effects of measurement error is critical to the appropriate interpretation of study results, there is, unfortunately, rather little that can be done to rectify such effects at the stage of data analysis unless one has done a validation substudy or has other information with which to correct for measurement error. Consequently, concerns over measurement error are most profitably addressed at the stages of planning a study and collecting the data. We therefore turn in the next two chapters to a consideration of techniques for the measurement of specific variables in epidemiologic research.

REFERENCES

Armstrong BK, White E, Saracci R. 1992. Principles of Exposure Measurement in Epidemiology. New York, Oxford University Press.

Bishop YMM, Fienberg SE, Holland PW. 1975. Discrete Multivariate Analysis. Cambridge, MA, M.I.T. Press.

Brenner H. 1993. Bias due to non-differential misclassification of polytomous confounders. *J Clin Epidemiol* 46:57–63.

Brenner H, Savitz DA, Jockel K-H, Greenland S. 1992. Effects of nondifferential exposure misclassification in ecologic studies. *Am J Epidemiol* 135:85–95.

Chavance M, Dellatolas G, Lellouch J. 1992. Correlated nondifferential misclassifications of disease and exposure: Application to a cross-sectional study of the relation between handedness and immune disorders. *Int J Epidemiol* 21:537–546.

Cohen J. 1960. A coefficient of agreement for nominal scales. *Educ Psychol Meas* 20:37–46.

Copeland KT, Checkoway H, McMichael AJ, Holbrook RH. 1977. Bias due to misclassification in the estimation of relative risk. *Am J Epidemiol* 105:488–495.

Dosemeci M, Wacholder S, Lubin JH. 1990. Does nondifferential misclassification of exposure always bias a true effect toward the null value? *Am J Epidemiol* 132:746–748.

Flegal KM, Keyl PM, Nieto J. 1991. Differential misclassification arising from nondifferential errors in exposure measurement. *Am J Epidemiol* 134:1233–1244.

Fleiss JL. 1975. Measuring agreement between two judges on the presence or absence of a trait. *Biometrics* 31:651–659.

Fleiss JL. 1981. Statistical Methods for Rates and Proportions. New York, Wiley.

Gammon MD, Thompson WD. 1990. Infertility and breast cancer: a population-based case-control study. *Am J Epidemiol* 132:708–716.

Green M. 1983. Use of predictive value to adjust relative risk estimates biased by misclassification of outcome status. *Am J Epidemiol* 117:98–105.

Greenland S. 1980. The effect of misclassification in the presence of covariates. *Am J Epidemiol* 112:564–569.

Greenland S. 1988. Statistical uncertainty due to misclassification: Implication for validation substudies. *J Clin Epidemiol* 41:1167–1174.

Greenland S. 1992. Divergent biases in ecologic and individual-level studies. *Stat Med* 11:1209–1223.

Gullen WH, Bearman JE, Johnson EA. 1968. Effects of misclassification in epidemiologic studies. *Public Health Rep* 83:914–918.

Kraemer HC. 1979. Ramifications of a population model for κ as a coefficient of reliability. *Psychometrika* 44:461–472.

Kristensen P. 1992. Bias from nondifferential but dependent misclassification of exposure and outcome. *Epidemiology* 3:210–215.

Marshall JR, Graham S. 1984. Use of dual responses to increase validity of case-control studies. *J Chron Dis* 37:125–136.

Newell DJ. 1962. Errors in the interpretation of errors in epidemiology. *Am J Public Health* 52:1925–1928.

Nunnally JC. 1978. *Psychometric Theory.* New York, McGraw-Hill.

Paganini-Hill A, Ross RK. 1982. Reliability of recall of drug usage and other health-related information. *Am J Epidemiol* 116:114–122.

Rosner B, Spiegelman D, Willett WC. 1990. Correction of logistic regression relative risk estimates and confidence intervals for measurement error: the case of multiple covariates measured with error. *Am J Epidemiol* 132:734–745.

Savitz DA, Baron AE. 1989. Estimating and correcting for confounder misclassification. *Am J Epidemiol* 129:1062–1071.

Thomas D, Stram D, Dwyer J. 1993. Exposure measurement error: Influences on exposure-disease relationships and methods of correction. *Annu Rev Public Health* 14:69–93.

Thompson WD. 1990. Kappa and attenuation of the odds ratio. *Epidemiology* 1:357–369.

Thompson WD, Walter SD. 1988. A reappraisal of the kappa coefficient. *J Clin Epidemiol* 41:947–958.

Wacholder S, Dosemeci M, Lubin J. 1991. Blind assignment of exposure does not always prevent misclassification. *Am J Epidemiol* 134:433–437.

Weinberg CR, Umbach DM, Greenland S. 1994. When will nondifferential misclassification of an exposure preserve the direction of a trend? *Am J Epidemiol* 140:565–571.

Willett W. 1989. An overview of issues related to the correction of non-differential exposure measurement error in epidemiologic studies. *Stat Med* 8:1031–1040.

EXERCISES

1. A brief written questionnaire concerning hearing deficits was used in a general population group. All of the participants were subsequently given thorough hearing

tests and were then classified with essentially no error as to whether they had a hearing deficit. The researchers were interested in evaluating the appropriateness of using the questionnaire as an inexpensive substitute for the definitive but costly hearing test in future epidemiologic studies. Of the total group, 15% had hearing deficits according to both the questionnaire and the hearing test, 10% had a deficit according to the questionnaire only, and 5% had a deficit according to the hearing test only. What are the sensitivity and specificity for the questionnaire?

2. In a case-control study, it is found that 20% of the cases have the exposure of interest as opposed to 15% of the controls. It is known from previous methodological work that the classification for exposure is subject to some error, which is nondifferential and independent with respect to case-control status. It is thought that the sensitivity is somewhere between 60% and 75% and that the specificity is somewhere between 90% and 95%. Calculate improved estimates of the odds ratio using this information on the accuracy of the exposure classification.

3. In order to assess the quality of data from death certificates, multiple coders have independently coded a large number of certificates using the rules of the International Classification of Diseases. The results of such methodological studies usually demonstrate a high level of agreement between coders as to the underlying cause of death. Comment on the value of these methodological studies for assessing the quality of data from death certificates.

4. Two equally accurate laboratory methods of testing for the presence of a specific chromosomal abnormality are available. Both tests are performed on each member of a case group and of a control group. It is known from extensive prior studies that neither of the tests yields any false positives but that 40% of abnormalities are missed by the first test and that 40% are missed by the second. How would you combine the results of the two tests into a single exposure variable for purposes of assessing the association between the abnormality and the disease under study? What is your rationale?

5. In a cohort study of the possible effects of a drug on the incidence of a rare blood disorder, 8 out of 10,000 exposed individuals actually develop the disorder, as opposed to 3 out of 10,000 unexposed individuals. What would be the observed risk ratio if, instead of using a completely accurate diagnostic technique, an investigator settled for one having a sensitivity of 99% and a specificity of 98%?

6. In a survey of upper respiratory infections, instructions to the people recording the data were to code "1" for the gender variable if the participant was a female and to code a "2" if the participant was a male. However, one of the people recording the data misread the instructions and coded "1" for males and "2" for females. Assuming that this error goes undetected, what effect would you expect to see on the odds ratio relating gender and prevalence of upper respiratory disease?

7. In a study by Paganini-Hill and Ross (1982), the medical charts of 50 out of 217 participants indicated some use of antihypertensives other than reserpine. During an interview, 44 of the 217 reported use of antihypertensives other than reserpine. There was no indication of any use of these drugs from either source of information for 154 women. Calculate the value of kappa for the agreement between medical charts and interview for this variable.

14

Measurement I: Questionnaires

Most epidemiologic studies use questionnaires to obtain at least some information from participants regarding their exposure to possible risk factors, their exposure to potential confounding variables, or the occurrence of the diseases of interest. For instance, cohort studies attempting to identify risk factors for coronary heart disease use questionnaires to obtain data on smoking habits as a possible risk factor or as a possible confounding variable when other associations are being considered; such studies also often obtain information by questionnaire on the occurrence of angina pectoris as one of the outcomes of interest. Case-control studies concerned with such exposures as smoking or use of oral contraceptives most often ascertain exposure to these possible risk factors by means of questionnaires. Even when information on the risk factor and disease of primary interest is obtained through laboratory measurement or through existing records, data on potential confounding variables may have to be determined by questionnaire. In addition, various symptoms, measures of disability, and other indicators of quality of life can be determined only by asking people. Thus, good methods of questionnaire design are of crucial importance to epidemiologists. Whereas statistical analysis can be repeated if done incorrectly initially, there is seldom a second chance to obtain information by questionnaire from large numbers of participants if the questionnaire was poorly constructed in the first place.

As with any method of measurement, data obtained by questionnaire should have a high degree of validity and reliability. *Validity* refers to the extent to which an instrument measures what it purports to measure, and *reliability* refers to the extent to which results obtained by a measurement procedure can be replicated. Measurement of validity and reliability and the consequences of failure to achieve a reasonable degree of reliability were covered in Chapter 13.

DEFINITIONS

Because different terms are used by various investigators to describe certain characteristics of questionnaires, the definitions to be followed in this book will be given here. A *questionnaire* will be considered to be the written document used to obtain information from respondents, regardless of whether it is self-administered or administered by an interviewer. When questions are asked by an interviewer, only *structured* (sometimes called standardized or formal) interviewing, in which the interviewer asks all participants the same questions in the same way, will be considered here. This contrasts with *unstructured* (sometimes called unstandardized or informal) interviewing, in which the questions asked of respondents may vary at the discretion of the interviewer. Although informal interviewing may be useful in clinical settings, it is of little value in epidemiologic studies in which the same data must be available on all respondents in order for the data to be properly quantified and analyzed.

Closed-ended questions will refer to those in which all possible answers to a given question are listed on the questionnaire, whereas the term *open-ended* will apply to questions in which the possible answers are not listed in advance. For continuously distributed variables, open-ended questions are usually necessary; for example, it would not generally be practical to list all possible answers in advance to the question, "What is your height?" For categorical variables, however, closed-ended questions are usually preferred because the possible answers are often easily precoded. *Precoded (or self-coded) questions* refer to those in which the number assigned to a given answer is printed next to the possible answer on the questionnaire, so that additional coding is not required. Precoded answers are desirable because this saves the time of assigning numbers (i.e., coding) later and because the additional step of assigning numbers later provides one more opportunity for errors. However, when all possible answers cannot be anticipated in advance, precoded questions may not be possible. When precoding is not feasible, the answers to the open-ended questions will have to be coded and quantified after the data have been collected, although a general plan for such coding should be specified in advance.

To illustrate the use of these terms, three different ways of asking about a person's legal marital status are presented:

Open-ended:

What is your current marital status?

Closed-ended, not precoded:

Are you currently (circle one)

married?

widowed?

divorced?

separated?

or have you never been married?

Closed-ended, precoded:

Are you currently (circle correct number)

married?	1
widowed?	2
divorced?	3
separated?	4
or have you never been married?	5

The open-ended version is the least desirable way of asking the question. Not only will the answer have to be coded later, thus adding to the expense of the study and increasing the likelihood of error, but some divorced, separated, widowed, and never married people may give the answer "single," and the investigator will not know what "single" really means. The closed-ended non-precoded version would probably elicit the correct answer, but would require coding at a later time, thus costing a coder's salary and adding to the likelihood of error. Therefore, the closed-ended precoded format is the preferred approach.

During the next several years, it is likely that more opportunities will become available to have answers submitted directly to a computer as they are given, thus further increasing efficiency. The use of computers by interviewers will be briefly discussed at the end of the section on interviewing by telephone. In clinical settings, favorable experience has been reported with direct entry of responses by the patient into a computer (O'Connor et al., 1989; Wong et al., 1986); direct entry by participants in epidemiologic studies may become more common in the future.

METHODS OF OBTAINING INFORMATION

The three common means of obtaining information through questionnaires are (a) by sending a questionnaire through the mail for the individual to fill out and return; (b) by having an interviewer administer a questionnaire over the telephone; and (c) by having an interviewer administer a questionnaire in person. Sometimes combinations of these methods are used. The next section will discuss some of the advantages and disadvantages of these three methods. For more detailed descriptions of postal questionnaires and personal and telephone interviewing, the reader is referred to other books and articles (Dillman, 1978; Groves and Kahn, 1979; Moser and Kalton, 1979; Siemiatycki, 1979; Weeks et al., 1983; Cartright, 1988; O'Toole et al., 1986; Rolnick et al., 1989).

Postal Questionnaires

The major advantage of sending a questionnaire through the mail is that compared to interviewing, it is inexpensive. In a postal survey second and third mailings may have to be used for initial nonrespondents, but the cost of postage is still much lower than the cost of paying for interviewers to locate participants and administer a questionnaire to them. Also, a study that collects information through the mail is likely to be completed much sooner than one that uses in-person interviewing. In many studies, all questionnaires can be sent out at once, and after a few weeks, second mailings and then third mailings can be sent to nonrespondents in order to try to achieve an acceptable response. Dillman (1978) recommends the following sequence after the original mailing:

> *One week after initial mailing:* Send a postcard reminder to everyone. This serves both to thank the respondents and to remind the nonrespondents in a courteous manner that their questionnaires have not yet been received.
> *Three weeks after initial mailing:* Send a letter and replacement questionnaire only to the nonrespondents. The covering letter is shorter; it informs nonrespondents that their questionnaires have not been received and appeals for their return.
> *Seven weeks after initial mailing:* Send a letter similar to the second one and a replacement questionnaire by certified mail in order to emphasize its importance.

Response rates can sometimes be raised further with follow-up by telephone of those still not responding, or, if the study is being undertaken in a relatively circumscribed geographic area, by in-person interviewing. All these additional steps take time and money, but the time and expense are not nearly so great as when *all* participants are contacted and interviewed one by one.

Because of the reduced cost per participant, a larger number of persons can be included with a postal questionnaire than with an interviewer-administered questionnaire, for a fixed total cost. Also, it is more feasible to include a wide geographic area. For instance, a study undertaken several years ago in England, Wales, and Scotland to determine whether air pollution increased the risk for chronic bronchitis (Lambert and Reid, 1970) has been mentioned in previous chapters. Because any effect of air pollution was likely to be small relative to the effect of cigarette smoking, a large number of participants was needed to provide sufficient power to detect any effect that air pollution might have. Also, it was important to cover a wide geographic area so as to have representation from communities with a variety of levels of air pollution. Although interviewers could have been recruited, trained, and supervised in all parts of the country, a postal questionnaire was much more practical.

Another circumstance favoring the use of postal questionnaires is when the respondent will need time to obtain the desired information. For instance, records of immunizations or of income may have to be sought. If information is being requested from a physician, time will usually be needed to locate the medical records. Some investigators report that questions that are sensitive or potentially embarrassing are more likely to be answered in a postal survey than in an interview (Siemiatycki, 1979); others do not find this (Cartright, 1988; Rolnick et al., 1989). A final potential advantage of self-administered questionnaires is that no opportunity exists for an interviewer to introduce bias into a study by the way he or she either asks questions or records answers.

On the other hand, postal questionnaires are associated with a number of potential disadvantages, many of which have been enumerated by Moser and Kalton (1979). Perhaps most important is that a substantial number of people do not return questionnaires. Typical response rates are 40% to the first mailing, and perhaps 60% after three mailings. Respondents almost inevitably differ systematically from nonrespondents. For instance, respondents tend to be better educated and more interested in the subject matter of the study. In addition to substantial nonresponse to the questionnaire as a whole, individual questions are frequently left unanswered.

Another limitation is that the questions and the instructions associated with them have to be relatively simple and straightforward. Often if a person says yes to one question, a certain series of questions is asked, and if the answer is no, another series of questions is asked. This can usually be done only to a limited extent if self-administered questionnaires are used; otherwise, the participants become confused. If a participant misunderstands a question, there is no interviewer around to repeat the question; in other words, the questionnaire is generally inflexible and the answers final. Exceptions to this occur when misunderstandings can be cleared up by follow-up telephone calls or personal visits.

If the order in which the questions are asked matters, then a self-administered questionnaire cannot be used because the respondent may read the entire questionnaire before answering the questions. Similarly, if it is important that the respondent not receive help from others in filling out the questionnaire, then a postal questionnaire cannot be used because the respondent has the opportunity to consult with anyone around. If spontaneous answers are desired, then postal questionnaires should not be used because the respondent would have ample time to think about the questions. Boring or tedious questions may be ignored by the respondent.

Postal questionnaires are also not appropriate when it is important to observe the setting in which the participant lives or if the participant is illiterate. Even if literate, some people just find it easier to talk than to write.

In general, however, low response rates remain the greatest problem. One way of preserving to a large extent the relatively low cost associated with postal surveys while increasing the response rate is to follow up nonrespondents with telephone interviews or home interviews. It has been shown that in many situations, this results in about as high a response rate as home interviewing alone (Siemiatycki, 1979). However, the comparability of the information obtained by the two methods must be assessed. Another approach to the nonresponse problem is to send a shorter questionnaire with certain key items to nonrespondents in the hope that they will be more likely to answer the shorter series of questions. Alternatively, if it is not essential to have all items answered by the same people, different parts of the same questionnaire may be sent to randomly selected groups of people in the hope that all the answers together will provide a composite picture.

Inclusion of a self-addressed stamped return envelope is obviously important. Higher response rates are also obtained when an actual postage stamp is used rather than a postage meter. Sponsorship and a convincing covering letter can affect response rates. "Selling" the study and questionnaire at the beginning of the covering letter is important. In the questionnaire itself, starting with questions of interest and concern to the respondents is desirable. A neat, clean, orderly format that makes it very easy for the respondent to follow the questions and record the answers is of the utmost importance. Monetary incentives (Perneger et al., 1993; Spry et al., 1989) and leaving messages on answering machines (Spry et al., 1989) may also increase response rates.

Nevertheless, because of the usual difficulty in obtaining acceptable response rates and because of the various other constraints, postal questionnaires are mainly used when other means of obtaining data are prohibitively expensive or in situations in which the target population is known to be highly motivated.

Telephone Interviewing

Interviewing over the telephone has been used with increasing frequency in recent years as a means of reducing the costs from what they would be if in-person interviewing were used, yet securing a higher response rate than is usually obtained with postal questionnaires. Some investigators have reported that a survey conducted by telephone costs about half of one that uses in-person interviewing (Groves and Kahn, 1979; Weeks et al., 1983), but others (O'Toole et al., 1986) report little difference in cost. In the past, telephone interviewing has occupied an intermediate position with respect to cost and response rate when compared to postal questionnaires and personal interviewing. Postal questionnaires are the least expensive, but people find it easy not to respond by simply discarding the questionnaire. In-person interviewing is the most expensive, but people find it harder to close the door in someone's face than to hang up the telephone. In recent years, however, this has been partly compensated for by the reluctance of people to open their doors to strangers, even if they do carry proper identification. It is of interest to note the finding of Groves and Kahn (1979) that telephone interviewing secures relatively higher response rates in cities, and in-person interviewing achieves relatively higher rates in rural areas. As of 1993, 94% of households in the United States had telephones (U.S. Bureau of the Census, 1994), so that although the poor are underrepresented among those with telephones (Jaffe, 1984; U.S. Bureau of the Census, 1994), bias from including only people with telephones is considerably reduced over what it used to be. Thus, the advantages of in-person interviewing over telephone interviewing may be less now than in the past.

Sending a cover letter before the initial telephone call tends to increase response rates. The introduction given over the telephone is crucial. Dillman (1978) suggests including the name of the interviewer, the name of the institution and city from which the call is being made, how the respondent's name was obtained, a brief statement of the purpose of the survey, an estimate of how many minutes the interview will take, and an opportunity for potential respondents to ask questions. Selection of interviewers who not only can ask the questions as instructed but who can also speak clearly, read questions fluently, be understood easily over the telephone, and deal with questions from the respondent is important. In addition, their voices should not be so loud or harsh as to interfere with other interviewers making telephone calls nearby. Careful training is needed. Many of the qualities desired for interviewers who will be interviewing participants in person, described in some detail in the next section, also pertain to telephone interviewers, except, of course, that appearance is not a concern.

Compared to in-person interviewing, telephone interviewing facilitates the inclusion of larger numbers of people over a wider geographic area over a much shorter period of time. Travel time is saved because interviewers can contact potential participants from one convenient location. Supervision and monitoring of interviewers is facilitated. It is less frustrating for the interviewer and less expensive when a telephone appointment is broken than when the interviewer has driven to someone's house. The interviewer is safer when telephoning, especially if evening interviews are necessary. The participant may feel more anonymity when the interview takes place over the telephone. In contrast to postal questionnaires, a telephone interview allows stated sources of confusion to be cleared up promptly, as long as the respondent feels comfortable admitting that he or she does not understand.

Telephone interviewing also has certain disadvantages. The respondents cannot be shown anything, such as pictures or lists of possible answers on cards, unless these are sent to the respondents in advance and are brought to the telephone for the interview. For instance, participants often find it easier to recognize pills they have taken by sight rather than by name. The setting in which a person lives cannot be observed over the telephone. More data are missing when telephone rather than in-person interviewing is used (Groves and Kahn, 1979). If specimens must be collected, such as blood or urine samples, telephone interviewing obviously will not suffice. Interviewers may find it more difficult to establish rapport with people over the telephone than in person, although this may vary from one interviewer to another. The interviewer may feel rushed over the telephone, since the interviewer may not know whether the respondent was in the middle of some other activity. It is easier for the telephone respondent than an individual being interviewed in person to terminate the interview, that is, by hanging up. People may be more suspicious if they cannot see the person to whom they are talking, and they may think their participation less important than if the interviewer has taken the time to make the trip to their home. The interviewer does not know if he or she has the full attention of the respondent and cannot see facial expressions of puzzlement. Thus, questions generally have to be simpler than when in-person interviewing is used. Finally, experience indicates that individuals who are ill can be interviewed more easily in person than by telephone.

In some studies, telephone interviewing may be used as a screening device to determine eligibility. If the person meets the study criteria as indicated by the questions asked over the telephone, then an appointment is made for a longer in-person interview. In a case-control study to identify occupations associated with a high risk of cancer of the larynx, the investigators wanted to match cases to hospital controls on age, gender, and smoking status (Zagraniski et al., 1986). Age and gender could be abstracted from hospital records, but smoking status, a potentially strong confounding variable, was not always included on the records. Accordingly, a short questionnaire administered over the telephone was used to determine whether the potential controls matched the cases on smoking habits. In a case-control study of prolapsed intervertebral discs, the investigators wanted to include only persons with symptoms of recent onset (Kelsey et al., 1984). Therefore, before in-person interviews were conducted, potential cases and controls were contacted by telephone whenever possible so that a short questionnaire could be administered and the nature and length of symptoms determined. The telephone screening saved considerable money by approximately halving the number of in-person interviews needed. In addition, many of the respondents were so pleased to have the opportunity to talk about their back pain that the telephone interviewing led to a higher response rate for the subsequent in-person interviewing than might otherwise have been obtained.

Another use of telephone interviewing mentioned in Chapter 8 was in random-digit dialing to find controls in case-control studies. Random-digit dialing may also be used as a means of identifying participants when a probability sample of the community is needed for a prevalence study. Sometimes the randomly selected individual is administered the entire interview over the telephone, but more often, a short questionnaire is given over the telephone in order to find out whether any household members are eligible for the study. The short questionnaire may seek to obtain a census of people living in the household according to age and gender, for instance. The entire questionnaire can subsequently be administered in person to eligible participants.

In summary, if nothing needs to be shown, if specimens do not have to be collected, and if interviewers skillful at securing cooperation over the telephone are used, telephone interviewing may be one way to reduce the cost and hazards associated with in-person interviewing. It may be particularly useful as a screening device.

Finally, computer-assisted telephone interviewing is being used with increasing frequency (Shanks et al., 1981). While administering the questionnaire, the interviewer uses a computer terminal, and when the questions appear on the screen and are asked of the respondent, the interviewer enters the responses directly into the terminal (Harlow et al., 1985). Range and logic checks can be built into the entry programs, so that only responses that pass the checks or that are manually overridden are entered. Other advantages include the ease with which complex question branching can be done for the interviewer; the ability of the computer to modify questions in a standardized way depending on answers to previous questions; ease of supervision of interviewers; reduction in the time needed for editing, coding, and other aspects of data management; and the facilitation of many aspects of survey management, such as sample selection, optimal scheduling of telephone calls, and frequent reports on sampling and field work performance (Wong et al., 1986). Disadvantages include the increased time needed to train interviewers the first time they use such a system; the lack of flexibility built into the system; and hardware and computer operator failures. Also important to keep in mind is the enormous investment of time and computer skills required to set up a computer-assisted interview system (Harlow et al., 1985; Shanks, 1983). The limited data presently available suggest that use of a computer does not affect response rates, the proportion of answers recorded as "don't know," or the quality of the interviews as judged by the interviewer. The interview may be slightly longer with a computer, and the number of recorded comments may be fewer (Harlow et al., 1985).

In-Person Interviewing

In-person interviewing, with properly trained and motivated interviewers, is still the most frequently used method of obtaining data in epidemiologic studies. It generally secures relatively high response rates, usually enables the best rapport to be established between the interviewer and participants, permits the participants to be shown samples and cards, and allows specimens to be collected. In-person interviewing also provides more flexibility because the interviewer is better able to sense when the respondent is confused, distracted, or otherwise unable to understand what is being asked. However, the allowance of more flexibility and the establishment of rapport can lead to lack of standardization, so that selection of interviewers and their training are highly important. Therefore, a few comments will first be made about the interviewer and the nature of his or her work.

The difficulty of the interviewer's job is often not recognized or appreciated, yet the quality of the interviewer's work has an enormous influence on the success of a study. In many situations a letter introducing the study is sent through the mail, and the interviewer's first task is to locate and make contact with the person. Finding potential participants, usually at home, is often time-consuming and difficult. Several visits to the home are often necessary, and if appointments are made in advance, they are broken much more frequently than one might expect.

Once the person is located, obtaining an interview can be challenging. People are busy, suspicious, and often do not want to "get involved." Over the past several years, response rates in studies using in-person interviewing have generally been decreasing. A letter indicating the sponsoring organization, explaining why the study is being done, and describing the potential participants' rights helps pave the way for the interviewer, and in fact is usually required by Institutional Review Boards. Interviewers should carry and show suitable identification. Politeness, of course, helps. The interviewer should be sufficiently sensitive to know when to be more assertive, when to be less assertive, when to offer to come back at another more convenient time, and when to try to obtain the interview on the spot. All the while, it must be kept in mind that the person does have the right not to participate, even though response rates that are too low raise questions about the validity of any results obtained.

After the person has agreed to be interviewed, the interviewer must ask the questions according to instructions. The interviewer thus should be someone who can follow instructions and who recognizes the need to ask questions in the same way of all participants. Many people cannot do this; they must be identified and dismissed as interviewers in a trial period before the actual study begins. One of the most common problems is for interviewers to put words in the respondent's mouth: "You didn't take this pill, did you?" rather than "Did you take this pill?" This is a particular temptation for interviewers when the respondent is struggling with an answer and the interviewer thinks he or she knows the answer.

Although interviewers should be as consistent as possible from one respondent to another and although a good questionnaire should make such standardization easy and natural, some situations occur in which an interviewer must reword a question or use "probes" to obtain information from a person who has not understood the question or who has not answered appropriately. Again, an interviewer should sense when this is necessary, should know that questions should be reworded only as a last resort, and should be carefully trained as to when and how this should be done. As an example, a respondent might answer "nothing" to the question, "What were you doing when your back started to hurt?" This is an unacceptable answer because "nothing" may mean any number of positions or activities, such as sitting, lying down, walking, or waking. An appropriate probe following such an answer would be "What do you mean by 'nothing?'" To use a probe such as "Do you mean you were sitting?" would bias respondents to say that they were sitting, so it is important that interviewers be trained to probe in a neutral manner and not to put words in people's mouths.

Another task of the interviewer is to record the answers according to specified instructions. Because an interviewer's job is often tiring and repetitious, errors can occur. Good questionnaire format is conducive to better recording. If for some reason the interviewer is uncertain as to how the respondent's answer should be handled, the response can always be recorded verbatim on the questionnaire and later called to the attention of the study director, who can decide how to quantify it.

Finally, the interviewer should check through the questionnaire, preferably before leaving the respondent, and clear up any discrepancies, ambiguities, omissions, or other problems. The interviewer's supervisor should also check through all completed questionnaires and promptly call to the interviewer's attention any errors or discrepancies.

As to what qualities one looks for when hiring interviewers, they should have the obvious characteristics of being tactful, careful, sensitive, polite, accurate, adaptable, interested, honest, assertive enough but not too assertive, perseverant, and able to withstand tiring work. (One eminent professor who was a reader of the first edition of this book commented that these are the very qualities that one seeks in a spouse.) In many studies, evening and weekend work is necessary. It is often impossible to tell what kind of an interviewer a person will be until he or she actually starts conducting interviews. The subjective impression prospective interviewers make when they are being interviewed for the job is one very good indicator of how they will do on the job, because in both situations they are trying to make a good impression and to persuade another person of either their own capabilities or of the importance of participation in the study.

Because of the repetitive nature of the work, part-time employment may be preferable to full-time employment. Job turnover among interviewers is high, and interviewers should in fact be encouraged to leave if they become bored or sloppy because such bad habits are not readily correctable. Varying the nature of their work, such as by giving them coding or other office tasks to do, can add some variety to their job.

Several weeks of training are often needed, including observing experienced interviewers, interviewing the project director and others around the office followed by critiques of the interview, and trial interviews with people similar to those who will actually be included in the study. Interviewing people who are like the actual participants is important because it is a big step from interviewing those with whom one feels reasonably comfortable to interviewing people who will answer and react in somewhat unpredictable ways. An interviewing manual should be prepared, covering both interviewing techniques in general and techniques and issues specific to the study being done. Included in the manual should be suggestions for neutral probes to be used in specific situations and instructions as to how to handle problems that may arise. Interviewers should review this manual periodically during the course of the study.

The supervisor should also observe each interviewer conducting actual interviews at stated intervals throughout the course of the study. Although an interviewer may be on his or her "best behavior" when being observed, any consistent or habitual deviations from what is desired may be detected and corrected. In some studies a sample of the people interviewed by each interviewer is recontacted by the supervisor to make certain that the interviews actually took place and to check on the consistency of answers to a few questions. As stated above, the supervisor should check each completed questionnaire for any omissions and obvious inaccuracies. Weekly meetings to review completed questionnaires individually with each interviewer are desirable, and meetings of all interviewers as a group should be held about once a month. Such meetings enable the supervisor to keep abreast of any unanticipated problems and enhance the morale of the interviewers, who can share problems and possible solutions and can be made to feel more a part of the overall effort.

COMMON PROBLEMS IN QUESTIONNAIRES

Construction of questionnaires almost always takes *much* longer than expected. Attention must of course be given to the general format, flow, and length of the questionnaire. An appropriate introduction must be developed, along with transitions from one subject to another. When possible, the questions of greatest interest to the participants should come at the beginning. Consideration must be given to whether the questionnaire is to be administered in person or by telephone, or is to be self-administered. However, deciding on how to ask individual questions is one of the biggest challenges in questionnaire design. The next section of this chapter will therefore categorize, with examples, some of the most common mistakes made in constructing individual questions.

Ambiguous Questions

An example of an ambiguous question was given earlier in this chapter: "Are you currently single, married, divorced, separated, or widowed?"

Here the intent is that only persons who have never been married classify themselves as single, yet many divorced, separated, or widowed persons also may consider themselves single. Therefore, if the investigator really wants to know if respondents have never been married, the question should be worded, "Are you currently married, divorced, separated, widowed, or have you never been married?"

"Have you ever smoked?"

What is meant by "smoked?" Does it mean cigarettes only, or marijuana, cigars, and pipes as well? Does "ever" mean even the one and only cigarette that many people tried when they were youngsters? Unless even this small amount of cigarette smoking is of interest, it is better to use a question such as "Have you ever smoked as much as one cigarette a day for as long as a year?"

"Do your menstrual cycles come at reasonably regular intervals?"

What is meant by "reasonably regular?" To some women, this may mean exactly every 28 days, and to others 28 days plus or minus 3 or 4 days. To others it may mean exactly every 33 days. The word "regular" is almost always ambiguous and should be avoided whenever possible. In the present context, it is not known whether "regular" refers to the so-called normal cycle of 28 days, to consistency in cycle length, be it 28 days, 23 days, or 35 days, or to both facets of periodicity. Also, it is unlikely that women will know what is considered normal variation in cycle length and what is not. Therefore, this question needs to be broken up into several more specific parts. Begin by asking how many days, on average, there are between the first day of one menstrual cycle and the first day of the next; then ask whether over the past 12 months (or other defined time period) these cycles have varied by less than 2 days, 3 to 5 days, 6 to 7 days, or greater than 7 days, on average. Even then, many women find this question difficult to answer.

Questions That Are Not Self-Explanatory

"What kind of home do you have?"

Different people have different frames of reference for this question. Some people might answer, "an apartment." Others might say, "a large one." Some might say, "a nice one," and still others, "a red-brick one." The question does not explain what category of answer is sought.

"How is heat delivered to your home?"

In this instance, the investigators were interested in whether heat was delivered in the form of hot air, hot water, steam, or other means. However, what people often said was that the heat was delivered in a fuel truck.

One way of dealing with this problem is, immediately after the question is asked, to read off the possible answers, such as (a) a one-family house, (b) a multiple-family house, (c) an apartment, (d) a room in someone else's house or apartment, (e) a condominium, (f) a trailer, or (g) some other type of home. Another approach is to hand the respondent a card with the possible answers:

1. hot air
2. hot water
3. steam
4. fireplace
5. stove
6. space heater
7. other _____ (Specify)
8. do not know

Two Questions in One

"Do you get out of breath when you walk up a hill?"

The problem here is that an answer of no may mean that the respondent does not walk up hills, or may mean that the respondent does walk up hills but does not get out of breath when doing so.

"Do you bring up phlegm when you cough?"

An answer of no may mean that the respondent does not cough or may mean that when he or she does cough, no phlegm is brought up.

The solution to this type of problem is to construct two different questions such that the second is asked only of respondents who answer yes to the first. For instance, the first question might be divided into "Do you walk up any incline or hill at least once a week?" People who answered yes to that question would then be asked whether they get out of breath when they do so.

Use of Words That Some Respondents Do Not Understand

"What was your age at menarche?"

Many women will not know what menarche is, so it is preferable to ask them how old they were when their menstrual periods started.

"Do you have lumbago?"

Although in England people apparently know that lumbago means low back pain, in an American study (Acheson, 1969) people reported having lumbago in their shoulders, heads, and elsewhere in addition to their low backs. This problem is easily taken care of by asking about low back pain rather than lumbago.

"Have you ever worked with polycyclic aromatic hydrocarbons?"

Most people will not know whether they have worked with polycyclic aromatic hydrocarbons, so that words that in fact are understood by participants must be substituted. Unfortunately, workers often do not know what specific agents they have been exposed to, and it is necessary to obtain such information by other means than merely asking the participants.

Asking About Events That Most People Will Not Remember

"How many times per week did you eat carrots when you were between the ages of 6 and 10?"

Investigators often engage in wishful thinking that people will actually be able to remember such activities. Furthermore, because people will frequently give some sort of answer (often in order to please the interviewer or to hasten the interview along), the investigator can be fooled into thinking that the answers are accurate. A critical look needs to be taken at any questions that relate to events that occurred long ago and that may not have had as much significance to the participants as to the investigator. As noted in Chapter 13, if no association is found between frequency of eating carrots during childhood and the disease under study, the investigator does not know whether measurement of carrot eating was so poor that a real association is obscured, or whether no association really exists between carrot consumption and the disease.

Hypothetical Questions

"Would you like to move to another place of residence?"

Almost everyone would answer yes to this question because, if money were not an issue, probably some improvement in a person's living situation could be made. In addition, answers to questions about what a person would do if put in a certain situation generally correlate poorly with what a person actually does in practice.

Insufficient Numbers of Categories

"When you go camping do you sleep in a camper, trailer, or tent?"

People who sleep in the open air without any of these forms of shelter have no category in which to place themselves. It would have been better to ask, "When you go camping, do you sleep in a camper, trailer, or tent, or do you usually sleep somewhere else?" If the answer is "somewhere else," the respondent should then be asked to specify what is meant, and this can be recorded on the questionnaire.

The use of this "other" category with instructions to specify exactly what is meant is important for any questions in which all possible answers are not given. For instance, in a case-control study of prolapsed lumbar discs (Kelsey and Hardy, 1975), cases and controls were asked what type of chair they usually sat in at work and were shown a card with pictures of various types of chairs. It turned out that the main difference between cases and controls in their answer to this question was that there was a large excess of cases compared to controls in the category, "other type of chair." When the investigators went back to the actual questionnaires, they found that this excess of "other type of chair" among the cases was attributable entirely to motor vehicle seats. This led to the finding, unanticipated when the study began but since confirmed in other epidemiologic and biomechanics studies, that driving of motor vehicles and exposure to vibration predispose to prolapsed intervertebral discs. If the "other" category had not been used, or if the respondents had not been asked to specify what "other" meant, this finding would have been missed.

Questions That Are Too Long, With Too Many Ideas

"Have you ever used birth control pills, estrogen replacement therapy, tranquilizers, or diuretics?"

Although this question appears straightforward, a great tendency exists among respondents to remember only the last item that is mentioned, which, in this instance, is "diuretics." Accordingly, respondents will tend to answer only regarding their diuretic use. Thus, each medication should be asked about separately.

"On this card are three types of household and leisure-time activities. Would you please tell me which one you spend the most time in and which the least."

1. Household chores and working in the yard (housework, repairs, washing dishes, etc.)
2. Social activities (visiting, entertaining, etc.)
3. Reading, watching television, or listening to the radio

The concept of ranking three types of activities is much too complicated and confusing for many participants. Again, each activity should be asked about separately rather than asking respondents to compare one type of activity with another.

Overlapping Intervals

"How many times a day do you lift objects weighing 25 pounds or more on the average? Never? 5 times or less per day? 5–25 times per day? 25 or more times per day?"

People lifting exactly 25 times per day, for instance, do not know in what category to place themselves. The question should be reworded to include the categories "never, less than 5 times per day, 5–24 times per day, and 25 or more times per day."

Questions That Require Too Much Detail

"Tell me each brand of cigarettes that you have smoked and for exactly how long you have smoked each one since you first started smoking."

One problem with this question is that respondents are being asked to keep several questions in mind at once. Furthermore, although people who have never smoked more than one or two brands may not find this question difficult, many people buy the brand that is on sale, or switch brands frequently for other reasons. Such people cannot possibly remember each brand smoked and for how long. The investigator is again engaging in wishful thinking. In addition, even if a respondent who had smoked many brands did in fact remember each brand, answering the question would be extremely tedious; not only would the accuracy of the answers be suspect, but it might make the respondent hostile to the remaining portions of the questionnaire. If such detailed information is absolutely crucial to a study, then it must be sought by means of a systematic series of questions; otherwise, such questions should be avoided.

Leading Questions

"Have you had any infectious disease in the past year, such as mononucleosis?"

Here the respondent is very likely to focus only on mononucleosis because this was the only disease specifically mentioned. The best approach to this question would be to read out to the respondent a list of infectious diseases, one at a time, and let him or her answer yes or no to each one. However, if there are too many questions with lists to be read off, and if the question under consideration is not highly important to the study, showing the respondent a card with the diseases listed is a good way to reduce the tedium without undue sacrifice of accuracy.

Degree of Accuracy Not Specified

"How tall are you?"

Some people will round to the nearest inch, whereas others will give their height to the nearest half inch or even smaller interval. This results in difficulties in subsequent quantification of the data for statistical analysis; this problem could be at least partially avoided if the degree of accuracy were specified. Because many people will not be able to give this information in finer intervals than inches, it makes sense to ask for the information in intervals of inches, not half inches. Even then, people who are five foot six and one half inches will not know whether to report themselves as five foot six or five foot seven. They need to be told whether to round up or round down.

Not Asking for Exactly the Information That Is Wanted

"Do you ever have a craving for certain foods?"

This question, asked in the course of trying to find out what people actually eat, may not elicit that information. Above and beyond the different meaning of the word "craving" to different people, some people may crave foods and eat them, whereas others may be able to resist the temptation. If frequent eating of large quantities of a food such as chocolate is the information that is desired, the question should be reworded to ask specifically about quantities of chocolate actually eaten.

Other Considerations

The use of cards for listing possible answers and to facilitate recognition has been mentioned several times in this chapter. Cards are a very useful device (provided the respondent can see and read) to save the time it would take the interviewer to read out possible answers and to assist the participant in learning what type of answer the interviewer wants. In addition, cards that show ranges of answers can reassure a respondent that only a rough estimate is expected. For instance, the question, "How many times a day do you lift objects weighing 25 pounds or more?" may make a respondent uncomfortable because he or she is unable to answer exactly. However, if a card is shown with the categories "never, less than 5 times per day, 5–24 times a day, and 25 or more times per day," the respondent realizes that an exact answer is not expected and can with some degree of certainty place himself or herself in one of these categories.

It should be emphasized that obtaining data on the exact number of times (or exact number of pounds) would be preferable to improve the precision of measurement, but, because the exact information is impossible to obtain, this rough grouping at least enables the investigator to have some information.

Cards may also be used when pictures can explain a concept better than words. For instance, if the investigator wants to find out whether a person has had low back pain, it is often not clear what is meant by "low." A picture depicting the various regions of the back (see Fig. 14–1) helps to ensure that all participants are really thinking of the low back when they answer this question.

SCALING

Finally, a brief summary of commonly used techniques to develop interval scales will be presented because a progressive graduated series of scores can often provide more useful information than less systematic ways of quantifying a variable. Textbooks on scaling cover the topic much more comprehensively (DeVillis, 1991; Streiner and Norman, 1989).

With *rating scales*, the respondent places himself or herself along a continuum according to the strength of his or her attitude. A range of attitudes could be constructed from feeling "strongly against" the use of fluoride in drinking water to being "strongly in favor" of fluoride in drinking water, for instance. Another option is to construct a rating scale with regular divisions marked on it and to ask the respondent to place himself or herself at the proper position. A respondent might be asked to rate the degree of pain he or she was experiencing along a scale:

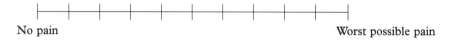

No pain   Worst possible pain

With *magnitude scaling,* the respondent is given a numeric score for one item, and then asked to give scores to other items in relation to the given item and score. For example, one way of obtaining an idea of the degree of stressfulness of various life events was to assign marriage a score of 500, and ask the respondent to give scores to other life events, such as death of a relative or loss of a job, in relation to the score of 500 for marriage.

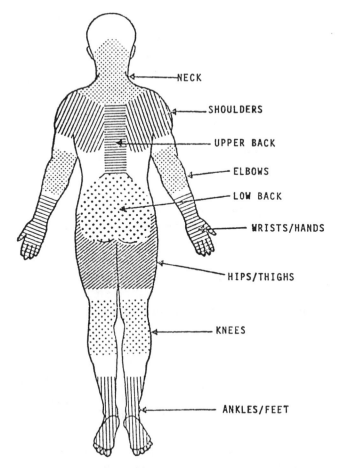

Figure 14–1. Diagram to assist respondents in specifying location of pain in study of low back pain. It illustrates the body regions mentioned in a questionnaire.

In a *Likert format,* for each item the respondent is asked to choose among several responses, not just whether he or she agrees or disagrees, so that an idea is obtained of the strength of agreement or disagreement. Typically, a respondent is asked whether he or she "strongly agrees," "agrees," "disagrees," "strongly disagrees," or is "undecided" about each of a series of statements. Each of these possible responses is assigned a score, and usually the sum of the scores for all the items is the respondent's score for that variable; occasionally the individual items may be differentially weighted and summed. In deciding which items to include from among many possible items, two procedures may be used to eliminate individual items that do not appear to measure the attribute being measured by the entire scale. First, correlation coefficients between scores for each item and the sum of scores for all items may be calculated. Items whose scores do not correlate well with the total score are then eliminated. A second means of eliminating items is to compare item scores for persons with total scores at either extreme of the attribute and to eliminate items that do not discriminate between the two groups.

Factor analysis is a statistical technique that can be used in selecting items for inclusion in scales and in data analysis. In factor analysis, a person's score on a scale item is assumed to consist of one or more components or factors, a factor being a latent, unobserved variable. Factor analysis involves estimation of factor scores from a knowledge of scores on individual items. The analysis provides estimates of *factor loadings,* which indicate the importance of a particular factor in a given item. A *general factor* is one that contributes to all items on the scale, a *group factor* contributes to more than one but not to all, and a *specific factor* contributes to only one item. Factors that contribute to both group and general factors are called *common factors.*

Factor analysis can be used in the construction of scales, such as a Likert scale. In the pilot study, a large number of items can be included and factor analysis used to identify items that make up a particular factor; this can help the investigator select items for scales to measure each of the dimensions of interest. Factor analysis is also sometimes used in data analysis to explore which items tend to group together into factors (exploratory factor analysis) or to confirm that individual items believed to have a common factor do in fact correlate with the sum of all the items believed a priori to share that factor (confirmatory factor analysis).

A *Guttman scale* is constructed by having a group of people respond to each of the items that are being considered for inclusion, and selecting the final items with the intent that every respondent agrees with all items less extreme than the most extreme one with which he or she agrees. On the final instrument thus constructed, the total number of items with which the respondent agrees then serves as the respondent's total score. In a properly developed Guttman scale, the *number* of items agreed to should indicate exactly *which* items were agreed to. If this is not the case, then the items are not unidimensional; that is, they are not reflecting different degrees of the same underlying quantity.

A FINAL WORD

The importance of trying out the questionnaire again and again and revising it until the questions are completely satisfactory cannot be overemphasized. Neophytes often plan to write out a questionnaire in one afternoon. However, good questionnaires require many, many drafts, and thus several months may be necessary for questionnaire development. Also, it is essential to try out the questionnaire on a variety of people, including those similar to the people who will actually be in the study.

REFERENCES

Acheson RM. 1969. Personal communication.

Cartright A. 1988. Interviews or postal questionnaires? Comparisons of data about women's experiences with maternity services. *Milbank Quarterly* 66:172–189.

DeVellis RF. 1991. Scale Development. Theory and Applications. Applied Social Research Methods Series Volume 26. Newbury Park, CA, Sage Publications.

Dillman PA. 1978. Mail and Telephone Surveys: The Total Design Method. New York, Wiley.

Groves RM, Kahn RL. 1979. Survey by Telephone. A National Comparison With Personal Interviews. New York, Academic Press.

Harlow BL, Rosenthal JF, Ziegler RG. 1985. A comparison of computer-assisted and hard copy telephone interviewing. *Am J Epidemiol* 122:335–340.

Jaffe AJ. 1984. Not everyone has a telephone at home. *The New York Statistician* 35:5–6.

Kelsey JL, Hardy RJ. 1975. Driving of motor vehicles as a risk factor for acute herniated lumbar intervertebral disc. *Am J Epidemiol* 102:63–73.

Kelsey JL, Githens PB, O'Connor T, Calogero JA, Weil U, Holford TR, White AA III, Walter SD, Ostfeld AM, Southwick WO. 1984. Acute prolapsed lumbar intervertebral disc: an epidemiologic study with special reference to driving automobiles and cigarette smoking. *Spine* 9:608–613.

Lambert PM, Reid DD. 1970. Smoking, air pollution, and bronchitis in Britain. *Lancet* 1:853–857.

Moser CA, Kalton G. 1979. Survey Methods in Social Investigation. London, Heinemann.

O'Connor KP, Hallam RS, Hinchcliffe R. 1989. Evaluation of a computer interview system for use with neuro-otology patients. *Clin Otolaryngol* 14:3–9.

O'Toole BI, Battistutta D, Long A, Crouch K. 1986. A comparison of costs and data quality of three health survey methods: mail, telephone and personal home interviews. *Am J Epidemiol* 124:317–328.

Perneger TV, Etter J-F, Rougemont A. 1993. Randomized trial of use of a monetary incentive and a reminder card to increase the response rate to a mailed health survey. *Am J Epidemiol* 138:714–722.

Rolnick SJ, Gross CR, Garrard J, Gibson RW. 1989. A comparison of response rate, data quality, and cost in the collection of data on sexual history and personal behaviors. *Am J Epidemiol* 129:1052–1061.

Shanks JM. 1983. The current status of computer-assisted telephone interviewing. *Soc Methods Res* 12:119–142.

Shanks JM, Nicolls WL II, Freeman HE. 1981. The California disability survey, design and execution of a computer-assisted telephone study. *Soc Methods Res* 10:123–140.

Siemiatycki J. 1979. A comparison of mail, telephone, and home interview strategies for household health surveys. *Am J Public Health* 69:238–245.

Spry VM, Howell MF, Sallis JG, Hofstetler CR, Elder JP, Molgaard CA. 1989. Recruiting survey respondents to mailed surveys: Controlled trials of incentives and prompts. *Am J Epidemiol* 130:166–172.

Streiner DL, Norman GR. 1989. Health Measurement Scales. A Practical Guide to their Development and Use. Oxford, Oxford University Press.

U.S. Bureau of the Census. 1994. Statistical Abstract of the United States: 1994. Washington, D.C.

Weeks MF, Kulka RA, Lessler JT, Whitmore RW. 1983. Personal versus telephone surveys for collecting household health data at the local level. *Am J Public Health* 73:1389–1394.

Wong WSF, Lee K-H, Chang MSA. 1986. A microcomputer based interview system for antenatal clinic. *Comput Biol Med* 16:453–463.

Zagraniski R, Kelsey JL, Walter SD. 1986. Occupational risk factors for laryngeal carcinoma: Connecticut, 1975–1980. *Am J Epidemiol* 124:67–76.

Exercises

1. The following questionnaire was used to obtain descriptive statistics to be presented at a tenth-year reunion of a large northeastern women's college. What are its inadequacies?

May, 1974

Tenth Reunion Questionnaire

( ) Check, circle, or fill in blanks applicable/answer yes or no

Where do you live?   country   suburbs   city   small town   outside USA
    In how many different towns have you lived since college? _____

Work   Paid _____ Volunteer _____ Hours per week _____ Salary _____
    Is the pay equal to that given men in a comparable position? _____
    How has work affected you? _____
    _____ Your family? _____
    _____

Describe your work _____
    _____
    _____

Occupations

Write F for you and M for him

Housefather _____	Mother _____
Teacher _____	Principal _____
Nurse _____	Doctor _____
Paralegal _____	Lawyer _____
Teller _____	Bank officer _____
Secretary _____	Executive _____
Keypunch _____	Systems analyst _____
Author _____	Editor _____
Lecturer _____	Professor _____
Research asst. _____	Scientist _____
Swimming instructor _____	Aquanaut _____
Cabin attendant _____	Pilot _____

Social worker _____   Psychiatrist _____
Other _____   Early childhood education _____

Total income (household):   under $10,000 10–20,000 20–30,000
    30–40,000 40–50,000 50–100,000 over 100,000 Percent inherited _____
Degrees attained since college _____
Degrees in progress _____
Honors, achievements, exhibits, publications _____
_____

If you could have any occupation, what would you do? _____
_____
_____

Avocation Involvement: strong   medium   weak
   Specify: Sports _____   Arts _____
            Cards _____   Crafts _____
            Flora _____   Fauna _____
            Cuisine: haute _____ bas _____ type _____
            Community/political involvement _____
            _____

Since college:
   Are you fatter _____ thinner _____ bustier _____ graying _____
   In better physical shape _____ More aware of politics _____
   More perceptive with regard to your motives and aspirations _____
   More frivolous _____ Less _____ Swapping mates _____
   Have you quit smoking _____ taken it up _____ kept right on _____
   Have you been depressed _____ seen a psychiatrist _____
   Have you been arrested _____ For what _____ Jailed _____
Since college:
   Have you had any sexual problems _____
   altered your sexual orientation _____
      to: hetero _____ homo _____ bisexual _____ indifferent _____
         opposed _____
   altered your sexual frequency (more, less) _____
   tried sex therapy _____

Since college:
   Have you returned to school _____ used dope _____ ridden to hounds _____ sold
   the ancestral estate _____ tried communal living _____ been invited to the White
   House _____ run for public office _____ been appointed/elected the only/first woman
   on _____
   been recognized in your community for achievement in _____
   _____

As to music, do you still play _____ only listen _____ live _____ tape/FM _____ rock __
   classic _____ other _____
What do you read?
   Nothing at all _____ books only _____ magazines only _____
   newspaper only _____
   Favorite magazines: _____
   Prefer: pornography _____ biography/autobiography _____ history _____
         gothic romances _____ philosophy _____ politics _____
         mysteries _____ best sellers _____ literary criticism _____
         recent favorite: _____

Do you consider yourself religious? _____ Do you participate in organized religion? _____
   Have you changed your religion since college? _____
   Why? _____ Have you kept a kosher home? _____

/ much TV do you watch? (hours per week) _____ Your children? _____
Program favorites: drama _____ news/documentary _____ PBS _____ other _____

Jo you have season tickets to: symphony _____ football _____ opera _____ repertory
theater _____ basketball _____ ice hockey _____ baseball _____ ballet _____
other _____

What do you spend your extra money on?
sculpture _____ painting _____ graphics _____ shrink _____ keeping a sailboat __
keeping a man _____ keeping a horse _____ designer clothes
_____ travel to _____ (China, Russia, other)

Do you go out? Sat. night only _____ much too often _____ very little _____ none at all _

Marital status: single _____ engaged _____ married _____ cohabiting _____ group
marriage _____ separated _____ divorced _____ widowed _____ No. of times
married: _____ Did you keep your maiden name after marriage? _____ Hyphenate? __
Resume it after divorce? _____ Did you walk out? _____ Extramarital affairs? _____
You only? _____ Him too? _____

Birth discouragement or promotion IUD _____ pill _____ rhythm _____
foam _____ diaphragm _____ condoms _____ coitus interruptus _____
abstention _____
Miscarriages _____ fertility pills _____ tubal ligation _____ vasectomy _____

Were you pregnant when you got married? _____ Have you had an abortion? _____
1 2 3 4 before marriage? _____ legal? _____ illegal? _____

Children How many? 0, 1, 2, 3, 4, . . . no. of girls _____ no. of boys _____
If zero, do you intend to remain a nonparent? _____
Birth date of eldest _____
Twins _____ triplets _____ quads or more _____ Number adopted _____
Interracial _____ Foreign: Vietnamese _____ other _____
Indicate number in each: public school _____ private school _____ nursery school __
parochial school _____ Montessori _____
free school _____ other _____
Have you changed your mind about the value of pre-kindergarten? _____
Any handicapped children? _____ mentally retarded? _____
physically? _____ other? _____
Are they at home? _____ Where else? _____

Household help What kind? gardener _____ cook _____ chauffeur _____ governess _
fille au pair _____
live-in _____ daily _____ weekly _____

Husbands, lovers, or boyfriends: Age _____
Does he: hold the door _____ drive when you're together _____ navigate as well __
tell you what a lousy driver you are ____ pay the bills _____
give you an allowance? for house _____ for yourself _____ other _____
apologize for cursing in your or another woman's presence _____ split the
housework 50–50, 80–20, 98–2 _____ go out for an evening with the boys? poker
_____ chess _____ bowling _____ string quartet _____
other _____
contribute to family income _____ diaper the baby _____ babysit _____
cook _____ do the dishes _____ stay home from work when you have key
meeting/when child is ill _____ put his razor back in the medicine cabinet _____
What does he do? _____
part time _____ full time _____ weekends too _____ wages _____ or salary/
fees _____ speculate on the stock market _____ allowance from his
mother/you _____

Is he independently wealthy? _____

Does he have: high school _____ college _____ post grad _____

Do you wish you had married the other fellow? _____ How does he feel about you? _____
_____ What's he doing now?_____
_____

Where did you meet?   in high school _____ at a party _____ at a frat house _____
at a mixer _____ in the lobby of your dormitory _____ blind date _____ in grad
school _____ at work _____ in a singles bar _____ in the Catskills _____
betrothal arranged by parents _____

Do you think Richard Milhous Nixon should
   be impeached _____   tough it out _____
   resign _____   none of the above_____

Whom do you prefer for the presidency in 1976?
   Jackson _____ Reagan _____ Mondale _____ Rockefeller _____ Ford _____
   Kennedy _____ Baker _____ Bayh _____ Other _____

Do you have charge accounts or loans in your own name? (specify) _____
_____

Have you experienced discrimination because you are a woman? _____
_____
_____

Have you been involved in women's liberation activities? _____
_____

   consciousness-raising group _____ Equal Rights Amendment _____
   other _____

Have you altered your perceptions of yourself? _____
_____

   your relationships with men? _____
   with women? _____

Your goals for yourself? _____
_____
_____

Should this college have gone coed? _____ Why?_____

Is there something that you wish you had learned or experienced at this college? _____
_____

Is your life pretty much as you expected or feared it would be? _____
_____
_____
_____

What have you done in the last 5 years that surprised you? _____
_____
_____

   that surprised your parents or spouse? _____
_____

How do you think your life is different from that of the majority of your classmates? _____
_____
_____
_____
_____

2. Design a questionnaire to be used in a case-control study of risk factors for hip fracture in persons of age 55 years and older. This could include established and possible risk factors for osteoporosis (e.g., gender, age, race, weight, use of estrogen replacement therapy, diet, smoking, alcohol consumption, physical activity, oophorectomy, reproductive history) and/or established and possible risk factors for falls (e.g., home environmental hazards, drugs and diseases affecting balance, alcohol consumption, physical activity).

15

Measurement II: Other Types of Measurement

The most common method of measurement used by epidemiologists has been the questionnaire. Undoubtedly, questionnaires will continue to be used extensively by epidemiologists, and, accordingly, Chapter 14 was devoted entirely to their design and administration. In the future, it is likely that an increasing number of studies will employ more direct methods of measurement, such as can be obtained by laboratory assays. Some of the issues involved in measurement by laboratory assay were covered in Chapter 10 in the context of serologic surveys. Other frequent methods of measurement include abstracting information from existing records, physical examination, and other clinical measures. This chapter discusses some of the issues involved in using these other types of measurement, and addresses some specific problems in perinatal epidemiology, epidemiologic studies in the elderly, occupational epidemiology, and psychosocial and psychiatric epidemiology, and in studies using biological markers.

RECORDS

Using existing records is usually much less expensive than making measurements oneself. In addition, measurements that cannot be made ethically for research purposes, such as by biopsy, may have been recorded on a medical record in the course of routine diagnosis or treatment. Measurements made in the past may be needed; when such measurements are available on records, a study that would not have been possible may become feasible. Often, however, the needed data have not been recorded, and if they have, the information may have been recorded by so many different people in such an incomplete and unstandardized way that it is of limited value. Before deciding to rely on records, it must be determined whether the data are sufficiently valid and reliable to be useful.

Perhaps the most common use of medical records is to establish that a person had the disease(s) under study, particularly in case-control studies.

exposure variables and on potential confounding variables are
atly obtained from medical records in case-control studies because
ata are generally not consistently recorded in the medical records of
institutions. Cigarette smoking habits, for instance, would usually be
rded for most patients with lung cancer, but not for individuals with an
ate condition believed to be unrelated to smoking, such as acute appen-
icitis. Thus, use of medical records to determine smoking habits could
lead to considerable differential misclassification (see Chapter 13). Furthermore, even when smoking habits are recorded, the degree of detail is
usually insufficient, because a record may categorize an individual as a
smoker or nonsmoker but will not indicate the number of cigarettes smoked
per day or the length of time a person has smoked. If the risk factor or
potential confounding variable is a demographic variable, such as age or
gender, or a diagnostic or medical procedure, the relevant information may
be recorded consistently enough to be useful, but for most other variables
this is not the case. Exceptions occur in institutions in which all patients
upon admission are given a short questionnaire in which data on smoking
habits and other variables of interest are routinely collected in a standardized manner. Also, in prepaid health care plans, pharmacy records may
enable an investigator to identify prescription drug use as a risk factor or
potentially confounding variable. In retrospective cohort studies, data on
past exposure are almost always obtained from records, such as from industrial records. As discussed in Chapter 5, this means that before such a study
is undertaken, an investigator must think long and hard about whether the
necessary data on possible risk factors and confounding variables were
recorded with enough consistency and in sufficient detail to make the study
worth doing.

PHYSICAL EXAMINATION AND OTHER CLINICAL MEASURES

When physical examinations are done in a standardized manner, they may
provide useful diagnostic information for epidemiologic studies. This requires careful training and monitoring of the individuals performing the examination. In the National Health and Nutrition Examination Survey I
(NHANES I), each new physician spent 1 to 3 days being trained by a Nutrition Medical Advisor (National Center for Health Statistics, 1973). Additional training was provided at the examination center in the field, and
retraining was provided during the course of the survey. In certain parts of
the survey, additional reliability testing was done. Dental advisors systematically repeated the measurements made by the field examiners for a subsample of examinees for the purpose of surveillance and on-the-spot re-

training. The dental advisors also periodically replicated the measurements made by each other. After the initial training period, ophthalmologists independently replicated the measurements of all the first day's examiners for each locale. Procedures such as these are essential to ensure that examinations are as standardized as possible.

Other specific clinical measures such as findings from x-rays, electrocardiograms, and respiratory function tests are also subject to variation. First of all, *physiologic variation* occurs in what is being measured; this variation may add to random error or may bring about bias. In the U.S. Health Examination Survey, the first blood pressure measurement was on the average higher than the others (National Center for Health Statistics, 1964), probably indicating lower levels as people relaxed. Height decreases slightly during the course of a day, so that systematically different height readings could be obtained in people measured at different times of day. *Pathologic variation* occurs too, as in diseases that become steadily worse over time. Other diseases may have periods of exacerbation and remission. Thus, one needs to be aware of these sources of variation, to establish standard conditions for measurement, and, when possible, to make measurements on more than one occasion.

Variation in the measuring instrument may occur. In taking blood pressure measurements, the application of the cuff and placement of the stethoscope may vary. A scale may change its zero point; a ruler may move. Thus, all such measuring instruments should be calibrated before, during, and at the end of an investigation, and provisions made to prevent lost of calibration. In some instances, it may be desirable to calibrate an instrument before each measurement is made.

Observer variation is common. People making blood pressure measurements may vary in their ability to hear sounds, to read a moving column of mercury, to remember what to write down, and to avoid digit preference (e.g., rounding to the nearest 0 or 5). Different people may see different lesions on x-rays. Accordingly, when feasible, two or more observers should make measurements independently and both intra- and interobserver variability be determined by the methods described in Chapter 13. Whenever possible, "hard," or "permanent," documents should be obtained. NHANES I (National Center for Health Statistics, 1973), for instance, used tape recorders, automatic recording of weights, photographs of height, x-rays, and magnetic tape for the recording of spirometry and electrocardiograms. With these hard documents, reading and interpretation can be done independently more than once. In a case-control study of fibrocystic breast disease (Berkowitz et al., 1984), one pathologist read all slides, and a second pathologist read slides from every eighth biopsy. The slides were classified as fibrocystic disease, fibroadenoma, or other benign breast dis-

Intraclass Correlation Coefficients[1] for Measurements of Shoulder,
d Midline Asymmetry Made by the Same and by a Different Rater

rement	Same Rater Twice	Two Raters Once Each
ction of one shoulder	0.79	0.58
vation of one hip	0.86	0.87
eviation of spine from midline of body	0.93	0.91

Source: Dieck et al. (1985).

ease. Slides for 34 patients were read a second time by both pathologists. When this procedure was used, the kappa statistics for intraobserver reliability were reasonably good (0.79 and 0.78 for the two pathologists), but the kappa for interobserver variability was only fair (0.64). On closer examination of the data, the pathologists differed in what they called "fibrocystic breast disease" and what they called "other benign breast disease." When such systematic differences occur, further training and discussion are needed.

In a study of the ability of measurements made from "posture pictures" in the teen years to predict the development of back pain in the adult years (Dieck et al., 1985), a random sample of 10% of the pictures was remeasured by the same observer and by a second observer. Intraclass correlation coefficients were calculated for measurements indicating elevation of one shoulder over the other, elevation of one hip over the other, and deviation of the spine from the midline of the body. Table 15–1 shows that measurement of shoulder asymmetry was considerably less reliable than measurement of hip or spine asymmetry, whether the measurements were made by the same observer or by two different observers. As a result, less confidence was put in associations relating shoulder asymmetry to back pain than in associations involving waist or spine asymmetry.

Before a study begins, standardized criteria and interpretation should be decided upon, and inexperienced observers should practice with more experienced observers. All observers need to be tested and corrected until good interobserver and intraobserver reliability are consistently achieved. During the course of a study, the observers need to be checked at frequent intervals and to be retrained and recertified if necessary. If large numbers of participants are available, the group can be randomly divided in half (or into smaller units), each half assigned to a different observer, and any systematic differences detected. Whenever possible, an observer should make measurements without knowledge of the person's status with respect to other variables of interest, such as whether a person is a case or a control. When "hard" data have been collected, such as slides or x-rays, several observers can make readings. Results from less experienced observers can be compared to those of one or more expert observers who read the slides without knowledge of the less experienced observer's findings. Conversely, known positive and negative (or normal and abnormal) specimens, as determined by an expert, can be given to all of the observers to measure independently without knowledge of the expert's classification.

One common reason for variation among observers is that when a measurement is dichotomized into present or absent, the observers may be uncertain as to how to categorize measurements that are truly borderline. Cutoff points should be clearly specified in advance, but nevertheless some observations may be difficult to dichotomize in practice. Use of a "borderline" category may be useful in this regard. Use of the measurement in its original form avoids the problem entirely.

Interactions involving the person being measured, the measuring instrument, and the observer also need to be considered. Concerning the respondent and instrument, the respondent may learn over time how to use an instrument properly, so that he or she may appear to have improved on respiratory function or grip strength, for instance, when the improvement is really attributable to familiarity with the instrument. Fatigue or boredom could produce the opposite effect. Blood pressure readings may be artificially high in people with large arms. Very large or very small values may be off the scale of an instrument.

Interactions between the observer and respondent may occur. Pulse rate may be decreased if an observer puts a respondent at ease. Measured height may vary if a tall person measures a short person or a short person measures a tall person. Blood pressure levels are on the average higher if taken by someone of the opposite gender.

An example of interaction involving the instrument and observer is digit preference, which may be minimized by having measurement scales with markings of uniform width and length:

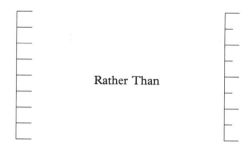

Rather Than

Interactions involving the respondent, observer, and instrument simultaneously are possible. For instance, when testing a respondent's knee jerk reflex with a reflex hammer, the observer may be hesitant to strike the knee briskly with the hammer in a respondent who appears delicate. To minimize all these potential interactions, awareness of their possible occurrence and careful training and monitoring of observers are essential.

MEASUREMENT IN PERINATAL EPIDEMIOLOGY

Special problems of measurement occur in studies of adverse reproductive outcomes. In cohort studies, measuring exposures before an abnormality develops in the fetus would be highly desirable in order to ensure that the exposure precedes the occurrence of the abnormality. However, a woman seldom knows she is pregnant at least until after the first menstrual period is missed, and many women do not seek medical care until much later in pregnancy. A highly sensitive and specific immunoradiometric assay for human chorionic gonadotropin (HCG) to detect pregnancy soon after implantation has been developed (Armstrong et al., 1984). Although this assay will undoubtedly prove useful in certain epidemiologic studies involving highly motivated women (Wilcox et al., 1988), most studies will continue to rely on more traditional methods of pregnancy detection at more usual times. Thus, even in most cohort studies, measurement of exposure status will occur at varying periods of time after the exposure occurred and, in some cases, after the disorder underlying an adverse outcome is present.

In case-control studies, women who have given birth to an infant with an abnormality often think extensively as to what might have caused it, thus increasing the likelihood of recall bias. Denial also may occur. Using mothers of infants with other abnormalities as a control group may help reduce the problem of recall bias.

Some exposures are important only if they occur at a precise time during the pregnancy, such as when a specific organ is forming. Agents that are related to the development of congenital heart disease probably have their effect at about the third to fourth week of embryonic life. Determining whether exposure occurred at exactly this time may be impossible because there may be no records documenting the time of exposure and the mother may not remember the precise timing. Therefore, exposure at any time during the early part of pregnancy is usually considered as a positive exposure, but since many such exposures are irrelevant because of inappropriate timing, any real association between the disease and an adverse reproductive outcome may be considerably diluted.

Ascertainment of all adverse outcomes of pregnancies is essentially impossible because early spontaneous abortions often occur before a woman knows she is pregnant; even if sophisticated pregnancy tests were applied to large numbers of women, pregnancy losses before implantation would not be detected. The precise incidence of fetal loss very early in pregnancy cannot be determined, but it is likely to be substantial. Kline and Stein (1985) have estimated that about 75% of fertilized ova may result in spontaneous abortions. Among pregnancies surviving to implantation, Wilcox and colleagues (1988), using the immunoradiometric assay mentioned above (Armstrong et al., 1984), found that 31% were lost, including 22% before the pregnancy was detected clinically.

Conceptions with defects often end in spontaneous abortions. Because most cohort studies identify only those defects diagnosed at birth, most of these studies provide data on the prevalence of conditions at birth rather than the theoretically desirable incidence of conditions among all pregnancies. Prevalence rates at birth may be a poor approximation of incidence rates and are influenced by factors that affect survival to birth as well as factors that affect the development of defects. Furthermore, it is possible that various detrimental exposures are mainly associated with early spontaneous abortions, making it difficult to detect them as risk factors in studies of full-term infants or perhaps even among recognized spontaneous abortions.

Prenatal screening tests such as amniocentesis are being used with increasing frequency. Positive results on such tests usually lead to induced abortions, further affecting rates of defects identified only at birth. For instance, because amniocentesis is undertaken much more frequently in older pregnant women than in younger pregnant women, not only will the prevalence rates of Down's syndrome at birth be affected, but certain features of the descriptive epidemiology will be altered as well. The increasing use of sonography, which can identify anomalies earlier in gestation, is intensifying this problem.

In addition to induced abortions for medical reasons, induced abortions for other reasons have occurred with high frequency. In large North American metropolitan areas such as New York City, about one-half of pregnancies end in induced abortion (Susser, 1981), so that full-term pregnancies are occurring in an increasingly select group of women. Thus, epidemiologic studies identifying adverse pregnancy outcomes at birth are focusing on infants whose mother elected not to terminate the pregnancy and who were able to survive to delivery. Because the proportion of pregnancies terminating in induced abortions varies from one subgroup of the population to another, risk ratios for adverse pregnancy outcomes such as spontaneous abortions may have to be adjusted according to the frequency of induced abortions in the subgroups of interest (Olsen, 1984).

MEASUREMENT IN EPIDEMIOLOGIC STUDIES OF THE ELDERLY

In epidemiologic studies in the elderly, many problems are encountered that occur to only a limited extent in studies of younger adults (Herzog and Rodgers, 1991; Kelsey et al., 1989; Kinard, 1990). For instance, starting at about 80 years of age, prevalence rates of severe cognitive impairment increase markedly. It has been estimated that 17% of non-institutionalized persons aged 85 and older have severe cognitive impairment (Weissman et al., 1985). Such individuals will not be able to answer a questionnaire. Cognitively impaired individuals may be excluded from an epidemiologic study, but this leaves out a significant proportion of the population to whom one would usually like to generalize results; also, participation rates will be substantially reduced. Therefore, interviews with proxy respondents (individuals who provide information on behalf of someone else) may be important. Issues involving the use of proxy respondents in epidemiologic studies are discussed in detail by Nelson et al. (1990, 1994) and by Magaziner (1991).

The quality of the information obtained from proxy respondents varies according to characteristics of the study subject (the person about whom it is desired to obtain information for the study), characteristics of the proxy respondent, the relationship of the proxy respondent to the study subject, and the nature of the information being requested. The length of time during which the study subject and proxy respondent have lived together and the frequency of contact if they do not live together are important determinants of the quality of the information obtained. For elderly persons living in households, the preferred proxy respondent is generally someone living in the same household, usually the spouse; for those living in institutions, the proxy respondent is often a caregiver or offspring of the study subject.

In studies in which information from proxy respondents has been compared with that obtained from study subjects themselves (although not necessarily elderly subjects), very good agreement has been found for chronic medical conditions, medication taken for chronic medical conditions, current smoking and alcohol consumption dichotomized as yes versus no, most recent job, and demographic characteristics. The reliability of data on number of cigarettes smoked, quantity of alcohol consumed, number of jobs held, height and weight, and current diet has generally been found to be fair to good; agreement on minor and non–life-threatening illnesses, overall health ratings, and private behavior such as ability to handle money has been poor. Objective questions that minimize judgment, interpretation, and opinion on the part of the proxy respondent are clearly preferable to subjective questions.

Generally, proxy respondents tend to underreport exposures relative to the study subjects themselves, although overreporting can also occur. Determining the reliability of information provided by proxy respondents relative to that provided by persons responding for themselves is important, either as a part of a pilot study or as a component of the main study. In case-control studies, for instance, a reliability study should be conducted to assess the consistency of data from proxy respondents and self-respondents for a subset of cases and controls. If the reliability cannot be determined for cases because, for instance, all cases are by definition demented or dead, then some indication of reliability can be obtained by comparing information from proxy respondents and self-respondents among the controls. As a minimum, data from these reliability studies can give an indication of the direction and extent of bias in measures of association from studies using proxy respondents. The data from such reliability studies can also sometimes be used to correct odds ratios and other measures of association by error-correction methods such as those described in Chapter 13. Magaziner (1991) has reviewed in more detail techniques for evaluating the extent of agreement and bias in studies using proxy respondents.

In the statistical analysis of epidemiologic studies with proxy respondents (Walker et al., 1988), data can first be stratified according to whether the information was obtained from the study subject himself/herself or a proxy respondent. (If a multivariate regression model is used, an interaction term involving type of respondent, the exposure of interest, and the disease can be examined.) If measures of association are similar in both strata (i.e., interaction is not present), then the results from the two types of respondents can be combined, with respondent status as a covariate; if not, then results from self-respondents and proxy respondents should be reported separately. It should be kept in mind that different results for self-respondents and proxy respondents may occur because of reporting error by proxy respondents, but may also be attributable to the reason(s) that the proxy respondents were needed (Magaziner, 1991). For instance, risk factors for hip fracture may actually be different in demented and nondemented individuals.

Missing data for individual items occur more frequently when proxy respondents are used than when an individual responds for himself/herself. One way to minimize the amount of missing data is to keep questions simple. Sometimes data from other sources can be used, such as from medical records. Methods of imputing values for missing data, discussed in Chapter 12, may also be used (Nelson et al., 1990).

Response rates in the elderly are often low, especially in those aged 85 years and older. Unlike younger individuals, older persons frequently give health and mental problems as reasons for not wanting to participate; this source of nonresponse has the potential to add a great deal of bias to studies concerned with health. Suggested ways of increasing response rates (Herzog and Rodgers, 1991; Kelsey et al., 1989; Kinard, 1990) include obtaining appropriate sponsorship and endorsement from organizations important to the elderly; obtaining cooperation from institutions such as nursing homes where some elderly will be living; providing special training to interviewers so that they can deal with problems presented by the elderly; perhaps using older interviewers; using mixed modes of interviewing when needed (that is, using telephone and postal questionnaires for respondents who are unwilling to participate in personal interviews); using proxy respondents or having relatives present to assist; and extending periods of data collection so that those feeling ill temporarily will have an opportunity to participate when they feel better. If physiologic data are to be collected or physical examinations are to be undertaken, better response rates will be obtained if they are done at the respondent's residence rather than at a central location.

When older people are interviewed, the questionnaire often has to be shorter than the investigator would prefer. In the very elderly, fatigue tends to set in after about half an hour. Although many older individuals can persevere for up to 45 minutes provided they are well motivated and in good health, interviews that are longer than 45 minutes are difficult. Sometimes the interview may have to be conducted on two separate occasions. The questions need to be relatively simple, and information may have to be obtained in less detail than desired. The elderly are more likely than young adults to have difficulty placing themselves in predetermined response categories, and missing data on individual questions are more frequent.

Other problems that are likely to occur with at least some respondents are difficulty understanding informed consent, vision and hearing impairment, rambling, and limitations in memory. For these and other reasons, interviews of the elderly on the average take considerably longer than interviews of younger individuals, and special training of interviewers to deal with problems of particular relevance to the elderly is desirable. Furthermore, over one-fifth of persons aged 85 years and older reside in nursing homes (National Center for Health Statistics, 1986). Arranging interviews in nursing homes and rehabilitation facilities requires still more time, since many different facilities are likely to be involved, each with its own procedures for obtaining permission to interview the participant. Often the legal guardian and primary physician are both required to give permission for the resident to be approached. If nursing home residents are not included, then generalizability is further diminished.

In summary, epidemiologic studies of the elderly are likely to be much more time-consuming and logistically complex than those in younger populations. The investigator needs to take this into account when planning studies.

MEASUREMENT OF OCCUPATIONAL EXPOSURES

Occupational Epidemiology, by Checkoway and colleagues (1989), is recommended to readers interested in a thorough coverage of issues related to the measurement of occupational exposures. Perhaps the first issue to keep in mind is that many people have no way of knowing what they are exposed to; they are often merely passive recipients of exposures of which they are not aware. If current exposures are of interest, the investigator can attempt to measure them. Usually, however, past exposures are important. Unless records of past exposure are available, current measures of exposure must be assumed to be measures of past exposure. Because exposure levels may change considerably over time, the validity of such extrapolation may be suspect. For instance, various improvements in the work environment have taken place in the United States to comply with Occupational Safety and Health Administration (OSHA) standards. Consultation with industrial hygiene experts about changes in technology over the period in question may lead to better estimates of exposure levels over time.

The investigator must keep in mind that failure to find an association may mean that no association exists or that measurement is too poor to permit detection of an association. Furthermore, the measured levels of environmental exposure may not be indicative of the levels actually inhaled, ingested, or absorbed, or of the concentrations that are biologically active in exposed individuals.

In cross-sectional, panel, or prospective cohort studies, information on exposure can generally be obtained directly from current records or from industrial hygiene measurements, either by area sampling or the wearing of personal monitors. Exposure data should be collected for the various places in which employees work. Depending on the study, it may be desirable to obtain information on whether a person was ever exposed to various substances, the total duration of exposure, the total duration times the average intensity of exposure, the peak intensity of exposure, the age at first exposure, the age at last exposure, which exposures occurred simultaneously, and the timing of the exposure relative to other exposures. In prospective cohort studies, estimates of dose-response relationships can usually be made with much greater accuracy than in case-control or retrospective cohort studies.

In retrospective cohort or case-control studies, records of where a person worked may be available from management or occasionally from unions. Many workers have changed jobs within a plant so many times, however, that collecting this information becomes tedious, time-consuming, and therefore expensive. Monson (1980) suggests that, as a minimum, date and age when employment in the plant started and total number of years worked there are desirable. When possible, it is also important to find out when and for how long a worker was employed in various departments within a plant. A decision must be made concerning the minimum duration of exposure that will be considered relevant. In most studies, for practical reasons, exposures of less than a year or sometimes less than 5 years are excluded, unless the dose is very high during that time or it is thought that the cumulative dose during a shorter time period is important. To the extent possible, abstracters should collect all information without knowledge of whether the individual has developed the disease of interest. Industrial hygienists who have been employed at the plant for many years can provide useful information about previous conditions and exposures. It is often desirable to analyze the data using several different measures of exposure.

Ascertainment of disease status may be subject to bias because a worker's known exposures may affect the diagnosis of a condition or what is listed as the cause of death. It is important to establish disease status in retired persons and terminated workers, since they may have retired, changed jobs, or moved because of health problems or because of exposures.

A recent article by Checkoway and Demers (1994) discusses various aspects of case-control studies focusing on occupational risk factors. In case-control studies, information on occupational history is frequently obtained by questionnaire. Routine records such as death certificates, tumor registry reports, and hospital records are of limited value because of the amount of misclassification and usual listing of only one job (Siemiatycki et al., 1989). Typically, in a questionnaire a respondent is first asked for his or her complete lifetime occupational history, including both the job and company of employment. Then, he or she may be asked about general exposures such as to dust or fumes, and finally about specific exposures to substances of interest, such as chromium or benzene. It must be kept in mind, however, that for most specific substances of interest, the vast majority of workers are not aware that they were exposed (Bond et al., 1988). Accordingly, sensitivity is likely to be quite low, although specificity may be acceptable (Joffe, 1992). Whether protective clothing or equipment was used should be determined. In addition, sometimes a checklist of putative high risk jobs is given to respondents. When possible, some categorization according to exposure level should be attempted, but often evaluation of dose-response relationships is not feasible.

From knowledge of the place of employment and nature of the job, the investigator may be able to obtain some information on possible exposures. Local sources of information are often helpful, but, in addition, the *Dictionary of Occupational Titles* (U.S. Department of Labor, 1977) and *Selected Characteristics of Occupations Defined in the Dictionary of Occupational Titles* (U.S. Employment Service, 1981) may be used to obtain descriptions of jobs and hazards typically associated with the jobs. Another approach for assessing exposure status is the job-exposure matrix (Hoar et al., 1980), in which each job a person has held is classified by industry and task and then linked with a list of suspected carcinogens. Classifying an exposure by probability of exposure, decade of exposure, and a more specific industrial-occupational coding system than is normally used can substantially increase the effectiveness of this method (Dosemeci et al., 1994). Other sources of information on specific exposures may be found in several references listed at the end of this chapter (Burgess, 1981; Considine, 1974; Cralley and Cralley, 1982; International Labour Office, 1983; Occupational Diseases, 1978). In addition, a trained team of chemists and/or industrial hygienists can be employed to infer exposures from the respondents' work histories (Siemiatycki et al., 1981; Siemiatycki, 1991).

Finally, although this section has focused on exposures in the workplace, many of the same issues as well as others present even greater problems in studies of health effects of environmental exposures outside the workplace. Examples are studies concerned with health effects of air pollution, water pollution, and toxic waste sites.

MEASUREMENT IN PSYCHOSOCIAL AND PSYCHIATRIC EPIDEMIOLOGY

The measurement of social, psychological, and cognitive processes is particularly important in those subareas of epidemiology known as psychosocial epidemiology and psychiatric epidemiology. Psychosocial epidemiology is concerned with the role of psychological and social processes in the etiology of diseases, whereas psychiatric epidemiology is concerned with understanding the causes of mental disorders and psychological impairment. These causes may include external physical, chemical, and biologic agents, genetic predisposition, and endogenous biochemical factors as well as social and psychological factors.

A particular problem in the measurement of psychosocial variables stems from the complex nature of what is being measured. There is often no obvious, straightforward way of quantifying the relevant variables. If the exposure of interest were lifetime ingestion of a physical agent such as saccharin, then although the problems of obtaining a valid and reliable method of measurement would be formidable, these problems would have less to do with what is meant by saccharin ingestion than with the logistic problems of collecting accurate information. That is, there would be relatively little disagreement among researchers as to how ingestion of saccharin might be measured under the best of possible circumstances, namely, by making direct measurements of the saccharin content of each food or beverage ingested over a person's lifetime, as well as direct measurements of the amount of each food or beverage ingested on a day-by-day basis. The primary area of disagreement would concern the choice of one or more of several more feasible but less than optimal methods for collecting such information. If, on the other hand, the exposure were some complex psychosocial factor such as stress, problems would be encountered at a conceptual level. The respondents themselves would not know exactly what is meant by stress, and different investigators have different definitions. When measuring a concrete variable such as saccharin use, investigators must be concerned with the reliability and validity of the way they measure saccharin use, but at least there is general agreement about what saccharin is. When studying psychosocial variables, however, one has to decide what a factor such as stress, anxiety, or demoralization is, in addition to being concerned about the reliability and validity of measuring what it is defined to be. Several of the scaling methods discussed in Chapter 14 can be used in constructing a measure of a psychosocial variable.

In psychosocial epidemiology, then, much effort must be devoted to constructing measures of the variables of interest. When setting out to measure a psychosocial variable, the investigator either has to use an existing measurement instrument or has to embark on an often lengthy process of developing and testing measures for reliability and validity. Let us take the concept of stress as an example. There is little consensus as to how, even in the absence of logistic or financial constraints, stress is most appropriately measured. Substantial differences of opinion exist regarding both concepts of the nature of stress and how these concepts should be implemented in empirical studies. Such fundamental decisions as to whether physiologic responses of the respondents have any relevance cannot be easily resolved.

One influential approach to the measurement of stress was the inventory of life events developed by Holmes and Rahe (1967). This approach illustrates some of the problems that are encountered when attempting to measure a complex psychosocial variable. The items listed in Table 15–2 are ranked according to ratings of the amount of readjustment they require of the individual. The events range from death of spouse, which is thought to require the greatest readjustment, to minor violations of the law, which are thought to require the least readjustment. A typical use of the Holmes-Rahe list has been to have a group of respondents indicate which of the events they have experienced within a specified time period, to sum the events (with or without weighing them according to severity), and then to relate this measure to a specific disease outcome.

The Holmes-Rahe approach to the study of the effects of stress obviously incorporates several assumptions about the nature of stress. A few of these assumptions are (a) that stress is additive, (b) that changes for the better are stressful in a way similar to changes for the worse, and (c) that the objective event and not the context in which it occurs or the response of the person to that event is what matters most. These and other assumptions

Table 15-2. Holmes-Rahe Life Events (1967)

Death of spouse	Trouble with in-laws
Divorce	Mortgage over $10,000
Marital separation	Start or end of work
Marriage	Outstanding personal achievement
Death of close family member	Begin or end of formal schooling
Jail term	Change in living conditions
Personal injury or illness	Trouble with boss
Fired at work	Revision of personal habits
Marital reconciliation	Change in work conditions
Retirement from work	Change in residence
Gain of new family member	Change in schools
Change in health of family member	Change in recreation
Sex difficulties	Change in social activities
Business adjustment	Change in church activities
Change of financial status	Mortgage or loan less than $10,000
Change to different line of work	Change in sleeping habits
Change in number of arguments with spouse	Change in family get-togethers
Pregnancy	Change in eating habits
Death of close friend	Vacation
Change in work responsibility	Christmas
Foreclosure of mortgage or loan	Minor violations of law
Son or daughter leaving home	

Source: Holmes and Rahe (1967).

have been questioned and have been the objects of considerable research (Dohrenwend and Dohrenwend, 1981; Rabkin and Streuning, 1976), but no closure has been reached concerning the most appropriate way to conceptualize stressful life events or how to measure them.

One consensus that has emerged in the area of research on stress and other psychosocial variables is to acknowledge whenever possible the complexity of the processes involved and to avoid combining diverse situations and responses. This has led some investigators to concentrate research on a single life event, such as job loss or retirement, so that contextual factors can be studied in detail, preferably with a prospective cohort design (Kasl et al., 1975; Minkler, 1981). There is increasing skepticism that scales designed to measure broad concepts such as stress or "feeling bad" (Lewis et al., 1984) are likely to provide important new insights (Kasl, 1984). In addition, narrowly defined concepts can be scaled more easily.

Broad areas of agreement have emerged concerning the measurement of psychiatric outcomes, but their measurement poses many conceptual and operational complexities similar to those encountered in the measurement of psychosocial risk factors for disease. Because there is currently no "hard" biologic basis for diagnosing psychiatric disorders as there is for the histologic diagnosis of cancers, the boundaries among various psychiatric disorders have often been difficult to draw. Historically, epidemiologic studies of psychiatric disorders have been hampered by the difficulty of transferring to a field setting the methods of clinical classification. Thus, early landmark studies in psychiatric epidemiology relied heavily on unidimensional scales of psychological impairment (Leighton et al., 1963; Scrole, 1962). Such scales often have little relevance to the variety of discrete diagnostic rubrics currently employed in clinical settings. This gap between measurement techniques used in psychiatric epidemiology and clinical classification systems has recently been bridged to a substantial extent. Official psychiatric nomenclature has been defined more objectively in terms of constellations of specific symptoms having a particular severity and duration (DSM III) (American Psychiatric Association, Committee on Nomenclature and Statistics, 1980). Simultaneously, interview instruments for collecting appropriate information in general population groups have been developed and refined (Dohrenwend et al., 1985; Endicott and Spitzer, 1978; Robins et al., 1981; Wing et al., 1974).

An area of research requiring special care in the design and interpretation of study results is that in which both psychosocial risk factors and psychiatric outcomes are of interest. Suppose, for instance, that one is interested in the relationship between stress and the incidence of major affective disorders. Because one of the life events on the Holmes-Rahe list, change in sleeping habits, is also a component of the criteria for major affective disorders (American Psychiatric Association, Committee on Nomenclature and Statistics, 1980), at least part of any observed association between stressful events and affective disorders would be a tautological one rather than an etiologic one. In such studies, especially close attention must often be paid to the conceptualization and measurement of the risk factor, and prospective designs are particularly important for addressing the complex issues of causal sequence that arise in these studies. However, because of the gradual onset of many psychiatric disorders, use of prospective designs does not guarantee clear identification of causal sequences.

BIOLOGICAL MARKERS

Biological markers may be defined as "cellular, biochemical, or molecular alterations that are measurable in biological media, such as human tissues, cells, or fluids" (Hulka et al., 1990). Biological markers such as antibodies as indicators of exposure to bacteria or viruses, or serum cholesterol as an indicator of risk for coronary heart disease, have been in use for many years. With the recent advances in molecular biology, a much wider array of markers that may provide more precise measures of biologic events has become available. Among the uses of biological markers in epidemiologic studies are as indicators of dose of exposure, dose of biologically effective exposure, biologic response, early disease, and host susceptibility (Hulka et al., 1990; Perera and Weinstein, 1982; Stein and Hatch, 1987; Hulka, 1991). Another book in this series, *Biological Markers in Epidemiology* (Hulka et al., 1990), is recommended to readers wanting more detailed coverage of this topic, particularly in regard to cancer epidemiology. Much of the material presented here regarding uses and limitations of biological markers is summarized from that book.

Biological markers may allow the investigator to improve considerably on measurement of exposure. At present, questionnaires are most often used to measure exposure status. For instance, in a previous section of this chapter it was mentioned that information on exposures in the environment or at the workplace are typically assessed by asking respondents about the presence or absence of the exposures of interest or by asking people what jobs they have held or where they have lived, and then assigning them exposure levels believed to be typical of that occupation or that area of residence. Both methods of assessment are likely to be inaccurate. However, if exposure status can be measured from a body tissue, then the classification of exposure may be more accurate. For instance, if blood lead levels are used as a marker of recent exposure to lead, more accurate classification of exposure is likely to be achieved than if people are asked about exposure to lead or if they are asked where they live or what their job is. In addition, information derived from questionnaires may provide a poor approximation of the dose reaching the target tissue because of individual variation in uptake or pharmacokinetics. Consequently, measurement of dose in the tissue of interest may be important.

Not all exposures are of biologic consequence, and some biological markers are used to detect biologically effective interactions of the exposure of interest with critical host tissue. For instance, if a chemical such as benzo(a)pyrene induces carcinogenesis by forming bonds with one or more DNA strands, then measurement of DNA adduct formation is a possible indicator of biologically effective exposure.

Biological markers of exposure can also be used to validate in small numbers of individuals measurements of exposures obtained from less expensive and more feasible methods such as questionnaires. Error correction methods (see Chapter 13) can then be applied.

Biological markers are used in various ways when effects of exposures are being considered. They may facilitate the detection of preclinical disease. For instance, serum alpha-fetoprotein level may be a marker for liver cancer, gastrointestinal diseases, and fetal neural tube defects. If the marker is highly correlated with the subsequent development of disease and can be measured before the disease becomes symptomatic or can be diagnosed, then prospective cohort studies can be completed more quickly than if one has to wait for the occurrence of symptomatic or diagnosed disease. Biomarkers can also be used in screening for preclinical disease, as in the use of the Papanicolaou test to identify precancerous lesions in the cervix.

Biological markers may permit better classification of disease. For instance, if chromosomal abnormalities are considered to be a marker of genetic damage, then spontaneous abortions in which chromosomal abnormalities are not found are likely to have different etiologies from spontaneous abortions in which they are found.

Biological markers of effect may be useful in suggesting mechanisms of action of exposures. For instance, in a study of effects of maternal stress during pregnancy, it was hypothesized that sustained elevations of catecholamines might, because of their vasoconstricting action, interfere with uteroplacental blood flow, which in turn could lead to vascular damage in the placenta and to decreased birthweight and other problems in the offspring (Hatch and Friedman-Jimenez, 1991). In addition to the traditional method of obtaining data from questionnaire on maternal psychosocial stress and from records on birth weight, the investigators collected maternal urine specimens for the measurement of catecholamine concentrations and placental specimens for identification of placental abnormalities. In this way, it is hoped that a better understanding will be achieved of the biology of psychosocial stress and the role of placental abnormalities in the pathogenesis of low birth weight and other adverse reproductive outcomes. Elucidation of mechanisms through biomarkers may be particularly helpful in providing evidence that weak associations found in other epidemiologic studies are real.

Biological markers may be used to identify people who are and who are not susceptible to a given disease. The susceptibility can be inherited or acquired. An example mentioned in Chapter 4 was lack of antibody as a marker of susceptibility to an infectious disease. A few markers of susceptibility may be found for diseases of noninfectious etiology as well, such as low alpha-anti-trypsin activity as a marker of risk for emphysema among smokers. It is expected that in the future more markers of susceptibility to noninfectious diseases will be identified. In addition to the usefulness of markers in identifying susceptible individuals for disease prevention programs, susceptibility markers can greatly increase precision and power in prospective cohort studies by permitting the exclusion of nonsusceptible people from the populations to be studied.

Finally, biological markers may be useful as measures of adherence or lack of adherence to a specified regimen in a randomized trial. Salivary or urinary cotinine may be used to measure whether a person is currently smoking, for instance.

Various limitations of the use of biological markers in epidemiology should also be kept in mind. First, the significance of many markers is uncertain. For instance, elevated levels of sister chromatid exchange (SCE) are thought to indicate that cells have been exposed to a mutagen. SCE occurs during cell replication when a chromosome duplicates its genetic material to form a pair of chromosomes (sister chromatids); through DNA breakage and rejoining, sister chromatids can exchange segments of DNA. Since mutagens are considered potential carcinogens, SCE may be used as a biological marker of exposure to potential carcinogens. At present, however, no long-term studies exist to show that risk for any cancers is increased among those with high levels of SCEs. Whether elevated levels of benzo(a)pyrene-DNA adducts are associated with a high risk for cancer of any site is also not known. We must await the results of cohort or nested case-control studies to answer such questions. Second, many laboratory assays are not ready for epidemiologic use because of high costs and lack of accuracy and precision, or because they are not acceptable to the study population. Third, the distribution of markers in the general population by such characteristics as age, gender, and race would be useful, since it is difficult to plan and interpret a study without such information. Fourth, many markers decrease or disappear after exposure ends, and more information is needed on variation in marker persistence among individuals. Some markers indicate only very recent exposures. Because of the short cycle of production and retention of urine, markers in urine are particularly susceptible to this problem. All of these potential limitations must be kept in mind when planning, carrying out, and interpreting the results of epidemiologic studies employing biological markers.

REFERENCES

American Psychiatric Association, Committee on Nomenclature and Statistics. 1980. Diagnostic and Statistical Manual of Mental Disorders. Washington, D.C., American Psychiatric Association.

Armstrong EG, Ehrlich PH, Birken S, Schlatterer JP, Siris E, Hembree WC, Canfield RE. 1984. Use of a highly sensitive and specific immunoradiometric assay for detection of human chorionic gonadotropin in urine of normal, nonpregnant, and pregnant individuals. *J Clin Endocrinol Metab* 59:867–874.

Berkowitz GS, Kelsey JL, LiVolsi VA, Holford TR, Merino M, Ort S, O'Connor TZ, Goldenberg IS, White C. 1984. Oral contraceptive use and fibrocystic breast disease among pre- and postmenopausal women. *Am J Epidemiol* 120:87–96.

Bond GD, Bodner KM, Sobel W, Shellenberger RJ, Flores GH. 1988. Validation of work histories obtained from interviews. *Am J Epidemiol* 128:343–351.

Burgess WA. 1981. Recognition of Health Hazards in Industry. A Review of Materials in Process. New York, Wiley.

Checkoway H, Demers PA. 1994. Occupational case-control studies. *Epidemiol Rev* 16:151–162.

Checkoway H, Pearce NE, Crawford-Brown DJ. 1989. Occupational Epidemiology. New York, Oxford University Press.

Considine DM. 1974. Chemical and Process Technology Encyclopedia. New York, McGraw-Hill.

Cralley LV, Cralley LJ. 1982. Industrial Hygiene Aspects of Plant Operations. New York, Macmillan.

Dieck GS, Kelsey JL, Goel VK, Panjabi MM, Walter SD, Laprade MH. 1985. An epidemiologic study of the relationship between postural asymmetry in the teen years and subsequent back and neck pain. *Spine* 10:872–877.

Dohrenwend BP, Levav I, Shrout PE. 1985. Screening scales from the Psychiatric Epidemiology Research Interview (PERI). In: JK Myers, MM Weissman, Eds. Epidemiologic Community Surveys. New Brunswick, New Jersey, Rutgers University Press.

Dohrenwend BS, Dohrenwend BP, Eds. 1981. Stressful Life Events and Their Contexts. New York, Prodist.

Dosemeci M, Cocco P, Gomez M, Stewart PA, Heineman EF. 1994. Effect of three features of a job-exposure matrix on risk estimates. *Epidemiology* 5:124–127.

Endicott J, Spitzer RL. 1978. A diagnostic interview: the schedule for affective disorders and schizophrenia. *Arch Gen Psychiatry* 35:837–844.

Hatch MC, Friedman-Jimenez G. 1991. Using reproductive effect markers to observe subclinical events, reduce misclassification and explore mechanism. *Environ Health Perspect* 90:255–259.

Herzog AR, Rodgers WL. 1991. The use of survey methods in research on older Americans. In: RB Wallace, RF Woolson, Eds. The Epidemiologic Study of the Elderly. New York, Oxford University Press, pp 60–90.

Hoar SK, Morrison AS, Cole P, Silverman DT. 1980. An occupation and exposure linkage system for the study of occupational carcinogens. *J Occup Med* 22:722–726.

Holmes TH, Rahe RH. 1967. The social readjustment rating scale. *J Psychosom Res* 11:213–218.

Hulka BS. 1991. Epidemiological studies using biological markers: Issues for epidemiologists. *Cancer Epidemiol Biomarkers Prev* 1:13–19.

Hulka BS, Wilcosky TC, Griffith JD. 1990. Biological Markers in Epidemiology. New York, Oxford University Press.

International Labour Office. 1983. Encyclopedia of Occupational Health and Safety. Geneva, International Labour Office.

Joffe M. 1992. Validity of exposure data derived from a structured questionnaire. *Am J Epidemiol* 135:564–570.

Kasl SV. 1984. When to welcome a new measure. *Am J Public Health* 74:106–107.

Kasl SV, Gore S, Cobb S. 1975. The experience of losing a job: Reported changes in health, symptoms and illness behavior. *Psychosom Med* 37:106–122.

Kelsey JL, O'Brien LA, Grisso JA, Hoffman S. 1989. Issues in carrying out epidemiologic research in the elderly. *Am J Epidemiol* 130:857–866.

Kinard M, Ed. 1990. Maximizing response rates. Network. Fall, 1990.

Kline J, Stein Z. 1985. Very early pregnancy. In: RL Dixon, Ed. Reproductive Toxicology. New York, Raven Press, pp 251–265.

Leighton DC, Harding JS, Macklin DB, Macmillan AM, Leighton AH. 1963. The Character of Danger. New York, Basic Books.

Lewis CE, Siegel JM, Lewis MA. 1984. Feeling bad: exploring sources of distress among pre-adolescent children. *Am J Public Health* 74:117–122.

Magaziner J. 1991. The use of proxy respondents in health studies of the aged. In: RB Wallace, RF Woolson, Eds. The Epidemiologic Study of the Elderly. New York, Oxford University Press, pp 120–129.

Minkler M. 1981. Research in the health effects of retirement: an uncertain legacy. *J Health Soc Behav* 22:117–130.

Monson RR. 1980. Occupational Epidemiology. Boca Raton, FL, CRC Press.

National Center for Health Statistics. 1964. Blood Pressure of Adults by Age and Sex, United States 1960–1962. Series 11, No. 4.

National Center for Health Statistics. 1973. Plan and Operation of the Health and Nutrition Examination Survey, United States 1971–1973. Series 1, No. 109.

National Center for Health Statistics. 1986. Health, United States, 1986. Washington, D.C., U.S. Government Printing Office, 1986. DHHS Publication No. (PHS) 87–1232, U.S. Public Health Service.

Nelson LM, Longstreth WT Jr, Koepsell TD, Checkoway H, van Belle G. 1994. Completeness and accuracy of interview data from proxy respondents: demographic, medical, and life-style factors. *Epidemiology* 5:204–217.

Nelson LM, Longstreth WT Jr, Koepsell TD, van Belle G. 1990. Proxy respondents in epidemiologic research. *Epidemiol Rev* 12:71–86.

Occupational Diseases. A Guide to Their Recognition. 1978. Washington, D.C., U.S. Government Printing Office. DHEW (NIOSH) Publication No. 77–181.

Olsen J. 1984. Calculating risk ratios for spontaneous abortions: the problems of induced abortions. *Int J Epidemiol* 13:347–350.

Perera FP, Weinstein IB. 1982. Molecular epidemiology and carcinogen-DNA adduct detection: new approaches to studies of human cancer causation. *J Chron Dis* 35:581–600.

Rabkin JG, Streuning EL. 1976. Life events, stress and illness. *Science* 194:1013–1020.

Robins LN, Helzer JE, Crougham R, Ratcliff KS. 1981. National Institute of Mental Health Diagnostic Interview Schedule: its history, characteristics, and validity. *Arch Gen Psychiatry* 38:381–389.

Scrole L. 1962. Mental Health in the Metropolis: the Midtown Manhattan Study. New York, McGraw-Hill.

Siemiatycki J. 1991. Risk Factors for Cancer in the Workplace. Boca Raton, CRC Press.

Siemiatycki J, Day NE, Fabry J, Cooper JA. 1981. Discovering carcinogens in the occupational environment: a novel epidemiologic approach. *J Natl Cancer Inst* 66:217–225.

Siemiatycki J, Dewar R, Richardson L. 1989. Costs and statistical power associated with five methods of collecting occupational exposure information for population-based case-control studies. *Am J Epidemiol* 130:1236–1246.

Stein Z, Hatch M. 1987. Biological markers in reproductive epidemiology: prospects and precautions. *Environ Health Perspect* 74:67–75.

Susser E. 1981. The Epidemiology of Spontaneous Abortion. M.P.H. Essay, Columbia University.

U.S. Department of Labor. 1977. Dictionary of Occupational Titles. Washington, D.C., U.S. Government Printing Office.

U.S. Employment Service. 1981. Selected Characteristics of Occupations Defined in the Dictionary of Occupational Titles. Washington, D.C., U.S. Government Printing Office.

Walker AM, Vatema JP, Robins JM. 1988. Analysis of case-control data derived in part from proxy respondents. *Am J Epidemiol* 129:905–914.

Weissman MM, Myers JK, Tischler GL, Holzer CE III, Leaf PJ, Oruashel H, Brody JA. 1985. Psychiatric disorders (DSM-III) and cognitive impairment among the elderly in a U.S. urban community. *Acta Psychiatr Scand* 71:366–379.

Wilcox AJ, Weinberg CR, O'Connor JF, Baird DD, Schlatterer JP, Canfield RE, Armstrong EG, Nisula BC. 1988. Incidence of early loss of pregnancy. *N Engl J Med* 319:189–194.

Wing JK, Cooper JE, Sartorius N. 1974. The Measurement and Classification of Psychiatric Symptoms. London, Cambridge University Press.

Exercises

1. In a study in which it is planned to measure weight and blood pressure, what steps would you take to maximize the reliability and accuracy of the measurements?

2. List the strengths and limitations inherent in (a) case-control studies and (b) prospective cohort studies trying to determine whether a causal relationship exists between maternal alcohol consumption during pregnancy and spontaneous abortions.

3. Select an occupational or environmental exposure that is measured as a dichotomous variable and could be considered a possible risk factor in a case-control study. Assume some reasonable levels of specificity, sensitivity, prevalence of the exposure in the control group, and expected true odds ratio, and use the methods of Chapter 13 to estimate the extent of attenuation in the odds ratio because of the (nondifferential and independent) error in measuring exposure.

4. List the information you would need in order to conduct a retrospective cohort study of the relationship between exposure to asbestos and risk for lung cancer.

5. Design a study to assess whether close social ties are related to the incidence of coronary heart disease in an elderly population. Carefully assess issues of causal sequence and indicate how your design may minimize problems in interpretation of the results.

NOTE

1. The intraclass correlation coefficient reflects differences in mean values as well as the degree of correlation between two sets of measures.

Index